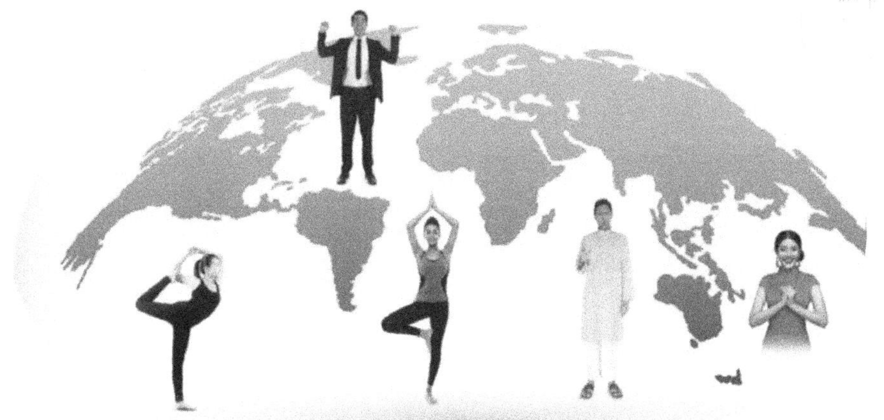

Yoga Concepts

For Global Application

A Primer for Beginners and Instructors

For those seeking deeper understanding of Yoga

For the Council for Yoga Accreditation International by:
C. Rajan Narayanan
Stephen Parker
Sanjeev Krishna
Idriss Raoua Ouedraogo
Ratna Nandakumar

Illustrations by Yolanda Chetwynd

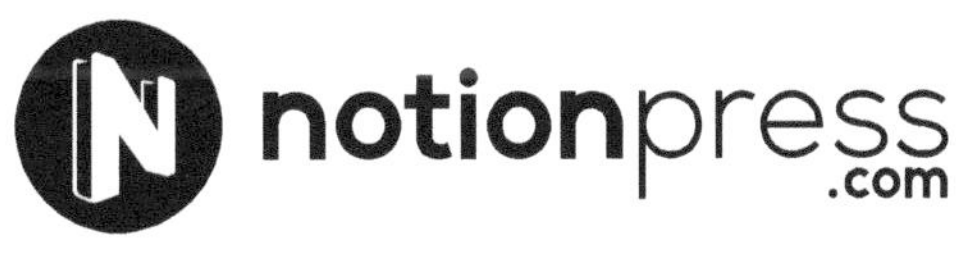

INDIA • SINGAPORE • MALAYSIA

ISBN
Hardcase 979-8-89588-971-8
Paperback 979-8-89588-366-2

WE DEDICATE THIS BOOK TO:

- Sage Patanjali, author of the Yoga Sutras, whose wisdom guides us;
- The Divinity, that guides the purpose of this book;
- To all of Humanity, whom we hope will benefit.

AUTHORS

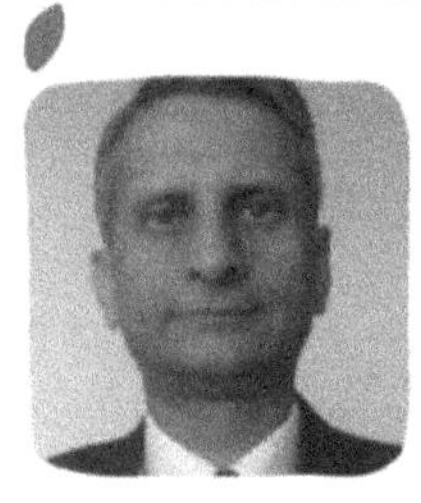	**C. Rajan Narayanan PhD, AYTh, former C-IAYT** Dr. Narayanan is the Executive Director of Life in Yoga Institute (https://lifeinyoga.org/) and the Chair of the Board of the Institute since 2022. He has been a spiritual guide and a trainer of yoga teachers and therapists and has conducted many training events since 1998. He has received recognition from major yoga institutions in India. He has developed the system of Measured Yoga Therapy whose essential approach is published as *Bioenergy and its Implication for Yoga Therapy* available at the website of the National Library of Medicine (https://pubmed.ncbi.nlm.nih.gov/29755226/). His main area of research interest is in the scientific understanding of intuition and tantra aspects of yoga.
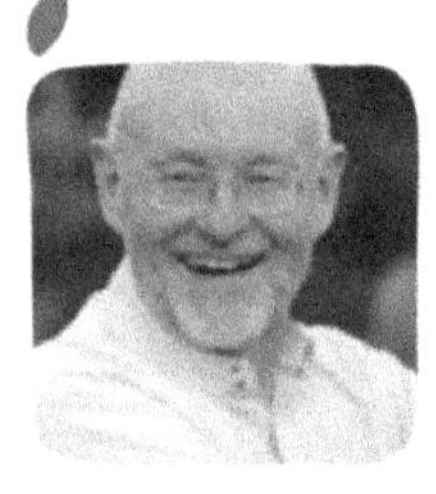	**Stephen Parker (Stoma) PsyD, LP, C-IAYT, AYTh** Dr. Parker is a spiritual guide, and a senior yoga teacher trainer in the Association of Himalayan Yoga Societies International (AHYMSIN). He has conducted workshops, seminars, and spiritual retreats in 15 countries around the world. He serves as the Chair of the Board of Council for Yoga Accreditation International since 2019. Dr. Parker is also a licensed psychologist and practiced psychology and psychotherapy for 35 years. His book, *Clearing the Path, The Yoga Way to a Clear and Pleasant Mind: Patanjali, Neuroscience and Emotion* was published in 2017, and he is the author of many book chapters and research articles.
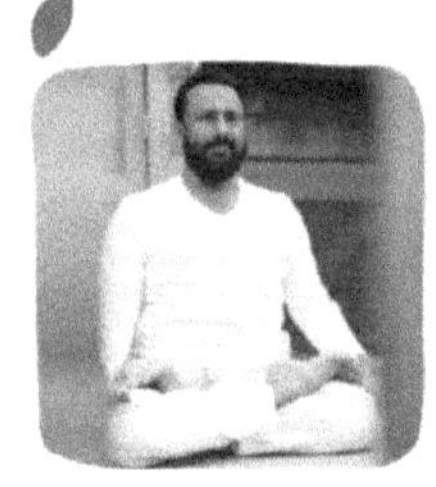	**Sanjeev Krishna, AYT** Mr. Krishna is the Founder and Yoga Acharya of Sanjeev Krishna Yoga in Dubai, UAE. Besides being on the CYAI Board, also serves on the Governing Council of ARYIC (Arab Region Yoga Instructors Council). He developed the Rhythm of Life program which has benefited thousands across the globe in physical, mental, and emotional health. He has worked closely on yoga with Knowledge and Human Development Authority of Dubai government. He was awarded Certificate of Appreciation by DOHMS (Department of Health and Medical Services) of Dubai in 2003. His organization became the First ISO 9001:2015 Certified Yoga center in the middle east. He is also a founder member for Rotary Club of Dubai Downtown.
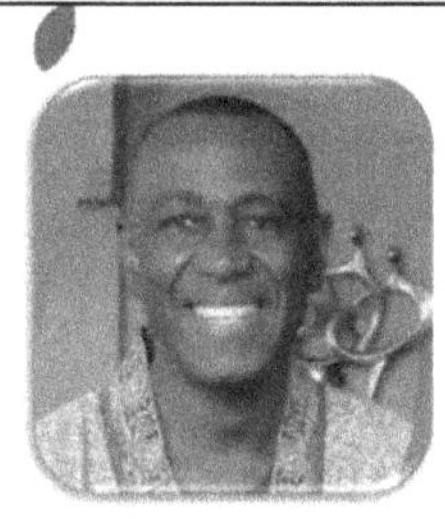	**Idriss Raoua Ouedraogo, AYT** Ambassador Ouedraogo is a diplomat for the country of Burkina Faso in West Africa, and has served as its ambassador in many countries of the world, including India. He also leads the West African Yoga Societies. While he has a background as an economist and financier, his true passion is in yoga, with long experience in teaching yoga and training yoga instructors. He has been a lead teacher of yoga for the Burkina Faso army. He teaches yoga therapy from a western point of view and as an adjunct to physiotherapy for people suffering from sickle cell disease, respiratory problems, physical disabilities, etc.
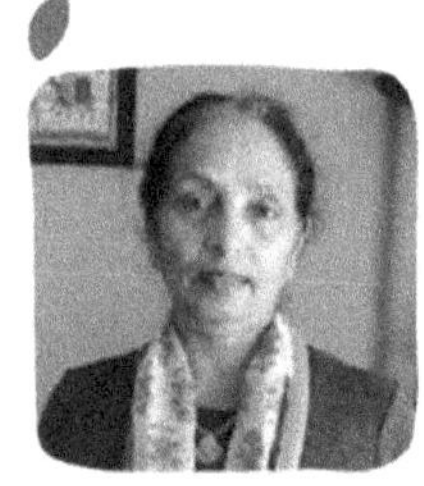	**Ratna Nandakumar PhD. AYI** Dr. Nandakumar is a Professor Emerita, University of Delaware. She is a certified yoga instructor and the coordinator of the Daily Online Yoga for Life in Yoga (lifeinyoga.org). She currently serves as the Chair of the Board of Life in Yoga Foundation and as Board Member of Council for Yoga Accreditation International. In addition, she contributes to the therapy, education, and research programs of Life in Yoga. Given her spiritual interest, over the years she developed familiarity with many different yoga traditions and practices finding the real core of yoga in the Yoga Sutras of Patanjali.

Guide to Transliteration of non-English Words

We have significant usage of non-English words, especially Sanskṛit, in the book. Academic style of diacritical marks is not commonly understood by all. Since this book is directed to both academic and non-academic readers, we make a slight compromise where phonetic representation of the English language that may be easier to pronounce is used in three exceptions to the academic rule. These are with respect to: **ś** which we present as **śh**, **ṣ** which we present as **ṣh** and **ñ** which is presented as **ñy**.

Accordingly, the transliteration pronunciation guide is as follows:

ā as long **a** sound like father.

a as **u** in cut or but.

e as in **e** in bed or bend

ī as in i in police or like **e** or east; in some instances, ee has been used in the text

i regularly written as in India

o as in bone

u as **u** in put or full

ū as in **oo** in boot; in some instances, **oo** has been used in the text

ṛa as in rum or rut (like Pitṛ**a)**

ṛi as in merrily (like Prakṛiti)

ṛī as in marine

ṅ as in sung

jñy as **nio** in bunion

ṇ as n in shun or none

ṭ as in Tom or torpedo

t as in **t** in thin

th as **th** in thick

ḍ as **d** in don't

d as **th** in they or those

śh as sh in shut or shame

ṣh as in dish

The remaining Sanskṛit alphabets are phonetically used as in English: ka, kha, ga, gha, ch, chh, ja, jha, pa, pha, ba, bha, ma, ya, ra, la, va, sa, ha.

Abbreviations Used

- YS refers to Yoga Sutras of Patanjali.
- Accordingly, YS:2.1, as an example would indicate first sutra of second *pāda* (chapter) of the Yoga Sutras of Patanjali.
- HP refers to the Haṭha Yoga Pradipikā
- GS refers to the Gheranḍa Samhitā

CONTENT

ACKNOWLEDGMENT

This is the inspired work of several people. We thank everyone who collaborated in this effort. Special specific thanks are noted here.

- Dr. Dilip Sarkar for reviewing and writing a Foreword for this book.
- Dr. Hansaji Yogendra, Dr. Ananda Balayogi Bhavanani, Dr. Aref Ali Nayed and Mr. Sunny Varkey for writing a reviewing of this book.
- Dr. Sundara Kulkarni of Seattle (formerly of Houston) who did a detailed proofing of the book and suggested an addition which we crafted in chapter 33, and provided insightful review that is incorporated in the back cover of the book.
- Dr. Hari Sharma of Columbus, Ohio, whose critical review of the first draft of this book resulted in significant changes including the addition of a chapter.
- Yolanda Chetwynd of Newark, Delaware, USA, who created most of the drawings in this book.
- Rajeev Jhanji of New Jersey, who provided critical guidance for publishing this book.
- Sreejith Kalam Chundayil who helped with the book header formatting in MS Word.
- Rashna Daroga of Toronto, Canada, who contributed the Zoroastrian segment in chapter 33.
- Dhanya Ratnam and Sanjeev Krishna of Dubai who contributed substantially to the pre-natal and post-natal yoga segments in chapter 6, in chapter 18 (on Asanas) and Islamic Salat in chapter 33.
- Idriss Raoua Ouedraogo of Burkina Faso, who made significant contributions in chapter 2 (Applications of Yoga) with a conflict resolution case, chapter 33 on Voodoo, and in chapter 13 (Bhramari).
- Stephen Parker of Minneapolis, Minnesota, who authored the entire content of chapter 37 (Functional and Ethical Requirements) and contributed significantly throughout the book with 'blue box' cases, and in chapter 33 (Bhakti Yoga and the Role of Religious Practices) specifically contributed on Śhri Vidyā, Christian practices, Turkish Mevlevis, Kabbala of Judaism.
- Rajan Narayanan has been the principal author of the book with editorial roles by Stephen Parker, Ratna Nandakumar, Sanjeev Krishna and Idriss Raoua Ouedraogo.

We cannot but feel that the above noted acknowledgement is incomplete. The inspiration from others and from meditation is significant. We only have God to thank for what has been produced in this book.

Council for Yoga Accreditation International

FOREWORD

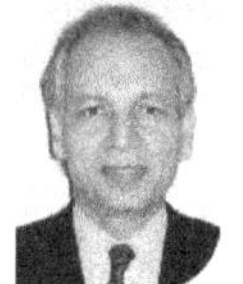

Dilip Sarkar, MD, FACS, D.Litt(yoga) writes:

In my journey of teaching yoga therapy to improve health and healing, I met Rajan Narayanan in a conference at NIH (National Institute of Health). He is an authority in yoga therapy, and we started teaching a CME (Continuing Medical Education) course together for the healthcare providers to integrate yoga therapy with the modern medicine. With his vast experience he wrote the book "Yoga Concepts for Global Application: A Primer for Beginners and Instructors" as the principal author with editorial roles by Stephen Parker, Ratna Nandakumar, Sanjeev Krishna and Idriss Raoua Quedraogo, a textbook for those seeking deeper understanding of yoga. The book explores the ancient wisdom of yoga and how it can be applied in today's modern world.

The book describes yoga as a spiritual practice and is experiential based on the personal experience and practice following the Yoga Sutra of Patanjali and Patanjali Aṣhṭānga Yoga. Yoga is a basic education like reading, writing and mathematics that promotes meaningful living and harmonious society.

The book covers a wide range of topics, including the history of yoga, the philosophy of yoga, the benefits of yoga, and the practical application of yoga in various areas of life. One of the unique features of this book is that it emphasizes that the meditative practices are the higher pathway of yoga and the need for a holistic approach to yoga, which considers the physical, mental, and spiritual aspects of the practice. This approach is particularly relevant in today's world where people are seeking holistic solutions to their health and well-being.

The book is written in a clear and concise style, making it accessible to both beginners and advanced practitioners of yoga. It also includes practical tips that readers can incorporate into their daily lives.

Overall, "Yoga Concepts for Global Application: A Primer for Beginners and Instructors" is a valuable resource for anyone interested in understanding the deeper aspects of yoga and how it can be applied in today's globalized world.

This book is a great addition to our yoga literature and highly recommended for yoga students, yoga teachers, yoga therapists, health care providers and scholars who are interested in the therapeutic and spiritual benefits of yoga and yoga therapy. They will find themselves coming back to the text time and time again for deeper study and practice.

Dilip Sarkar, MD, FACS, D.Litt(yoga)

REVIEW

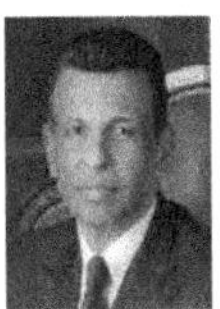

Sunny Varkey - An Education Visionary with Six Decades of legacy in transforming Education, UNESCO Goodwill Ambassador, Member of Harvard University's Global Advisory Council writes:

"Yoga Concepts for Global Application" by the Council for Yoga Accreditation International is a very noble initiative and an apt book for all yoga enthusiasts. This book covers the entire concepts of this deep science that is applicable to humanity for health, peace, harmony, and wellbeing.

The step-by-step integration of yoga system in universal applications and the culmination of all religious concepts brings unity in diversity. Such knowledge is very essential in this world today.

I do wish success for your endeavor in bringing this global application of true yoga.

I am sure the readers will find the best value for their investments.

Sunny Varkey
Chairman, Gems Global
Founder – Varkey Foundation and Gems Education

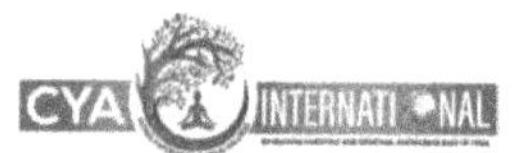

PREFACE

Commercial and religious interests can sometimes distort the development and dissemination of knowledge. Further, inertia and conventions can sustain such distortions. This has been the unfortunate state in the field of yoga. This book is an effort to correct this distortion and disorientation in the knowledge of yoga. Accordingly, the target audience for this book are two-fold:

- Those who want to teach yoga to others – such people should not distort the knowledge. For such people, this book serves as an introductory level textbook. Yoga schools and universities that offer yoga certification programs may consider adopting this book as their primary textbook. To serve this purpose, every chapter ends with questions and items for discussion.
- Those who seek to know about yoga even if they don't intend to teach others.

Setting Right the Distortions

Following are the key points of correction conveyed in this book:

1. Yoga is about connecting into the zone before birth and after death of the body and realizing the nature of existence in the temporal and spiritual plane. Yoga is a spiritual philosophy.
2. Yoga is NOT merely a set of exercises or practices.
3. Practices that promote the yogic experience and realization are essentially NOT physical as portrayed by images in the public space and yoga studios. Real yoga practices belong in the deeper realm of vibrations within, reduction of mental reactivity, and promotion of inner awareness.
4. Yoga is anchored on an ancient text called the Yoga Sutras of Patanjali and is NOT correctly reflected in later texts influenced by non-theistic and occult doctrines that present it more as physical as in Haṭha Yoga.
5. Yoga philosophy is like religious philosophies but does not have rituals and beliefs that are required in religions. People of all religions can engage in yoga practices even while adhering to their religious traditions. Yoga embodies the spiritual content of all religions. Yoga is experiential and is not based on beliefs.
6. Yoga is a personal experience. However, it has significant positive consequences in society and environment, engendering a soulful and ethical way of living.

7. Yoga elements can be measured scientifically. However, without a model of cosmic existence that yoga suggests, current research orientation that measures correlations portrays yoga as something for physical and mental health and helps to limit and disorient the real understanding of yoga.
8. Yoga should be viewed as basic education like reading, writing, and mathematics, that promote meaningful living and harmonious societies.
9. Meditative practices are the higher pathways of yoga.

Suggestion on How to Read this Book

This book endeavors to provide comprehensive overview of all aspects of yoga. Accordingly, to appreciate the place of different types of yoga practices, this book anchors the discussion around Patanjali's philosophical model of cosmic existence of yoga, and the mechanism of yoga. Such an approach that integrates historical influences and scientific studies provides clear perspective of different yoga approaches. However, integrative understanding for readers can be difficult depending on their background, and exposure to information and disinformation in yoga.

To keep the assimilation of information presented in this book tractable and building in stages for an interested reader with minimal exposure to yoga, the book unfolds in nine parts. However, for novice or leisure readers, this may still be challenging. For many readers, the footnotes, references, and terms related to research may engender searches on the internet to ensure adequate understanding. Further, grasping the model may take time. Thus, this book may be slow reading for many, and may require multiple readings.

Following may be a schema for readers who are not guided by a course faculty using this textbook.

- Begin from chapter 1, and then review the last chapter 38 that provides a comprehensive overview of the book.
- Next read all the chapters in part I of the book through chapter 7. Beginners in yoga should devote enough time to read and reflect on chapter 5 to ensure it is well assimilated before proceeding to the later sections.
- Then the following chapters can be read in clusters that are independent and may be read in any order: (a) chapters 8-14 in part II on breathing practices; (b) chapters 16-17 in part III on summarized view of physiology to avoid stress, and Haṭha Yoga; (c) chapters 22 and 26 in part IV on Tantra Yoga; (d) chapters 28, 29 and 31 in part VI about meditation.
- Thereafter, chapters 32-36 in part VII can be read for integrative understanding of yoga in daily life.
- Only thereafter should the other chapters be considered for learning.

We think such a reading schema may make it easier to assimilate.

The nine parts of this book can be summarized as follows:

I. **What is Yoga** is the first part consisting of seven chapters that provides an overview of yoga with introduction to the mechanism of yoga in the fifth chapter.

II. **The Power of Breath in Yoga** serves to make the point that breath is a key ingredient for the body's energy production and by learning to direct the energy with simple breathing practices it can have both physical and metaphysical benefits. Without energy that sustains this body-mind complex it cannot sense the metaphysical experiences and realization of yoga in the spiritual domain.

III. **Haṭha Yoga** is the third part of this book. Since the physical aspects of yoga is most popular, the roots and traditions of this practice are explained. Readers who have some background in yoga may quickly find that current day, popular physical practices of yoga may appear to be significantly modified from the root texts. The point is noted that the age of the Haṭha Yoga texts is only about a thousand years or less compared to the Yoga Sutras that go back more than 5,000 years. The inconsistencies with the Yoga Sutras suggest influences by non-theistic philosophies and occult traditions that came after the Yoga Sutras. Therefore, traditional Haṭha Yoga texts may suffer from some corruption of yogic knowledge.

IV. **Tantra Approach to Yoga,** working in the vibrational domain, is the key bridge to the higher meditative practices of yoga. While the conceptual element of Tantra is key to the higher realization of yoga, some of its popular representation in various literature and propagated by many may not be valid. This is clarified and the essential elements of Tantra and its ethical application is noted.

V. **The Source of All Knowledge in Yoga** is the culmination of the conceptual understanding of the mechanism, process, and purpose of yoga.

VI. **Meditative Approaches to Yoga** is a review of approaches and practices of yoga that can be adopted by a seeker or applied in teaching yoga. Distinction of mindfulness meditation and transcendental meditation is noted.

VII. **Integrative Understanding of Yoga in Daily Life** points to application of mindful, ethical living in every aspect of life. It can be part of one's own religious or non-religious routines. Special note is made about group effects and relevance for health. To note the relevance for society and the environment, a separate chapter is dedicated to societal imbalances and how yoga's spiritual orientation can restore the balance.

VIII. **Functional and Ethical Requirements in Leading a Yoga Class** is guidance for those who plan to teach yoga to others and is presented in a single chapter.

IX. **Conclusion** is a single chapter summary of the main points of the book. Some readers may find it useful to begin their reading from Chapter 38 in this section. It may provide motivation and direction to the content of this book.

We hope the readers of this book will find its content meaningful to serve their interest in yoga. We welcome input from those knowledgeable in yoga to enhance the content in future editions. Suggestions may be sent to narayanan@lifeinyoga.org.

With Best Wishes,

C. Rajan Narayanan
Stephen Parker
Sanjeev Krishna
Idriss Raoua Ouedraogo
Ratna Nandakumar

July 13, 2023

CYAI.ORG is a non-profit [501(c)6] organization that seeks to promote and standardize authentic knowledge of yoga. It offers membership to any individual or institution interested in promoting yoga and its benefits to mankind. Individuals who seek to be certified in yoga may take certification examinations for instructor, teacher, and/or therapist levels. Institutions offering educational programs in yoga whose mission is to uphold authentic standards in yoga may also seek accreditation. Please visit https://cyai.org/ .

PART 1 – WHAT IS YOGA?

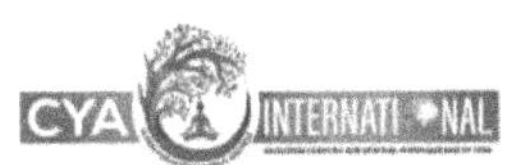

CHAPTER 1:

Understanding the Nature of Yoga

Yoga as understood today is mostly certain practices. However, the real meaning of yoga is integration of the "body, mind, and spirit" as said in common parlance, whereby one's meaning of life and nature of existence unfolds within oneself, in an intuitive way. Practices that promote such an achievement in gradual steps have come to be known as yoga, although it would be more correct to call them yoga practices.

With such an enunciation of yoga for a beginner, the natural questions that come to mind are the following:

- How do you know whether a practice can be called a Yoga practice?
- There are so many yoga practices around, each with a name of a founder or type of practice? Are they all valid? How should we assess any claimed practice of yoga?
- Where is the documentation to understand this?
- This business of 'spirit' enters the domain of religion and religious philosophies. Yoga is not supposed to be religious. Is there a relationship?

To answer these questions, we need a systematic approach.

Roots of Yoga

Yoga's roots lie in the human quest to know what life is – people (and other animate beings) are born, grow, age, and die. What is the meaning of this life? What is it that enters the body that gives life to an entity at conception or birth? What is it that leaves the body, upon which the person is said to be dead? This question of "Who am I and what is this world all about" has been the quest of the thinking human being from time immemorial.

Every religion speaks to its own view of the answers to these questions. They are further clothed with rituals and dogmas, often within the culture of its geographic origins or molded by other cultures that adopt it, with each one claiming a superiority in their views and approaches over others. Whatever may be the premise, every religion harbors some component of yoga since the quest of every religion is the same as that of yoga. But unlike yoga, in religion one can get lost in the woods of rituals, dogmas and culture, while in yoga the focus is clearly on comprehensive experiential principles. For the discerning person, while observing religious practices, it will be easy to separate the cultural cloaking and religious dogmas from essentials of yoga.

So, while every religion was engaged in different types of yoga practices within the cloak of rituals, an enlightened sage in ancient India, by name Patanjali, wrote a text called the Yoga Sutras. There, he systematically unfolded the yogic principles that lead to experiencing the higher reality and answers to all questions.

HOW CONFUSING CAN YOGA GET?

The proliferation of yoga around the world as gym exercise, and each with different name, also creates an environment where one can get lost trying to understand yoga. The world of yoga today is no better than religions competing and claiming greater superiority. It must be understood Yoga is One. The principles are clear. One may approach in different ways. That makes them different ***yoga practices***, but not different **yoga**.

Yoga Philosophy

The Yoga Philosophy enunciated in the Yoga Sutras by the sage Patanjali, is a theistic philosophy. It is addressed to the seeker to answer the questions stated earlier. Patanjali presents it systematically in four *pādas* or Quarters (colloquially called chapters).

In the first *pāda*, Patanjali points out that when one associates oneself with external stimulations, one is far away from yoga. When one is unaffected by external stimulations, the stillness within evokes understanding of the higher reality. Attainment of the higher reality may appear difficult for many people, but it can be approached in stages. With daily meditative practice, one can slowly transcend the reactivity to external stimulations and begin to develop intuitive awareness, and eventually cosmic wisdom.

The second *pāda* explains the programmed nature of each being, and the systematic process of attaining the yogic state. Here, the often quoted, eight-fold (*Aṣhṭānga*) yoga is introduced.

LIMBS OF THE EIGHT-FOLD *AṢHṬĀNGA YOGA*

The limbs of eight-fold (*Aṣhṭānga*) Yoga are stated as *Yama*, *Niyama*, *Āsana*, *Prāṇāyāma*, *Pratyāhāra*, *Dhāraṇā*, *Dhyāna*, and *Samādhi*. A short description of each is the following.

1. *Yama* – understood as being true to one's conscience.
2. *Niyama* – understood as having regularity in living.
3. *Āsana* – understood as physical alignment that permits optimal nerve communication that affects energy flow.
4. *Prāṇāyāma* – understood as regulation of vitality with breathing practices that allows one to fulfill the purpose of life and move towards spiritual purification.
5. *Pratyāhāra* – understood as ability to sense and direct internal vibrations that control the body-mind complex.
6. *Dhāraṇā* – understood as one-pointed focus to lead towards meditation.
7. *Dhyāna* – understood as going beyond the mind . . . state of mindlessness.
8. *Samādhi* – understood as balance of the intellect that is enabled by connection into the cosmic intelligence in an intuitive way that can provide answer to any question that may be the focus of *Dhāraṇā*.

The third *pāda* continues the unfolding of the systematic yoga process and deals with the last three of the eight-fold yoga process, which yield enhanced intuition and abilities. Patanjali provides these details so that a person will not get confused on the way to higher realization if such experiences manifest.

The fourth *pāda* addresses the nature of creation, the role of the individual within the context of all of creation, and the final state of liberation.

Thus, while the first three *pādas* serve as guide to individual practice, with details of the principles of yoga practices and yoga attainment, the fourth *pāda* is designed to complete the philosophical understanding of existence.

SUMMARY OF THE PHILOSOPHY OF YOGA

All of creation comes from one source – a dynamic program unleashed by a single force, which to fulfill its program intent creates several small units, each as a programmed entity. Each entity in performing its function contributes to this cosmic flow. Thus, the cosmos is like a distributed computing system.[1] When an entity, like a human being, endowed with the sense organs and ability to think, gets carried away by what it observes through its senses (from external stimulations), it defines itself by those sensory and reactive experiences. However, when one lets the program flow without reacting, except where one's active engagement is required to meet the cosmic need, one begins to realize one's true self.

This requires regular introspective meditative practices, designed to train one to be less reactive and more receptive to the inner recognition of where active engagement may be needed. When discriminative awareness comes, one intuitively understands where one's engagement lies, and where one should not react. Such inner anchor can also lead to intuitive experiences that go beyond the physical world that reveals the nature of existence beyond what is seen. In the highest realization, each person understands that we are only instruments of the cosmic flow.

One can also attain enhanced abilities that are not common in normal living. The philosophy clearly emphasizes that a person attaining such experiences and abilities should never consider himself or herself superior to other beings. After all, each individual is only an instrument of the cosmic flow.

---

[1] The concept of a distributed computing system originates from the concept of 'parallel computing.' In this conception, a computer needs to perform an enormous task. Within its processing capacity alone, its execution may be too slow or not effective enough. To enable the outcome, the computer intelligently distributes the program load among other computers, which are connected in its network, which do part of the job so that all the computers together are able to do the task more effectively and much faster.

Practice Approaches to Yoga

In the Yoga Sutras of Patanjali, often referred as the document of *Rāja* Yoga[2] or System of Yoga, Patanjali covers all approaches to yoga. Most approaches to yoga practices can be categorized as *Haṭha Yoga*, *Tantra Yoga* and *Bhakti Yoga*.

- ***Haṭha Yoga*** or Physical Yoga has an approach of beginning with the physical body as the stepping-stone for higher realization. This approach incorporates *āsanas* or postures and the six 'cleansing' techniques called *Ṣhaṭkriyās* (described in detail in the *Haṭha Yoga* Part of this book). These practices are considered the beginning step towards training oneself to be less affected by external stimulations, to eventually become a pure observer (called *Laya Yoga* in this tradition). The highest experience in this tradition is called *nāda anusandhāna* or experiencing the cosmic vibration.

- ***Tantra Yoga*** approach is to work with gross and subtle vibrations. It incorporates breath and sensory awareness in physical movements. It also incorporates mantras/sounds, power of intention and visualization techniques in meditative practices. Associated with *Tantra Yoga* are the pathways of vibration communications (called *nādis*).

- ***Bhakti Yoga*** approach is the faith-based path of surrender to God that is present in all theistic religions. One learns to live a life with every moment surrendered to God. This is completely in the mental-attitudinal domain in higher awareness, and God is understood beyond name, form, and attributes, except for the characterization as the unmanifest source of everything. However, in lower awareness it can manifest as rituals and beliefs associated with religions.

Popular schools of yoga largely focus on Haṭha Yoga practices. However, a more integrative and holistic yoga approach coming from a comprehensive *Rāja* Yoga tradition includes all the three approaches noted above. The goal of all these practices is to transcend the reactivity to external stimulations in all aspects of daily living, which is understood as the process of purification. This approach to living where all actions are performed without reactivity is often described as Yoga of Selfless Action or *Karma Yoga*. In effect, one surrenders all intent of action to the cosmic flow or God. It is also closely related to leading a disciplined life with strong ethics, being true to one's conscience, with an attitude of surrender to God.

---

[2] *Rāja* Yoga has been described by some as the approach of meditation instead of the comprehensive system of yoga that incorporates all aspects of yoga. This view cannot be validated based on the correct interpretation of the Yoga Sutras.

CONCEPT OF GOD IN THE YOGA SUTRAS

In the text of the Yoga Sutras, ***Īśhvara*** and ***Prabhu*** are two words, that are interpreted as God.[3] *Īśhvara* literally means Lord and Controller. *Prabhu* means the Creator.

Sutras 1:23-29 define the nature of *Īśhvara* in the following ways:

- Surrender to *Īśhvara* leads to the highest yogic realization;
- *Īśhvara* is untouched by any impurity and is outside the '*karma* cycle' of birth and death;
- *Īśhvara* is the unsurpassed source of all knowledge;
- Unbroken by time, *Īśhvara* is the Guru (teacher) of all;
- Om is the vibration that connects *Īśhvara* to all of creation and is the communicating mechanism with sentient beings.

Sutra 4:18 speaks to *Prabhu* as the all-knowing Creator who is fully aware that matter is the same, no matter how it is expressed in different forms and beings, while the same understanding may not be apparent to the created.

All these yoga approaches are included in the Yoga Sutras stated in different ways. *Karma Yoga* or Yoga of Selfless Action is referred as *Kriyā Yoga*[4]. *Bhakti Yoga* is referred as *Īśhvara Praṇidhāna* or 'Surrender to God'. The *Tantra Yoga* approach is embedded in the meditation techniques described in the last part of the first *pāda* and the third *pāda*. *Haṭha Yoga* is embedded in segments of the eight-fold (*Aṣhṭānga*) yoga approach.

Another approach discussed in *Vedānta* expositions is called *Jñyāna Yoga*. The best way to understand this from the Yoga Sutras is that one must seek to receive the wisdom. This is described as *Samyama* in the Yoga Sutras which consists of three steps: inquiry, contemplation and receiving the wisdom intuitively. However, this is accessible only after adequate purification, which is the initial focus of yoga practices. Hence *Jñyāna* yoga may be considered as the higher-level outcome of yoga practices of the three approaches noted above that lead to purification.

Role of Guru in Yoga

According to the Yoga Sutras **God is the Guru of everyone at all times**, and every created being (including every person) is only an instrument of the cosmic flow. So, what is this meaning of Gurus in the field of yoga?

---

[3] One other word used is *Sattva-Puruṣha* meaning the Pure *Puruṣha*. The word *Puruṣha* suggests unmanifest or inner cause. In common usage the gender male is also referred as *Puruṣha*. The implication is that a male is the unmanifest or inner cause of a new-born. In this introductory section, to avoid confusion the use of the word *Puruṣha* is avoided.

[4] *Kriyā* Yoga as used in this book is specific to the usage as in the Yoga Sutras. This should not be confused with a school of yoga that calls their practice as *Kriyā Yoga*.

Patanjali also notes a meditative practice focusing on a purified being that can lead to a higher experience in meditation.[5] Further, such beings can affect the vibrations of others by their mere physical presence or intention or touch. These highly cosmically connected beings can also provide powerful blessings. This is the role of priests in any tradition, who are supposed to be more connected and convey the intent to the cosmic intelligence on behalf of the seeker. Such is the impact of Yogis who have higher awareness, whose influence makes others treat them as Gurus.

Yet, the truly realized Yogi will never see himself or herself as a Guru, but simply as an instrument of the divine flow doing their job as a cosmic duty to help those on the spiritual path. Patanjali warns that any yogi who starts to feel self-importance, as superior to others, has not had full realization of the nature of existence. Where there is commercial intent, pressure and a person wanting to be on a pedestal, we can safely assume yoga has been compromised.

Mechanism of Yoga

In the philosophical exposition of yoga noted in the previous sections, it is abundantly clear that all of creation, including each entity in creation, is a programmed entity. There are three underlying components that contribute to understand the mechanism of yoga.

1. ***Processor*** of the programmed entity is called ***chitta***. By the nature of any computing system, it only receives input and delivers output. It has no intention of its own.
2. ***Programs*** that work through the *chitta* are called ***kleśha* and *karma*** in the Yoga Sutras.[6] *Kleśha* are the initial programs of creation embedded in each entity. These programs have intention. They work through the *chitta* to make the entity function, as ordained by creation, when facing external stimulations which are received as input by the *chitta*. For entities with ability to think, like human beings, reactivity to external stimulations creates new programs which are called *karma*. [Creation of *karma,* by judgemental

---

[5] In religious practices, this is called invocation.

[6] *Chitta* is described in *Sāṅkhya* philosophy as in the nature of '*sattva*' (unchanging) with no intention of its own. Yoga Sutras 4:4 describes *chitta* as in nature of *asmitā* or being a pure observer. The next sutra 4:5 says that to accommodate different needs of creation, from the one *chitta* emerges many. Thus, we understand there is a Cosmic *Chitta* and an individual *chitta*, both of which are simply processors without individual intent. The cosmic *chitta* processes the intent of *mahat* (as per *Sāṅkhya* philosophy) which manifests as the program of the cosmic flow, while the individual *chitta* processes the individual's *Karma-Kleśha* which are the components of the cosmic program allocated to a particular *chitta*. In this sense, the description allows latitude to think of *chitta* as the container of the programs (*Karma-Kleśha*) that it processes. The outcome, *chitta vritti* in the Yoga Sutras, are the experiences of the individual. Judging and reacting to these experiences is the job of the mind. The mind is conditioned by the inner programs and hence functions through the *chitta* in both judging and reacting to experiences. In this sense, *chitta* is considered as the mind-field or mind-system implying the system through which the mind works. The *chitta* is also described by some as consciousness which connotes the activity potential of a processor.

reaction to external stimulations, can be considered as learning by observation as in the artificial intelligence paradigm in the field of Computer Sciences.]

3. ***Channels of communication,*** called ***nādis,*** serve as conduits to *chitta* for input and output. Sensory stimulations are carried by the *nādis* into *chitta* as input. The output from the *chitta* is carried as vibrations that manifest in the activations – every aspect of living – of the entity.

Thus, **Yoga works with our *chitta***, and the communication system between the *chitta* and the trillions of cells of the body. Since each one of us and everything created is part of the larger cosmic flow, our individual *chitta* works in sync with a larger cosmic processor, the **Cosmic *Chitta***. The Yoga Sutras states that the One Cosmic *Chitta* projects many (smaller) *chittas* (like us) to fulfill the purpose of creation. Even beyond the Cosmic *Chitta* is its source and the seed of creation (called *Īśhvara* or *Prabhu* in the Yoga Sutras, interpreted as God), and connecting into THAT source is said to be the highest realization of yoga. [These concepts may be difficult to comprehend for a novice. Chapter 5 and 27 provide more details with flows and connections illustrated with diagrams.]

The individual *chitta's* communications upon entering the three-dimensional world come as vibrations and waves as they enter the physical elements of creation. Within the body, the communication channels, *nādis*, are actively assessed in traditional medicine systems (e.g. Ayurveda and Chinese Medicine) for diagnosing dysfunctionality in the system. The *nādis* also work with hubs where multiple *nādis* converge and are called *chakras*.

Outside the body, the vibrations and waves result in experiences beyond the body including intuitive perceptions.

When one is less reactive to external stimulations, less new *karmas* are formed and more of the embedded programs (*karma* and *kleśha*) deplete. It reduces the program load within the *chitta* and the communication load in the *nādis.*[7] [This is the process of *Kriyā* Yoga.] Such purification enables enhanced communication within and outside the body. This is the intermediate goal of yoga, a key stepping-stone towards intuitively realizing the nature of existence through cosmic connectivity. More details of *nādis* are in chapter 5 and higher-level applications are reserved for teacher level and therapy level training.

Recognizing Real Yoga Practices

Any practice that claims to call itself a yoga practice cannot violate the yogic principles laid down in the Yoga Sutras of Patanjali. Yoga's mechanism is through *nādi* communication. Specifically, it is gentle stimulation of the nādis without strain. Strain creates an overload in

---

[7] The reduction in the program load of the *chitta* is sometimes referred as purification of the *chitta* or *nādis*. More accurately it can be said to be the purification of the Causal Body referred in Chapter 5. However, since the *chitta* must work with the programs, some view all of it as in the domain of the *chitta* and use the term "purification of the *chitta* or *nādis*."

communication and always blocks *nādis*. Only when the mind is relaxed – the idea of 'let it be done' as opposed to 'I have to do' – can the *nādis* function optimally. Where there are fast movements and strained activity (seeking a 'work-out'), there is no yoga. Such yoga practices that are viewed as an extension of gym-based exercises are false yoga.

Religious practices may have yoga elements embedded. There may also be occult elements which may or may not be yoga. When daily prayers or meditative practices are done for no reason other than connecting into the spiritual domain to understand life and its purpose, irrespective of religion, they are all yoga practices. When occult practices are intended to fulfill individual desires that are not consistent with the cosmic flow, while they establish the connection beyond the physical domain, they cannot be considered as consistent with yoga principles.

Thus, practices such as swimming, walking, dancing, knitting done with focus – in fact any activity done with meditative engrossment – has a yoga effect. The examples in the blue box below illustrate this point.

THE REAL NATURE OF YOGA PRACTICES
– A Story of Music Yoga and Swimming-Sauna Yoga

On Thursday, March 9, 2006, about 4 pm, a yogi was beginning a Yoga-Meditation class conducted as free session organized by one of the student clubs at the University of Maryland. Among the students, the yogi perceived two of them as having developed some level of yogic alignment – purification of the *nādis* that allows for intuitive potential. Accordingly, he asked them, a male and a female student, what meditative practices they did. Both denied doing any meditative practices.

The yogi intuitively perceived that the female student had been in this state for a few years, whereas the male student had begun to experience the transformation only three days back. So, he asked the male student what had changed in his daily routine about three days back.

The student noted that he had started a new campus job from Monday and had developed a new daily routine. During the lunch break, he would take an hour off, in which he did about 20 minutes of lap swimming followed by 10 minutes seated in the sauna, and then he would pick-up some lunch from a cafeteria and would return to his work-desk. Reflecting on this, he started noting that after the swim of continuous laps, when he was in the sauna he would go into a mindless, transcendental state. This had been happening the last three days. He had not realized until this moment he had been engaging in a meditative practice.

With the female student the yogi intuitively sensed that in the evening hours her meditative nature was subdued, while it was more active during the mid-day period. The female student revealed that she went to bed late and woke up late. However, she would never get out of bed immediately upon waking up. For the past several years, upon waking up, she would reach her hand out to a music player by the side of her bed and begin playing it – the same music she had been playing for years. While the music played, she would go into a meditative state and would not know when the music stopped. She would probably be ready to get out of bed about an hour later. This is how she began the day around 10 or 11 in the morning, every day for the past several years.

Purpose of Yoga in One's Life

It is clear from the above discussion, that the **purpose of yoga is to experience the "body-mind-spirit" integration, that leads to the realization of the nature of existence and the understanding that one is only an instrument of the cosmic flow.**

However, for the average person, yoga practices are about deep relaxation, clearing the mind, finding renewed vitality, finding a focus in life, and also for overcoming physical or mental health issues.

For spiritual seekers and those philosophically oriented, yoga is about realizing that this body has been given by the cosmic intelligence to play our role as per our inner program to contribute towards the divinely planned cosmic flow. Not playing one's role would be considered going against yoga. Being in sync with one's cosmic plan can lead to liberation beyond rebirth when all the programs within dissipate. However, that requires playing one's role with the attitude of an observer and only reacting where one needs to do one's cosmic duty and not reacting to outcomes of our actions. Thus, from a philosophical perspective, the yoga approach would be considered *Dharma Śhāstra* (system of living life to support the cosmic flow – the art of living) that leads to *mokśha* (or release).

A mistaken view by some seekers is that yoga is just *Mokśha Śhāstra* (system of release) without recognizing the special role of each birth for fulfilling the purpose of the cosmic flow. This results in misguided attempts to escape from participation in normal aspects of living that contribute to the cosmic plan.

Larger View of the Term: Yoga

The word, yoga, comes from the root word *yuj*, which means to connect. In usage of the term, there are the following different connotations and contexts from a top-down view.

- ***Nature of Creation*** – As noted the entire cosmic flow is a connected dynamics of everything in existence. Therefore, ***all of existence is in yoga***, i.e., connected.
- ***Self-Realization*** is a term used for an individual seeker to connect into the higher reality and imbibe the intuitive knowledge of all of existence – what we have called the integration of the "body, mind, and spirit" earlier in this chapter that reveals the nature of existence. The ***state of that highest connectivity is yoga***, and such a connected person is called a yogi.
- ***Natural Unfolding of Events in Life*** is ***said to be connected in yoga***. What is meant to happen is often said to have yoga connection and what did not happen had no yoga connection to make it happen. This type of usage is related to the understanding of the cosmic interconnection of everything.
- ***Practices*** referred as yoga rather than yoga practices is the most common usage and the most incorrect usage.

It is worth noting that the Yoga Sutras explains that in our natural state we are in **yoga** – as connected with the cosmic existence. However, when the mind takes over, we get disconnected.

Questions and Discussion Topics

1. When you come across different types of yoga, how will you recognize what really is true yoga?
2. Can you be religious and a yoga aspirant at the same time?
3. Can you be non-religious and a yoga aspirant at the same time?
4. When one is able to connect beyond the body, and use the power of intention for successful attainment of what one wishes, can it be considered yoga?
5. Is yoga only about going beyond *karma* and the rebirth cycle (*mokśha*)?

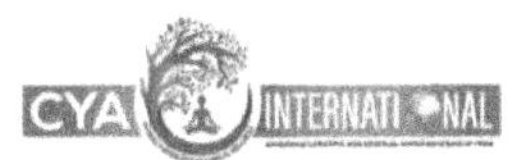

CHAPTER 2:

Application of Yoga

While the Yoga Sutras of Patanjali serve as a guide for the spiritual seeker, in the fourth *pāda* it also discusses the larger creation beyond the individual. The nature of creation and existence revealed in the fourth *pāda* of the Yoga Sutras suggests that yoga is not only the process of cosmic creation and dissolution, but also the dynamics of cosmic sustenance. Thus, the application of yoga spans the individual, society, and the cosmic spectrum.

For the Individual

For the individual, by allowing the integration of the "body, mind and spirit," yoga enables enhanced intuition that facilitates the following:

- Health Maintenance – Keen sense of what is good for the body and mind, and what is not – thereby allowing oneself to have a lifestyle that is in sync with one's nature, and consequently be in good health.
- Health Restoration – The same keen sense and regular practices helping to overcome health inadequacies.
- Finding Ones Calling – The intuitive sense guides one towards finding one's true purpose in life – that which fulfills the individual being while satisfying the flow of the cosmic program.
- Social Integration and Emotional Balance – The realization of cosmic integration allows one to be socially useful, an endearing team player, and a heartful contributor for others. This realization of the cosmic dynamics through intuitive awareness also allows one to take the ups and downs of life with emotional equipoise.
- Finding Fulfillment and Happiness in Life until the day one departs from the body is the natural outcome of the above four points.
- Highest Realization of Yoga, whereby one can connect with the source of all knowledge and become fully Self-Realized, is a distinct possibility for those in the path of yoga.

Beyond the Individual

The philosophy of yoga, that describes the nature of creation whereby the one dynamic program multiplies into many to fulfill the cosmic goal, makes it obvious that everything in existence is interrelated. The yoga mechanism of this interrelationship is explained by the Standard Model of physics, consisting of the four forces, and quantum theories, at least at the high level of interplanetary and intra-planetary movements of nature and the lowest level of the smallest particles. From a yogic standpoint we also go into the dimensionality of people and social forces.

Whether it be the role of the sun and stars and the planetary systems which stay on its course, or impact of sunspots and solar radiation on earth's magnetic field, or the climate and weather patterns on earth affected by the electromagnetic field of the earth, or the role of moon's gravitation on ocean tides, or the extinction or mutation of species, or the interpersonal impact of individuals or in groups and the consequent impact on sociopolitical outcomes, all of these are part of this interrelationship phenomenon.

Following are some examples of such interrelationships:

- Interdependence of Species – We are learning about how species influence each other – whether by food chain links or external influences like by-products. Bees pollinating flowers and flowers giving the nectar for honey is one example. However, ecologists have identified hundreds of such interrelationships. Thus, when some species are destroyed, we recognize today that it could have unwanted effects on others. Desertification has been found to be related to loss of soil organisms by destructive overuse.
- Interdependence of Matter and Energy and its Consequences – Not only is Einstein's theory of matter and energy equivalence validated, but we also know that every matter, in certain forms, has desirable impact on some and undesirable impact on others, and that the entire world is in an ecological balance. For example, nuclear energy is a great source of energy, but with inappropriate application is also toxic and dangerous. Similarly, every medicine, in pharmacology, is known to be a poison; however, the poison is used as an antidote to the poison within.
- Role of Environment – Sunlight, climate, weather, and tides are all governed by inter-related forces and have led to substantial understanding of weather patterns and predictions. The scientific community has established the correlation between atmospheric increment in some gases (carbon dioxide, methane, etc.) and its impact on global warming.
- Agricultural Productivity is affected by everything around us including environmental factors and development of technological advances.
- Evolution of Societies, Societal Governance and Political Thinking is affected by all the above. Even the concept of thinking, communicating ideas, and the sense of feeling and imbibing, have vibrational basis. They result in such phenomena as gun ownership[8], religious extremism, charitable orientations, etc. This also creates oppression in

---

[8] https://worldpopulationreview.com/country-rankings/gun-ownership-by-country For instance in the United States there are 393 milion guns privately held relative to a population of 330 million, i.e. 1.2 guns per person, adult and child included. Whereas, the next highest is Falkland Islands at 0.6, and a comparable colonized country like Canada has 0.3.

societies and gives rise to extraordinary people who rise to the occasion and find solutions.

- Menstrual Cycle research has shown that when many women in child-bearing ages cohabit, over a period of time, all the women develop the same menstrual cycle.

Thus, yoga philosophy helps us to understand interrelationships in all aspects of living. This can provide guidance for bringing global harmony. This harmony emanates from individual levels that build up into communities, nations, the globe, and even the cosmos.

- Individual harmony by individual yogic way of life
- Societal harmony as the collective of individuals
- Environmental harmony with appropriate use of global resources
- Cosmic harmony by being in sync with the cosmic flow.

EXAMPLES OF INFLUENCE OF YOGA IN WORLD DYNAMICS

Integrative medicine, that has become a popular notion in medical practice, is just another way to understand the integrative nature of the body parts and its relationship with the environment. A key contributor to this thinking, besides the influence of traditional medicine systems, is the advent of Yoga Therapy, which is well recognized now, all over the world. While Integrative Medicine is in the yogic direction compared to Allopathic medicine, too often reductionism in application loses the deeper yogic principles.

Management Development principles largely emanate from yogic principles and then get diluted into non-yogic goals. They begin with ideas like: (a) fitting into one's role, being satisfied and fulfilled in one's role; (b) being empathetic to others: one's work contributing to others and roles of others contributing to the overall functioning of the organization, and thus working with sharing of knowledge and helping others, as opposed to working with selfish interest. However, the tragedy of the material orientation towards running a business is that at some point the focus becomes mere productivity and business value as measured in monetary terms, where employees get measured on individual productivity. The overall impact on employee satisfaction, the organization, and society as a whole, which represent the higher dimensionalities of cosmic existence, are compromised.

Concept of 'Good Corporate Citizen' emanates from the understanding of interrelationships across society. However there too, often it goes towards strategic philanthropy and gaining political influence rather than the common good.

Meditative Introspection to Resolve Conflicts – This is an approach that has been used in conflicting situations where toning down emotions (from judgmental reactions) and quiet meditative reflection have revealed other options that may be agreeable to the conflicted parties. In instances where a conflict cannot be fully resolved, this approach helps to maintain the relationship so that people can agree to disagree without breaking the relationship. While this is extensively used in world diplomacy, following are a few examples encountered in social interactions.

EXAMPLES OF MEDITATIVE INTROSPECTION TO RESOLVE CONFLICTS

Example 1 - Once an organizational issue arose in a church congregation. The conflicting views had resulted in extensive discussion and processing but showed little progress. There was great concern that the membership of the church might fracture. Swami Veda Bharati (AHYMSIN) suggested that the people involved sit together at the Meditation Center. Everyone joined for a one-hour guided meditation session. Afterwards the emotional edges of the conflict had been smoothed and the relationships eased so that people's emotional disturbance did not contribute so much to the friction in peoples' interaction. A fracture, which had happened in a previous conflict, was avoided.

Example 2 - In 2006, at the capital of Burkina Faso, Ouagadougou, there was a strike of teachers in the school system, where teachers refused to conduct a required preliminary exam without additional resources. Communication between the teachers and the school director had collapsed. The Minister of Education became involved to find a solution. As Finance Director, Idriss Raoua Ouedraogo was called to lead the meeting. He opened the meeting with meditative equipoise that lowered the emotions and allowed the teachers and school administrators to state the problem. He found that the reason for the problem was that the teachers were never involved in the budgeting process for the schools, but rather the school director made up the budget without teacher consultation and had not allocated money for the exams. Idriss suggested that in future the teachers must be involved in preparing the budget with allocation of money for every prioritized activity. This resolved the strike, and the teachers went back to their schools and found their resources to conduct the exam.

CAN YOGA-MEDITATION REDUCE CRIME RATE?

A yogi can connect within and also beyond into everything. The concept of connectivity is how the Universe hangs together. Maharishi Mahesh Yogi is known to have said that if enough meditators were in synchronistic meditation, they can transform the consciousness of geographic areas and reduce crimes. About 15 studies were done and it is claimed that with 1% of the population doing meditation, crime can be reduced.

Mental Health Application – A Special Need of Our Times

Worldwide, the approach of individualism, lack of empathy, and materialism has created emotional upheaval from the perception of success and failure for individuals, resulting in suicides and other erratic and destructive social behaviors, including gun violence. Polar opposite has been adherence to narrow religious views in an attempt to find spiritual meaning to one's existence, and thereby developing a sense of self-righteousness that leads to unhealthy social behavior, including unwanted violence, inciting social unrest and even wars. The role of yoga can be thought as the process of 'growing up' for everyone – expanding one's horizon and seeing the cosmic purpose of one's temporal existence – and thus bring a long-term solution to this mental health pandemic that the world suffers today.

Commonly people think about mental health as the province of mental health experts. Furthermore, there is a tendency to blame modern technology, social media, and other external influences. However, stability of the mind begins at home – the influence of family members and social relationships.

Yoga provides the basis for self awareness in a larger sense to understand that we, as a family and society, come together to fulfill a cosmic purpose. This is the way to overcome individualistic and materialistic thinking.

Many people describe the COVID pandemic as stressful because they were forced to make a change in their way of living: dealing with their family members more than they had planned; limiting vacation plans and social gatherings; having a different kind of interaction with colleagues at work, etc. However, a positive side has been the soul searching to find the meaning of life. This has led many people in affluent countries to quit from the work force to find greater satisfaction within the individual and the family relationship.

A study from Australia based on a sampling of 2,130 parents notes the following:[9]

> "Overall, the findings demonstrated a breadth of responses. Messages around loss and challenge were predominant, with many families reporting mental health difficulties and strained family relationships. However, not all families were negatively impacted by the restrictions, with some families reporting positive benefits and meaning, including opportunities for strengthening relationships, finding new hobbies, and developing positive characteristics such as appreciation, gratitude, and tolerance."

A report from US Census data found a positive impact from COVID, reported as follows:[10]

> "The Covid-19 pandemic upended many family dynamics but one positive consequence of this upheaval: Parents shared more dinners and read to their children more often, according to the U.S. Census Bureau's 2020 Survey of Income and Program Participation (SIPP)."

The experience of COVID, in these reports, clearly demonstrates how the people who expanded their consciousness by introspection improved their quality of life, while those who remained stressful were probably embedded in their individualism and materialism. [In yoga we say that

---

[9] Subhadra Evans et. al (Deakin University, Geelong, Australia) From "It Has Stopped Our Lives" to "Spending More Time Together Has Strengthened Bonds": The Varied Experiences of Australian Families During COVID-19. (Front. Psychol., 20 October 2020): https://doi.org/10.3389/fpsyg.2020.588667

[10] YERÍS MAYOL-GARCÍA Pandemic Brought Parents and Children Closer: More Family Dinners, More Reading to Young Children, JANUARY 03, 2022 https://www.census.gov/library/stories/2022/01/parents-and-children-interacted-more-during-covid-19.html

such difficult situations become catalysts for the spiritual quest. Some expand and find higher realization, and others fail and succumb to the stress.]

Reflecting on earlier generations, one can develop insight into how societies kept the mental health balance by adherence to customs and beliefs. Daily prayers and ritualistic living were part of the meditative introspection. Further, roles of family and community, and roles of priest for spiritual guidance were all part of this support system. However, at times it also engendered rigidity, which created abuse and resistance. Today, yoga has this special role for individuals, families, and the society as a whole. And when yoga is understood in its larger dimension, there can be no rigidity in yoga.

Questions and Discussion Topics

1. Reflect on the effect of yoga on your life. Review the five points noted in the application of yoga for the individual. Have you personally experienced any one or more of them? Explain.
2. People who have made big contributions to society, and have become well-known, are often described as having yogic components in their daily living. Pick any individual and review their daily ritualistic way of living and explain their yogic component.
3. Can you describe any traditional way of living, including religious living, that has created rigidity? If so, analyze the pros and cons of such traditional living. Further consider how such unwanted elements of rigidity can be avoided and how yoga can show the way.

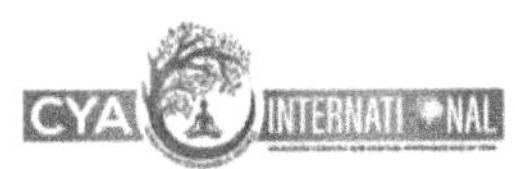

CHAPTER 3:

History of Systematic Development of Yoga

As noted earlier, yoga is essentially about spiritual realization. It is as old as humanity's quest for the meaning of life and death. Therefore, to put a timeline on development of yoga and yoga practices is impossible. While yogic thoughts and practices may have emerged from many traditions around the world, it was systematically developed and documented as a spiritual system in ancient India.

The academic world timelines, related to Indian philosophical thoughts and Vedic hymns, are much colored by the Oxford University approach of the British colonial era. They appear to be based on comparative assessments of Egyptian and Mesopotamian civilizations, with the assumption that these biblical civilizations were the oldest. Modern day availability of scientific methods, including carbon dating of fossils, luminescence dating of pottery/ceramics artifacts, climatic evolution dating from polar ice core drillings, sea-bed plankton deposits and rings in the trunks of ancient, fossilized trees, and ancient global migration studies based on genetic mutation, provide a different and more ancient view of the history of the human race and civilization in the Indian sub-continent. Astronomical analysis of astral observations made in the Indian epics of Rāmāyana and Mahābhārata, attempted by Nilesh Oak[11] and others, also places the Indian civilization as far more ancient than that suggested by the Oxford school. Based on multiple methods of scientific dating it is well-recognized today that the Vedic civilization is much older than 5,000 years and the Mahabharata war likely occurred more that 5,000 years ago. Hence, it is best to avoid specific dates, and instead focus on sequence of chronological developments without specific dates, anchoring on the Yoga Sutras of Patanjali and Vyāsa. Vyāsa is known to be the compiler of the Vedas and author of the Mahābhārata. [Bhagavad Gitā[12] is a segment within the Mahābhārata.]

Following are some interesting points of chronology about the ancient development of yoga:

- ***Yoga known before Patanjali*** - Yoga Sutras, authored by Patanjali more than five thousand years ago, serves as the summary and systematic enunciation of yoga. In other words, yoga was known before Patanjali. This is evident in the way Patanjali refers to

---

[11] Nilesh Nilkanth Oak: When Did The Mahabharata War Happen? : The Mystery of Arundhati, 2011, ISBN-13:978-0983034407; ISBN-10:0983034400

[12] While Yoga Sutras of Patanjali is the defining document of yoga, several yoga schools use the philosophical content of Bhagavada Gita for instructional purposes.

chakras and *nādis* in the third *pāda* without discussing them, as if they were common knowledge.

- ***Yoga Philosophy of Patanjali predates Vyāsa's Vedānta Philosophy*** - In the ancient Indian philosophical system, there are six ancient philosophies which in chronological order are: *Sāṅkhya*, *Nyāya*, *Vaisheṣhika*, *Mimāmsa*, Yoga and Vedānta. Vedānta is the philosophy written by Vyāsa, culled from the Upaniṣhads of the Vedas (which he compiled), as the final message of the Vedas.
- ***Yoga and Vedas cannot be separated in evolution*** - Vyāsa compiled the Vedas from the hymns of 33 religious systems of ancient India and established a Vedic religion.[13] He knitted the message of the Upaniṣhads, which is the philosophical content of the Vedas, to establish the Vedānta philosophy. Prior to that Patanjali had authored the Yoga Sutras to establish the yoga philosophy. Vyāsa also wrote a commentary on the Yoga Sutras establishing the parity of the two philosophies. It is enough to conclude that both Patanjali and Vyāsa lived during the times when uncompiled Vedic knowledge was known. While Patanjali focused on the spiritual component alone, Vyāsa focused both on the religious and spiritual components.

From that era, after many centuries or millennia, the next generation of thinking came with the emergence of Jainism and Buddhism in ancient India. Buddhism being non-theistic, its influence developed a later yoga philosophy called *Sāṅkhya-Yoga*, that took components of *Sāṅkhya* and Yoga and enunciated it as non-theistic. This new philosophy led to the emergence of Buddhist yoga practices.[14] When we are focused on the Yoga Sutras, we don't need to digress there.

In the post Buddhist period, the ritualistic ancient system of living, based on faith in what was beyond the temporal world, ensured acceptance of things that could not be controlled. The following approaches to Yoga emerged:

- Daily meditative rituals with faith in God within organized societies,
- *Haṭha Yoga* practices among those who were in the hilly and mountainous terrain of the Himalayas, often associated with asceticism,
- Occult practices of *Tantra Yoga* associated with the Vedic religion. [Such occult practices are also observed in other parts of the world, like Voodoo in Africa, Shamanism in native America, Paganism in Europe, etc.]

---

[13] While this is not much talked about, the evidence of it lies in two specific places: (i) there are 33 forms of temple worship in various parts of India (28 associated with *Śhiva* family, 3 with *Vaiṣhnava*, and 2 with *Devi*); (ii) in the compilation of the Vedas by Vyāsa, he includes in the twelfth stanza of *Chamakam* the acceptance of the 33. [*Chamakam* follows after *Namakam* of *Rudra Praśhna* that is popularly used in temple worship, which asks for blessing of everything worldly and spiritual and ends with asking for all the 33, which we interpret as the forms of temple worship.]

[14] The Buddhist yoga influence from *Sāṅkhya-Yoga* philosophy may be observed in may practices like zen meditation and other practices within the South Asian Buddhist traditions.

These were probably influenced by the revival of the Vedic tradition (by Shankarācharya[15]) in the post Buddhist period.

The emergence of European colonialism with a high focus on materialism and physical strength probably resulted in the emergence of *Haṭha Yoga* as the most popular form of yoga over the last century. The story of Krishnamacharya, spanning the twentieth century, tells us that a significant percentage of his students came from the elites of the western world, and his prominent Indian students, BKS Iyengar and Pattabhi Jois, went on to propagate and emphasize the physical dimensions of yoga, namely *Haṭha Yoga*. Unlike the other propagators of yoga who came from monkhood, this tradition expanded more into yoga studios.

Another approach to yoga was brought as Kriyā Yoga by Yogananda to North America in the 1950s. This system has not propagated as widely as the others.

The *Tantra* side came mainly from Swami Rama and Maharishi Mahesh Yogi, where Swami Rama was more holistic in integrating all aspects of yoga while the Maharishi was more focused on Mantra-based meditation.

Another major influence was that of Ramakrishna,[16] whose disciples went on to establish a worldwide network that included Vedāntic studies and meditative practices.

Another branch that tried to integrate *Haṭha Yoga* and Vedānta came from the Divine Life Society established by Swami Sivananda in the early twentieth century. [Swami Sivananda was a practicing physician before he became a monk, and that may explain his focus on *Haṭha Yoga* on one side, and Vedāntic philosophy on the other side.] Today, the branches are called Sivananda Ashrams and are established in many parts of the world.

Aurobindo Ghosh who started as a freedom fighter in India, in his isolation in British jails had the deeper experiences of yoga in meditation. His main approach was meditation.

Another major influencer was Prabhupada who brought Krishna Consciousness with his organization ISKON. His focus was the idea of 'Surrender to God' – *Bhakti Yoga.*

These were the main influences of yoga in most of the twentieth century. Late in the twentieth century and then emerging into the twenty-first century, we see many more schools.

---

[15] Shankarācharya is thought to have had a short lifespan of about 32 to 33 years between the 8th and 10th century CE. While there is controversy on the precise dating, he is credited to have revived the Vedic religion by establishing many monasteries around India and creating an order of monkhood. It is recognized that because of his influence the predominant presence of Buddhism in India faded into nominal and negligible status.

[16] Ramakrishna's principal disciple Swami Vivekananda is credited to have created an organization called Ramakrishna Mission that now has network in many parts of the world. Ramakrishna, often referred as Ramakrishna Paramahamsa was a temple priest from Bengal in India from the 19th century. His spiritual experiences are documented in the text called The Gospel of Sri Ramakrishna.

It is sufficient to note here that integrative approach to yoga requires inclusion of all the different elements of yoga. Although in initial stages of yogic practice focusing on one approach is helpful to build discipline, focus on one approach alone usually creates narrowness in thinking. That results in incompleteness in the spiritual journey. Because yoga is the discipline of experiential realization, it requires one to approach practices with no assumptions with openness to consider all approaches.

INFLUENCE OF *SĀṄKHYA-YOGA* PHILOSOPHY ON MAINSTREAM YOGA

The emergence of *Sāṅkhya-Yoga* as a non-theistic philosophy, a few thousand years after the Yoga Sutras, had a profound influence on the later exposition of yoga, especially *Haṭha Yoga*. For example, the term *brahmacharya* was interpreted as celibacy. In earlier times, it was understood as "curiosity to learn" based on the root meaning. Vyāsa (the author of the Vedānta philosophy) in his commentary on the Yoga Sutras describes *brahmacharya* to mean activation or elevation of the mind, which he describes as the eleventh sense organ, which matches the root meaning of *brahmacharya* as movement or exploration of all that is created. [*brahma* refers to all that is created and *charya* to mean movement within it.]

The emergence of such understanding of *brahmacharya* in *Haṭha Yoga* can be explained as follows. The non-theistic view of *Sāṅkhya-Yoga* and Buddhism viewed liberation from the cycle of rebirth (created by *karma*) as the goal of life. Engagement in activities of life is thought to create desires, adding *karma*, and perpetuating rebirth. Hence, they negated the idea of procreation and sexual intercourse as driven by desire. Thus, a new interpretation of *brahmacharya* was evolved in this era that meant celibacy. *Haṭha Yoga* texts, having emerged in the post *Sāṅkhya-Yoga* era (a few thousand years after the Yoga Sutras), tend to adopt some of the *Sāṅkhya-Yoga* elements, like celibacy, while also integrating the *Tantra* concept of *Śhiva* and *Śhaktī*. [Mahāyāna Buddhism uses *Tantra* concepts as well.]

Questions and Discussion Topics

1. Is it important to determine the origins of yoga? If so, why or why not? Consider arguments for both sides.
2. You will come across people who say yoga does not involve any belief in God and those who will say that yoga is a theistic philosophy. In a debating forum how will you defend both sides?
3. Pick any school of yoga and analyze its approach and examine its level of completeness as a yoga system that leads to the highest realization.

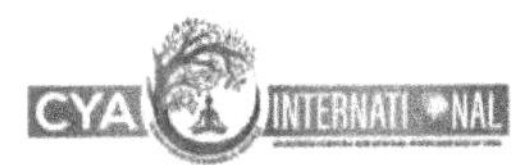

CHAPTER 4:

Becoming an Instructor in Yoga

The requirement of Instructor level certification is that one must be able to lead a yoga practice session effectively and safely.

Effectiveness in Leading a Session

To be effective in leading any type of yoga practice session there are some requirements, with varying levels of competency, that come over time. Following is a description of these considerations:

- ***Having significant competency in the type of yoga practices that one instructs*** – This comes from regular personal practice over many months where one is able to sense the impact of the practice within oneself and understand subtle nuances. And this regular practice, which may modify and mature over time, must be maintained throughout one's life to be effective as a yoga instructor.

- ***Ability to sense or observe indicators of effectiveness in others*** – Such indicators can be internal or external. Internal assessment is possible only when a yoga instructor has attained the ability to be intuitive. External assessment happens through indicators like posture alignments, speed of breath and body movement, expression on the face, and sound vibration when one speaks or chants.

- ***Internal transformation must occur for an instructor***. This is observed in terms of less reactivity – being an observer more often and selectively interacting with external engagements. It often shows as a more peaceful demeanor, measured in language and expression, having a greater understanding and a more forgiving nature towards follies of normal living. This happens with internal programs (*karma-kleśha*) dissipating as they activate, and one remains non-reactive.

  Observing participants in regular yoga sessions, and following up with the same group over time, can be instructive for the instructor. During each session, there would be a temporary transformation among the participants, which an instructor may sense. With regular practice the participants' transformation becomes second nature to them. This is what the instructor would have attained through regular practice over many months. By observing the changes in the participants, the instructor becomes more aware about her/his own personal transformation.

- ***Appropriate environment is another important consideration for effectiveness.*** Environmental vibrations must be peaceful and conducive for yoga practice. This is addressed in greater detail in chapter 37 (eighth part of the book) that addresses functional and ethical requirements.

> INTERNAL TRANSFORMATION MUST BE PERCEIVED BY PEOPLE AROUND YOU
>
> In the AHYMSIN training program, trainees used to ask Swami Veda Bharati if he perceived progress in them. He would respond saying, they should ask their spouse if they had transformed enough to make it easier to live with. At times he would even suggest they should ask their mother-in-law.
>
> The point is that if one is truly on the path of yoga, transformation must occur!

Safety

Safety issues arise mainly because of the inability to sense and adhere to a basic principle enunciated in the Yoga Sutras – all practices must be done with ease and with light effort (i.e., with no strain whatsoever). When ease is lost, one always exposes oneself to potential injuries.

A second area of safety relates to the mundane elements of the physical environment that is addressed in chapter 37 (eighth part of the book).

A third area of safety relates to sensitivity in dealing with people and ensuring that one does not violate ethical requirements. Many people get attracted to yoga because they are in a state of imbalance. As they begin to experience the benefits of yoga, they may develop attachment to their teachers. Keeping ethical requirements in mind, it is important to keep one's distance to avoid untoward incidents.[17]

Becoming an Instructor is only the First Step

Aspiring to be a yoga instructor may have different motivations, for different people, expressed in different ways. It generally begins with a profound personal benefit from yoga practice. Very often people facing difficult circumstances in life, whether physical or mental, find significant relief from regular yoga practice of one type or the other. The profound benefit serves as a motivator to learn more, and for some it becomes a passion to learn more to help others. This motivates one to pursue yoga instructor training.

---

[17] People in states of mental imbalances can hallucinate and later may develop attachment to the teacher. It is important that the teacher recognize this potential and ensure safe distance in interactions.

Yogis understand that difficult circumstances that bring one to yoga is the cosmic conspiracy to show the path of spirituality when the soul is ready. Learning to become a yoga instructor is only the first step towards advancement in yoga. It begins with discipline in one's personal practice. Then as one shares with others, in time, deeper understanding emerges.

While many yoga schools consider such certification as an enabler to earn income, that focus will necessarily become a barrier to advancement in yoga. We recommend that yoga instructors should have their own separate source of income and conducting yoga sessions as an instructor should be viewed as fostering the deeper experience of yoga – after all yoga is the experience and not the practice. The key realization is that each one of us is not a separated entity from others around, but rather we are an integrated cosmos. As you teach, it will teach you more. The receiver is blessed, and you are twice blessed.

Since there are many approaches to yoga practices, selecting any one as the starting point and developing depth and mastery in the practice should be the initial goal. It will automatically open the door for exploring other practices until the true nature of yoga is experienced and realized.

Meditation is the core component of yoga. Experiences in meditation are individual and varied, with some experiencing profound revelations. Common experiences are quietening the mind, deep silence within, and progressive development of inner awareness. This is the building block towards the higher experiences of yoga.

Regular daily practice of at least an hour that includes a minimum of 30 minutes of meditative practice is required for systematic advancement in yoga. As you continue with your regularity, you will soon find ways to make many more aspects of your life – in fact, every aspect of your life – into a yoga activity. By letting every activity be in a natural flow, without expectation, and most of the time as an observer with inner awareness, makes every activity into a yoga activity – whether it is walking, talking, writing, or cooking. In a religious sense, one begins to just feel like an instrument of the cosmic flow to serve God's purpose.

Caution in Expectations

For progress in yoga, one needs to be a pure observer. That means one cannot have expectations. Whatever one is meant to experience will unfold in time. Having expectations in the progress of yoga will itself prevent progress.

One may hear of yogis or come across such yogis who can sense people by mere thought or from a picture, or even with ability to transcend time. The third *pāda* (quarter) of the Yoga Sutras note extraordinary and enhanced abilities that may come from the realization of yoga. However, one may or may not experience any such abilities even with decades of practice. It is important to note that these abilities are NOT the purpose of yoga.

In the Yoga Sutras, sage Patanjali explains that enhanced abilities come only to fulfill the purpose of one's existence (one's *Sva-dharma*) for the sake of the cosmic flow. If such abilities come, they should never be used except when there is inner spiritual guidance, that is untainted by desires. When there is spiritual guidance, it will only be for a greater good and not for a selfish interest.

Questions and Discussion Topics

1. State what motivated you to begin a yoga instructor training program. Then review the four considerations for effectiveness in leading a yoga session noted in this chapter, and then prioritize them with adequate justification. Also feel free to add additional considerations if you wish.
2. Assess yourself, as you are currently, with respect to capacity to lead a yoga session? Compile a prioritized list of what you need to develop to become a better yoga instructor.
3. If you are ready to begin leading a yoga session, what would be your checklist to ensure safety of those who participate in your session? Prioritize the list with adequate justification.

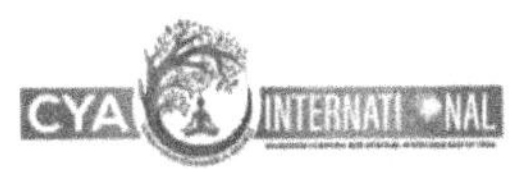

CHAPTER 5:

The Underlying Mechanism of All Yoga Approaches

As noted in chapter 1, there are various approaches to yoga practices, even though yoga itself is only one. The mechanism of all yoga practices is through the communication system of the *nādis* working through one's *chitta*, as noted in chapter 1. [Please review the terms *chitta* and *nādis* in the Mechanism of Yoga section in chapter 1.] Because the *chitta* is the processor of our entire programmed being, activation of the *chitta* impacts all our psychosomatic elements. Further, as cosmic beings, the interrelationship is established between our individual *chitta* and the cosmic *Chitta*, whose interaction governs the cosmic flow. The Yoga Sutras also recognizes that the individual *chitta* of living (sentient) beings has a separate direct connection to the cosmic intelligence, which is the unmanifest and supreme source of everything, *Īśhvara* (God). All yoga approaches work most of the time in the domain of the individual and cosmic *Chitta*, and in the stillness of meditation the individual *chitta* accesses *Īśhvara* to imbibe cosmic intelligence and understand the nature of existence.

The following topics address in detail the internally conceived and externally observed mechanism of yoga:

- ***Notion of Three Bodies*** – the yogic view of the physical and subtle elements within
- ***Karma Cycle Concept*** – the nature of reactivity
- ***Nādis and Marmas*** – the mechanism of channels of internal communication
- ***Concept of Five Levels of Communication, Left and Right Sides and Chakras*** – types of communication and their pathways
- ***Process Leading to Samādhi***
- ***Power of Intention, Intuition and Role of Dharma***
- ***External Monitors of Beneficial Yoga Practice***
- ***Physiology View of Yoga Practices***
- ***Stress Reduction and Balance*** – as understood by the yoga mechanism.

Notion of Three Bodies

In the tradition of yoga, three levels of the body are recognized. The physical elements of the body are referred as the ***gross body***. Activation of the gross body is enabled by vibrations, which upon ceasing the person is dead. These vibrations constitute the ***subtle body.*** The channels of these vibrations, *nādis* in Yoga and Ayurveda, are called *Mai* in Chinese Medicine (which is anglicized as meridians or bio-meridians). Underlying the subtle body is the repository of programs (like software in our computers) which cannot manifest without the gross body and energy flowing in it. These programs constitute the ***causal body***.

Another way to understand is that out of the cosmic intelligence of *Īśhvara* comes *Prakṛiti,* the primordial energy of subtle and manifest creation.[18] *Prakṛiti* creates and triggers activation of the cosmic *Chitta,* along with its intent in the form of programs to create the cosmic flow. The cosmic *Chitta* creates individual *chittas* with assigned program content (called *kleśha* in yoga) to each individual *chitta* to fulfill the intent of the cosmic flow. The assigned program content constitutes the causal body of each individual *chitta.* The individual *chitta* processes the programs of the causal body, which create vibrations forming the subtle body, whose expression manifests as the gross body as illustrated in Figure 5.1 on the next page. Each individual *chitta* (of living beings) also has a separate connection to *Īśhvara* (God) that is called ***chetanā*** in Yoga. That *chetanā* connecting to the unmanifest source of everything is called the ***Puruṣha*** element and can be thought as the soul.

Figure 5.1 represents the most accurate description of the psychosomatic being. Y**ou may now realize that our informal usage of the term "body, mind and spirit" is only a convenient common usage and is not exactly accurate**. The mind is only the reactive element, in the subtle body, of the functioning of the composite of the three levels of bodies. Its reactions *(karma)* get embedded as new program elements in the causal body (in addition to the remaining *kleśha*) facilitated by one's *chitta.*[19] In common usage, the spirit essentially refers to the causal body.

While the gross body and the vibrations of the subtle body (upon entering the electromagnetic spectrum) are amenable to measurement, the causal body and the *chittas* are purely in the psychic domain and are considered not measurable with currently available scientific tools. They can only be sensed intuitively by yogis. Measured assessments through their expression in the vibrations of the subtle body[20] and the state of the gross body only provide some insights. [The cosmic *Chitta* can only be intuitively sensed in a very high level of *Samādhi* through the cosmic intelligence of *Īśhvara* – discussed in a later section.]

---

[18] *Prakṛiti* is explained in more detail in chapter 22 (Concept of Tantra and its Application). The same word *Prakṛiti* in the Ayurvedic context of Doshas noted in chapter 19 on *Ṣhatkriyās* refers to the microcosm – the individual person who is part of the manifestation of the subtle and gross dimensions – which is different from the whole cosmic creation.

[19] When the mind ceases to react, it feels like the *chitta* [YS 4:22]. In that stillness of the *chitta*, the Soul/*Puruṣha's* connection can potentially access the cosmic intelligence of *Īshvara*.

[20] The vibrations are measured in traditional medicine systems with three-finger assessment of the pulse vibrations and also with Electro-photonic Imaging. [See next section on *nādis* and *marmas*.]

Figure 5.1:
THE THREE BODIES AND THE EXPRESSION OF THE CHITTA

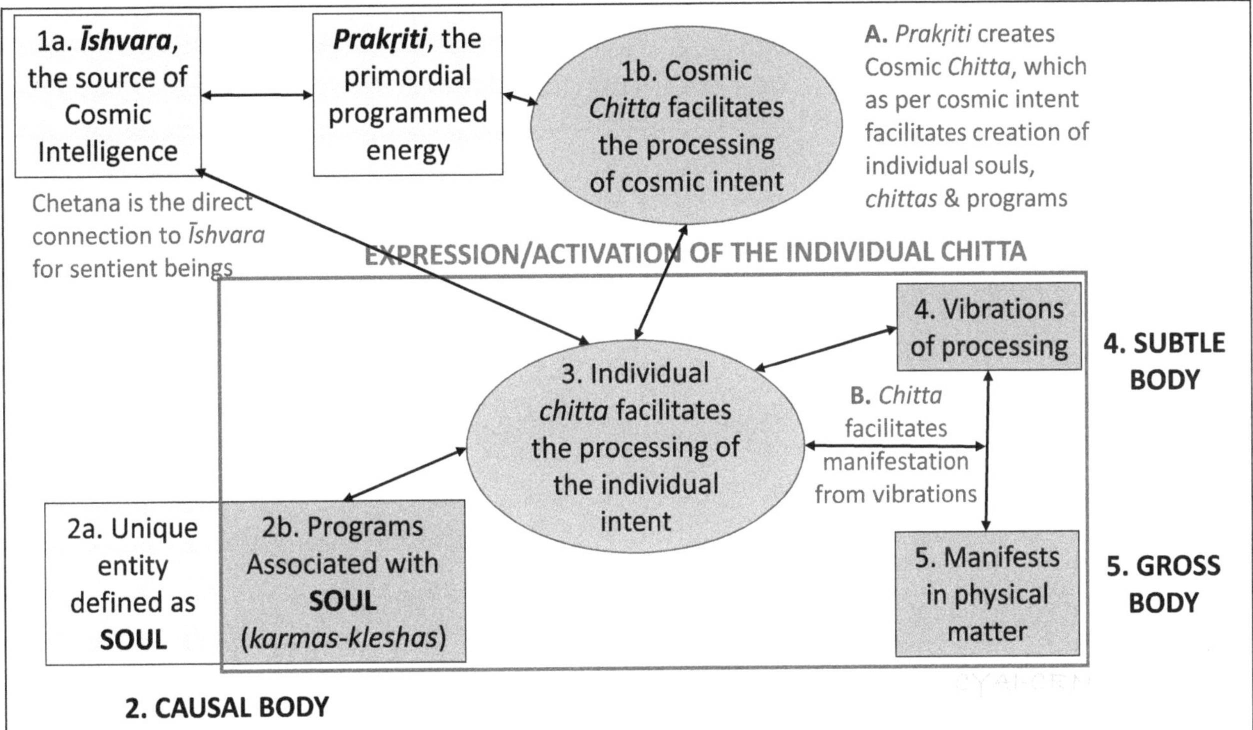

In the diagram above, all the arrows are bi-directional indicating communication both ways. While vibrations of the Subtle Body (4 above) affect the Gross Body (5), physical stimulations of the Gross Body (5) affect the vibrations of the Subtle Body (4). While the programs of the Causal Body (2) operating through the individual *chitta* (3) create vibrations of the Subtle Body (4), the reactive vibrations from the Subtle Body (4) are processed by the *chitta* (3) as new programs called *karma*. In effect, the programs (2b) and individual *chitta* (3), create the expression/activation of the *chitta* in the Subtle Body (4) and Gross Body (5), referred as *chitta* vritti of the Yoga Sutras. The mind is the reactive element of the Subtle Body. The Cosmic Intelligence of *Īśhvara* (1a) can directly access and be accessed by the individual *chitta* (3) of sentient beings (with soul) that is called *Chetanā*. Thus, each sentient being has a dual connection through the individual *chitta* into the Cosmic *Chitta* of *Prakṛiti* and *Īśhvara* concurrently. [A more detailed view is in Figure 27.1 in Chapter 27.]

Karma Cycle Concept

The reaction of the mind creates new programs, like the artificial intelligence learning paradigm. These are called *karmas* as explained earlier in chapter 1 in the *Mechanism of Yoga* section. These *karmas* are impediments to higher spiritual realization and are considered to be the perpetuators of rebirth in eastern philosophies even when the *kleśha* element is fully dissipated. *Karmas* and *kleśha* work through the same mechanism of *chitta* and the *nādis* until one overcomes them through the yogic process.

Nādis and *Marmas*

In traditional medicine systems, the nature of vibrations of the subtle body, that indicate the activation along the *nādis* or bio-meridians, is assessed by sensing the pulsation with three fingers in the forearm just below the wrist. Using different levels of pressure and sensing the drift of the pulse Ayurvedic and Chinese medical practitioners assess disorders in the system. This process is called *nādi* assessment displayed in Figure 5.2 below. [Please see blue box at the end of this chapter that reports how a Tibetan physician examined a patient in a hospital in the United States.]

Figure 5.2:
PICTURE OF THREE FINGER ASSESSSMENT

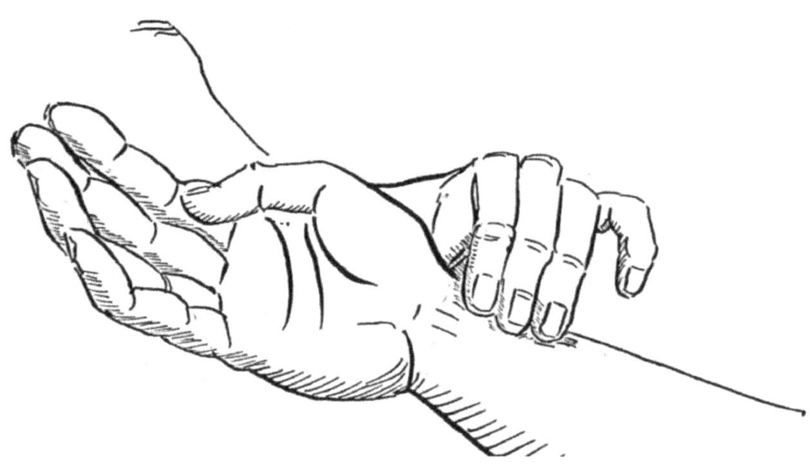

Russian and German researchers have developed electromagnetic tools to objectively measure these vibrations. Very few yoga institutions currently conduct pre-post assessment in conjunction with any yoga protocol to measure the impact of such practices for yoga therapy. [21]

The Chinese configured the bio-meridian system with over 2,000 acupuncture points in the body[22], most of which are internal and require a needle to access. In the Yoga-Ayurveda system there is an understanding of 107 ***marma*** points[23] that can be accessed by epidermal finger pressure. Points of the acupuncture system and *marmas* of Ayurveda are generally thought to lie along the *nādis*, and are useful for specific stimulation related to healing.

---

[21] One such instrument is called the Bio-well developed by Professor Konstantin Korotkov that is used extensively by Life in Yoga Institute. https://www.youtube.com/watch?v=RxHLv1_90fM

[22] Some claim over 5,000 points. 2,000+ acupuncture points as published by Johns Hopkins Medical School - https://www.hopkinsmedicine.org/health/wellness-and-prevention/acupuncture#:~:text=Traditional%20Chinese%20medicine%20practitioners%20believe,is%20responsible%20for%20overall%20health.

[23] This is referred in the *Suśhruta Samhitā*, the ancient surgery manual of Ayurveda.

Concept of Five Levels of Communication, Left and Right Sides and *Chakras*

In Ayurvedic and Vedic systems, the five aspects of communication in the *nādis* are called ***Prāṇā, Apāna, Vyāna, Udāna*** and ***Samāna***. In conventional Ayurveda, these are not connected relationally with the Chinese and modern medicine systems. Life in Yoga Institute's integrative approach of mapping Ayurveda with the Chinese and modern medicine systems offers the following understanding.

Prāṇa refers to the vibrations that communicate to control energy regulation of the body that sustains life. This view makes *Prāṇa* more than simple oxygen intake.[24] From a medical sciences perspective, at a gross level, it relates to the activity of the Nervous System that controls passive respiratory rate, the heart rate, and hence the circulatory system. This results in the distribution of nutrients to different parts of the body for energy production in each cell of the body (cellular respiration), that supports all the organ systems. Thus, *Prāṇa* is considered the most important level of communication, without which none of the other *nādi* communications can enter the gross body. At the instructor level, most yoga practices are designed to optimize the flow of *Prāṇa.*

Balancing the flow of *Prāṇa* between the left and right sides of the body is a concept unique to yoga and traditional medicine systems, where the left is considered our inner programmed entity and the right is considered the interaction and influence of the external environment. The left and right interacting together stimulated by *Prāṇa* make us who we are at each living moment and serve us to fulfill our purpose of creation as an integrated element of the cosmos. The communication related to this is called ***Samāna***. In a modern medical sense, the inner programmed entity can be thought as the genes and the external influences as the epigenetic factors, which combined creates the gene expression on a moment-by-moment basis.

In yoga, the main channel of communication in the left side of the body is called ***Idā Nādi*** and the one on the right side is called ***Piṅgalā Nādi,*** and the interaction of the two are said to communicate through the ***Suṣhumnā Nādi*** which expresses the ***Samāna***. In conventional Ayurveda, it is said that ***Samāna*** is responsible for digestion – of food and thoughts – and is associated with fire and the navel *chakra*. In other words, it is the integration of the internal program dealing with the external environmental needs, which is the idea of gene expression.

In yoga, directing energy to the functionality makes the functionality possible. This is the role of *Prāṇā,* the regulator of vitality. From an anatomical perspective the brain as part of the

[24] Yogic view of *Prāṇa* is discussed in this article: https://www.frontiersin.org/articles/10.3389/fpsyt.2014.00167/full Shirley Telles, Nilkamal Singh, Acharya Balakrishna. Role of respiration in mind-body practices: concepts from contemporary science and traditional yoga texts. Front. Psychiatry, 25 November 2014, Sec. Psychological Therapy and Psychosomatics, https://doi.org/10.3389/fpsyt.2014.00167

nervous system is the controller of the vitality flow through its control of the respiratory and the circulatory systems. Therefore, the Alternate Nostril Breathing technique is used to balance the two hemispheres of the brain which control energy regulation to the opposite sides of the body. Thus, the ***Samāna*** is balanced in the ***Suṣhumnā Nādi*** by the influence of the ***Idā*** and ***Piṅgalā Nādis***.

Along the ***Suṣhumnā Nādi*** which is in the middle of the body from the perineum to the top of the middle of the head, there are seven hubs of communication. These are referred as the ***seven chakras***. [See Figure 5.3 below.] Of these, the five *chakras* (other than the topmost and bottommost) have one end of their hub connected to the spine for access to the energy regulation of *Prāṇa*. And from these hubs there are communications to the musculature of the body called ***Apāna***, and to the fluid circulation of the body called ***Vyāna***. In conventional Ayurveda ***Apāna*** is considered responsible for excretion (which happens by muscle control).

Figure 5.3:
PLACEMENT OF *CHAKRAS*

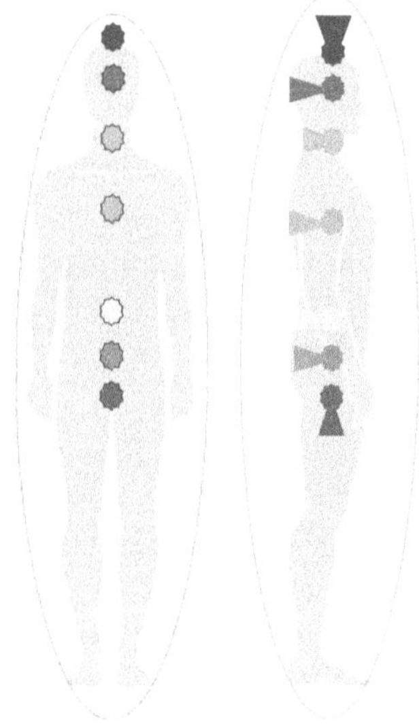

A fifth level of communication called ***Udāna*** refers to cosmic communication. From a medical system perspective, it can be associated with the source of immunity in the body; and from a yogic perspective it is also the gateway, through the seventh *chakra* on the top of the head, for experience beyond the body.[25] In conventional Ayurveda, it is related to organs in the head.

[25] The Yoga Sutras [YS 3:40] describes *Udāna* as allowing one to glide over thorns and bogs, possibly implying that cosmic connectivity can change the body's electromagnetic field to make it lighter and gently glide.

Udāna communicates along the ***Ātma Nādi***[26], which in deep sleep can download the daily dose of 'immune system and program' updates[27], from the cosmic intelligence (through the *chitta*), for the body to keep it functioning well. In modern medicine, immunity is divided into two categories – innate immunity and adaptive immunity. Innate immunity is the resident memory in the white blood cells. Adaptive immunity is the new immunity information that is created (typically associated with vaccines) that is also associated with adequate deep sleep. The ***Ātma Nādi*** mostly flows along the front middle of the body below the skin. [See Figure 5.4.] Along the ***Ātma Nādi***, just inside the lowermost part of the sternum, is our soul (*Purușha* element) connectivity or 'cosmic wireless transmitter-receiver.' This is described in a Vedic hymn called the *Nārāyana Sūktam*[28]. The Yoga Sutras refers to it as ***Hṛidaya*** (meaning the hidden core); we call it the ***Ātma Chakra;*** and some people use the word *'spiritual heart'*.

---

[26] *Ātma Nādi* is not known to be written in any common yoga texts, but it is something that is experienced by yogis, and elements of it can be gleaned from the Vedas.

[27] In modern medicine, deep sleep is associated primarily with the immune system that is regarded as the fighting mechanism to prevent unwanted elements invading the body. In yoga and traditional medicine systems, the role of deep sleep equally emphasizes ability to repair all the functions of the body that we refer as program updates, along with the immune system enhancement.

[28] Unfortunately, the words from thousands of years ago attempting to describe the concept of transmitter-receiver, which was unknown at that time, fail for adequate interpretation among normal people. However, yogis who have experienced it see the depth of the description in these ancient scriptures. The following verse from the *Nārāyana Sūktam* describes the cosmic transmitter-receiver within us as follows:

adho niṣṭyā vitastyānte nābhyām-upari tiṣṭhtati |अधो निष्ट्या वितस्यान्ते नाभ्यां उपरि तिष्ठति

jvālamālā-kulaṃ bhātī viśvasyāyatanaṃ mahat ||ज्वाला माला कुलं भाति विश्वस्यायतनं महत्

From the Adams apple, at the distance of an extended finger-span, above the navel, is established the great presence with lustre of concentric rings of fire (waves transmission) that reaches the entire Universe.

The exact words are the following:

Word	Meaning
adho अधो	Downward
niṣṭyā निष्ट्या	From the Adams apple
Vitastyānte वितस्यान्ते	Distance of stretch from the tip of thumb to tip of little finger with the hand fully stretched
nābhyām-upari नाभ्यां उपरि	Above the navel
tiṣṭhtati तिष्ठति	Is established
jvālamālā-kulaṃ bhātī ज्वाला माला कुलं भाति	Jvālamālā is ring or garland of fire; kulam is family or collection indicating plurality of the ring or garland of fire; bhāti is lustre or luminescence; Full translation could be '<u>emanation of concentric rings of fire</u>' ***referring to waves of a transmitter-receiver.***
viśvasyāyatanaṃ विश्वस्यायतनं	Reach of the entire Universe – viśva means universe
Mahat महत्	Of importance or greatness

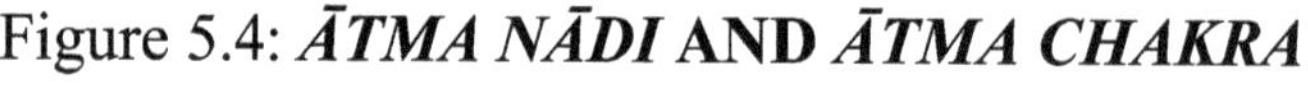

Figure 5.4: ***ĀTMA NĀDI* AND *ĀTMA CHAKRA***

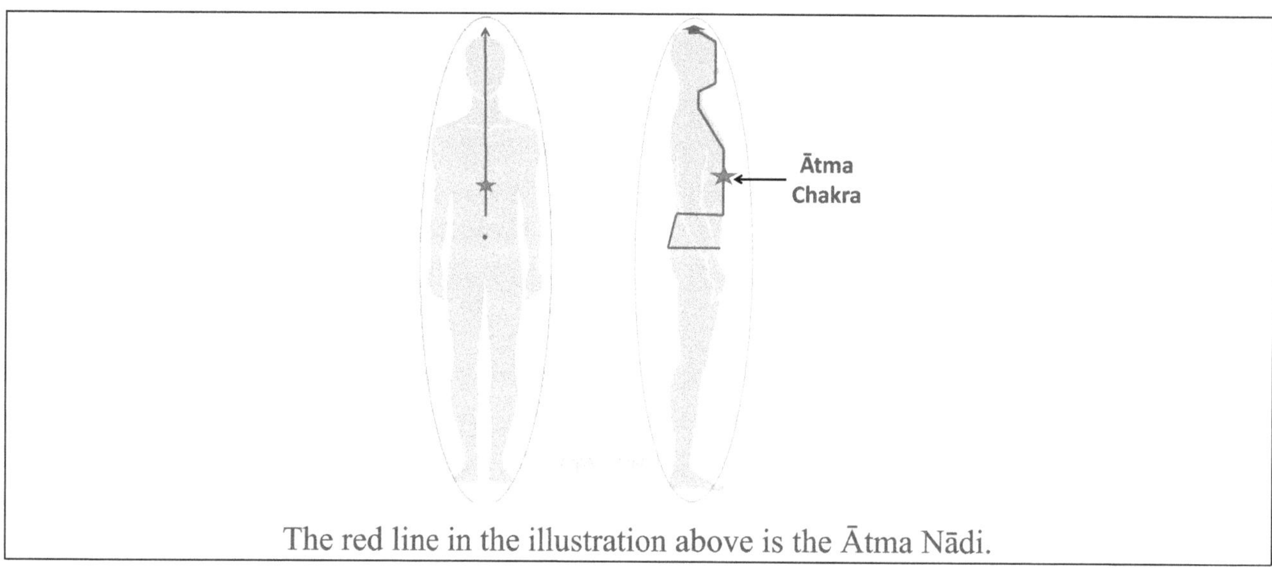

The red line in the illustration above is the Ātma Nādi.

REDUCTIONISTIC AYURVEDIC VIEW OF THE FIVE LEVELS OFCOMMUNICATION

Although the roots of Ayurveda are embedded in spiritual understanding, a rule-based approach was developed to train and dispense the health recommendations. Any such reductionistic approach has limitations in representing the spiritual understanding.

In rule-based Ayurveda, the five communications (*Pancha-Prāṇa*) are associated with regions of the body and cannot be correlated with modern medicine or Chinese Medicine systems.

Following is the often-described view of the five *Prāṇas*:
- *Udāna* functions above the throat, in the face and head region.
- *Prāṇa* functions between the throat and the diaphragm. All organs of the thorax including heart and lungs are maintained by *Prāṇa.*
- *Samāna* operates between the navel and the diaphragm. *Samāna* is responsible for digestion and assimilation – of everything consumed including food and thoughts.
- *Apāna* controls organs situated between the navel and the perineum. It is primarily responsible for elimination and stimulates the downward movement of the wastes.
- *Vyāna* is associated with the circulatory system that carries the nutrients to every cell of the body. As students of Swami Rama of the Himalayan Institute recall, he has noted that Vyāna permeates skin and all the physical tissues including the nervous system. This would imply the integrative functionality of the blood circulation, lymphatic circulation and also nerve stimulation.

In the Vedic literature associated with yoga as explained by some yoga schools, there is often a conception of five layers or sheaths of our existence. [29] While this is often mentioned in popular yoga literature, there is no systematic way to measure it or use it effectively even in traditional

[29] *Taittriya* Upaniṣhad section called *Bhriguvalli*. See Chapter 7.

medicine systems. It is an individual experiential element from Vedānta philosophy that one may find inspiring that is addressed in Chapter 7.

Process Leading to *Samādhi*

The five aspects of *nādi* communications indicate the state of a person, whether the person is in balance or imbalance, whether reactive or non-reactive. The ideal for any person is to engage with the activations of the programs (*kleśha* and *karma*) without reactivity. This is called fulfilling one's cosmic plan without creating new *karma*. When the program load of the causal body eventually becomes very light, or when a yogic practice (like mantras) temporarily stops the flow of the programs, the stillness of the *chitta* gives a glimpse of the higher reality of the cosmic intelligence.

Figure 5.5:
CHITTA CONNECTING TO COSMIC INTELLIGENCE IN THE STATE OF STILLNESS

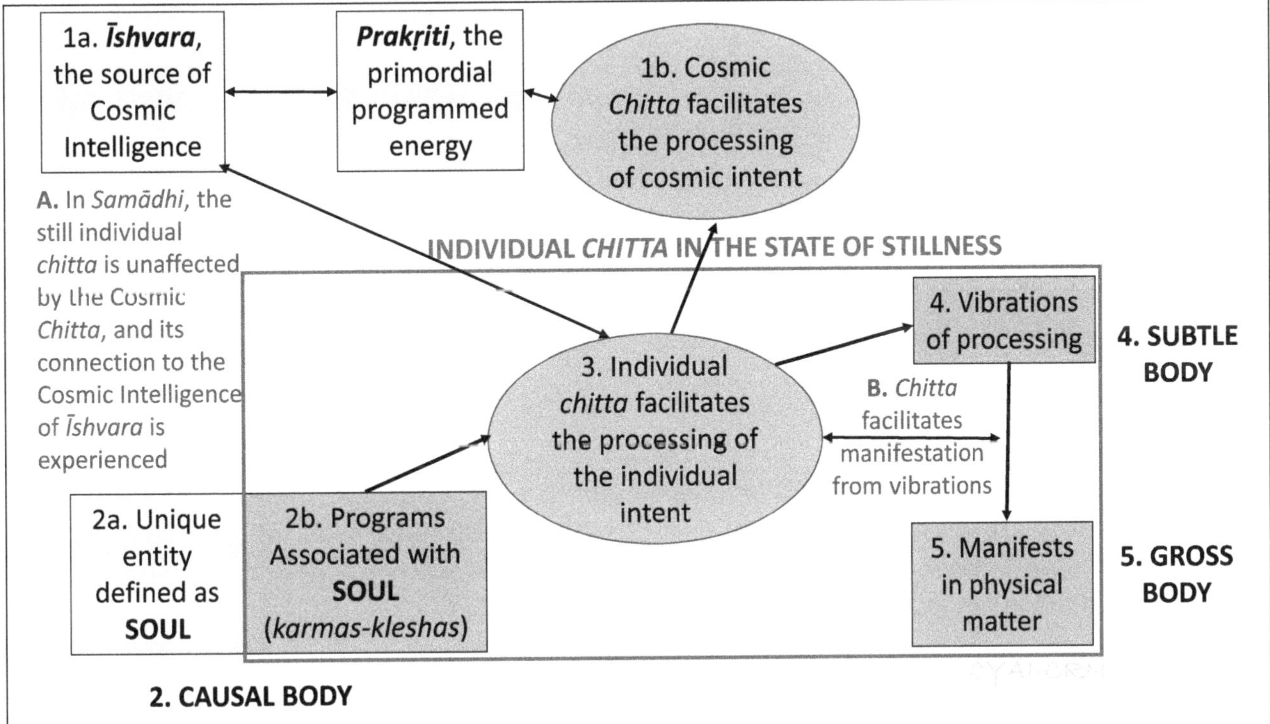

In the diagram above, all the arrows are unidirectional, except A and B (and the connection between *Īśhvara*, *Prakṛiti* and the Cosmic *Chitta*). In A, the still Individual *chitta* (3) connects into the Cosmic Intelligence of *Īśhvara* and its perception is transmitted by B into the Gross Body (of the yogi) in the state of *Samādhi*.

Figure 5.5 is the process of *Samādhi* described in the Yoga Sutras. Chapter 27 provides further details of *Samādhi* and Self-Realization.

Power of Intention, Intuition and Role of *Dharma*

Figures 5.1 and 5.5 in the previous pages map the relationship between the individual, the cosmic flow, and the cosmic intelligence (*Īśhvara*). Intention (like the power of positive thinking) and intuition work through the connectivity beyond the body and has an impact on *Dharma*. *Dharma* is the natural flow of activity that is consistent with the ordained cosmic flow. Thus, *Dharma* is said to support the cosmic flow. Violation of *Dharma* – activities that go against the cosmic flow – has its consequences.

Intuition happens in the stillness of the individual *chitta* when it can access the cosmic intelligence (of *Īśhvara*). It is a response from the cosmic intelligence to a query, that one may carry in one's mind, that is activated through the individual *chitta*. If there are no assumptions or preconceived biases in the query, in a high level of meditation or in deep sleep when the other active programs take a break, the '*Samādhi*-like' state provides the answer to the query intuitively. If there are assumptions or preconceived biases, the individual *chitta* never attains the stillness needed to elicit the intuition, but rather one's own biases are reflected in answer to the query.

Intention arising out of one's intuition that are unaffected by external observations or conditioning of an opinionated mind are in sync with the flow of *Dharma* – in other words, in sync with one's innate purpose of life.[30] When such is not the case, the conflict with *Dharma* happens inflicting consequences on the causal body (through the cosmic *Chitta*). When people seek to heal others or offer blessings with their intention, if there is a conflict with the cosmic *Dharma*, it will have negative consequences for the person's causal body. This is the reason advanced yogis always offer healing and blessings as per the cosmic intent. This is a reminder for all in the field of yoga that they are only instruments of the cosmic flow.

External Monitors of Beneficial Yoga Practices

There are multiple ways to monitor attendees during a yoga session. Advanced yogis may intuitively assess them. Those trained in *nādi* pulsation do the same with the three-finger pulse reading. Unlike them, for a beginning yoga instructor the externally visible symptoms of the *chitta's* expression are the only indicators available.

Following are external elements of the expression of the *chitta* that can be observed during a yoga session to ensure that the practice is safe and beneficial:

- ***Physical alignment*** – In every yoga practice, particular attention is paid to the spine – it should not bend or slouch. It may be vertical and erect, or in supine lying down position, or in any inclined way where the natural alignment of the spine is not bent or twisted. This is understandable since general yoga practices focus on optimization of energy

---

[30] Such intuition without biases providing guidance for one's life purpose is called Pure *Sankalpa* in the blue-box in chapter 22 (Concept of Tantra and its Application) on *Sankalpha Śhaktī*.

regulation and the spine is part of the Central Nervous System (CNS). The brain which is part of the CNS controls the energy regulation of the body by taking the nervous system input of the needs of the body, and accordingly controls the involuntary breath rate (oxygen input) and heart rate. The spine has a very important role in this nervous system communication.

In the *Haṭha Yoga* system, particularly in some schools, careful attention is paid to the alignment of muscles in all parts of the body, especially in the hands and legs. The intent is the alignment of *nādis*, that correlate anatomically with the stimulation of the Peripheral Nervous System.

- ***Ease of practice and peaceful expression on the face are important indicators***. This follows directly from the Yoga Sutras, which states that all practices must be done with mild effort so that the ease is conducive for meditative focus. It also implies that communication of the flow through *nādis* is optimal when effort is mild, i.e., mild stimulation – in effect there is no stress in the system.

  Perhaps the most indicative elements in this assessment are the breathing and expression on the face. Anytime when the body is disturbed, breath will be disturbed. It will either be too fast or irregular. If there is pain it will show on the face. At the time of practice, breath and facial expression become very important indicators of appropriate and beneficial practice of yoga. Breath must flow slowly and smoothly, and the face should look peaceful.

- ***Feedback from participants is another important measure for assessment***. Typically, the feeling of wellness manifests in the forms of disappearance of mild pains in the system, emergence of greater vitality, better quality of sleep, and a joyful approach to living.

Physiology View of Yoga Practices

While a yoga instructor should focus on the yoga process working through the *chitta*, modern medicine approach with its limited understanding of life and existence has done significant research on the physiological impact of yoga practices that are worth knowing. Key among them is the deep relaxation response (often called parasympathetic tone) that pervades the psychosomatic span from the state of the mind to gene expression, neurotransmitter, organs, muscles, and tissues.

Another allied field called Exercise Physiology, that focuses on physical exercising, has examined the health aspects of different kinds of exercises. The four health aspects of exercising are considered to be flexibility, muscle strengthening, cardiac-fitness and fat reduction. Flexibility and muscle toning are considered very important to avoid injuries, especially as one ages. Muscle and bone health are related to isometric, pressure-based or weight-bearing exercises. The desirability of cardio-respiratory fitness and appropriate BMI (Body Mass Index) are well-known and need no explanation. Spine health is also considered very important as explained earlier with respect to the CNS and the energy regulation of the body.

This physiological perspective can be viewed in common yoga practices in the following way.

In yoga postures, spinal alignment (functioning of the CNS), flexibility, muscle strengthening, and balancing aspects can be viewed from a physiological angle. As we flex in yoga postures, muscles that are not normally used frequently get more blood flow and this eases the tensions in these muscles. Associated with flexibility is joint mobility and specifically the role of pelvic flexibility which also impacts the CNS. Staying in a position and keeping consistent pressure on the musculoskeletal structure strengthens the muscles. Lastly it is recognized that balancing exercises have an important impact on the brain. With regular practice (of anything newly learned) the brain is thought to make new connections within itself – the process is called neuroplasticity. Balancing exercises are thought to be effective in addressing or preventing aging-related neurological disorders.

Breathing exercises, from the perspective of modern physiology, are viewed in terms of air exchange and its impact on vitality, and the relaxing effect called parasympathetic tone. The concept of impact on left and right is not known in modern physiology.

The role of vibrations (mantras) and ***the role of thoughts*** are understood as affecting neurotransmitters and hormones.[31] However, it is not frequently used as a therapeutic intervention in conventional medical treatment.

Stress-Reduction and Balance

At an instructor level the objective of any yoga session is to relieve stress and restore balance in the system. The concept of stress and balance is different in yoga from conventional psychological or physiological views.[32]

---

[31] Infante JR, Peran F, Rayo JI, Serrano J, Domínguez ML, Garcia L, Duran C, Roldan A. Levels of immune cells in transcendental meditation practitioners. Int J Yoga. 2014 Jul;7(2):147-51. doi: 10.4103/0973-6131.133899. PMID: 25035626; PMCID: PMC4097901.

Muehsam D, Ventura C. Life rhythm as a symphony of oscillatory patterns: electromagnetic energy and sound vibration modulates gene expression for biological signaling and healing. Glob Adv Health Med. 2014 Mar;3(2):40-55. doi: 10.7453/gahmj.2014.008. PMID: 24808981; PMCID: PMC4010966.

[32] In conventional view of psychology and physiology there is a concept of good stress (eustress) and bad stress (distress). Eustress is associated with the idea of happy events like falling in love and getting married, or getting a new desired job, resulting in one getting involved in more activities that consume more energy and therefore resulting in physical stress. This happy stress is considered motivational and energizing. By the same token breaking up of a marriage or being laid-off from a job with loss of income can create unhappy stress (distress) that is depressing and saps energy. In the yogic view, being in sync with the cosmic flow, the cosmos provides enough energy to do the cosmic job done through the person. Stress is involved when the mind takes over, resists the natural flow based on a strong sense of likes and dislikes, and thus goes against the cosmic flow.

Stress in yoga is defined in two ways, where functionally there may be an overlap:

- ***Energy Utilization Impact*** – Stress is activated when demands on the energy of the body is more than the available supply of energy, resulting in *nādi* communication blocks or overloads. This is sometimes referred as the allostatic overload in modern medicine. It is important to note that the mind – thinking, and its association with the brain – is the biggest consumer of energy, and confused thinking (or worrying) causes blocks in the channels of communications.

- ***Imbalance between Left and Right Brain*** – Stress comes on when logical and creative thinking are not in balance. In yoga terms, we say this happens when external affectations and internal being are not well synchronized to serve one's purpose of life.

De-stressing involves one or more of four approaches:

- ***Remove communication blocks*** in the *nādis* by holding firmly and releasing in yoga postures.

- ***Reduce energy demands*** primarily by lessening the activity of the mind, and secondarily by resting the body.

- ***Increase supply of energy*** primarily with more air exchange in the lungs, and for advanced yogis through other esoteric methods of yoga.

- ***Improve balance between left and right*** by multiple methods of awareness with and without breath.

For example, in the *Haṭha Yoga* approach of holding postures, and then releasing and relaxing removes communication blocks in the *nādis*. At the same time, it reduces energy demand by mindful holding of postures and relaxation of the mind as a pure observer. In the *Tantra Yoga* approach, movement and breath integrates all the four approaches of de-stressing mentioned above. However, it is gentler than *Haṭha Yoga* and can be slower in the manifestation of results, unless mantras are used.

Breathing practice like the Alternate Nostril Breathing are designed to balance the left and right. Slow breathing of 4 to 6 breaths per minute is designed to evoke relaxation (called parasympathetic tone in physiology) and reduces energy demands. Deep bellows-type breathing is designed to increase more air exchange and oxygen availability in the body, to increase the supply of energy.[33]

Questions and Discussion Topics

1. Explain the notion of the three bodies, and its relevance in yogic or health assessments.
2. What is the significance of the left and right sides? Reflect on cultural practices that orient one to be right-handed and explore any correlation with the spiritual sense.
3. What is the role of the nervous system in the body?
4. How does modern medical sciences explain the benefits of yoga practices like postures and breathing in physiological terms?
5. What is the yoga view of stress and how does it compare with physiological view of stress?
6. What are the five types of communications along the *nādis* and what are their roles?

---

[33] From a respiratory physiology standpoint, increased oxygen in the system is not accepted. This is because theoretically the maximum buffering of oxygen in the red blood cells is the limit. The implication is that deep breathing beyond a certain point does not lead to oxygen absorption, but it is dumb breathing without additional oxygen absorption (eventually fainting from respiratory alkalosis). However, there is a fallacy in this understanding since the brain may also release the excess oxygen for functionalities beyond its normal release. We see this all the time. For example, for those with arthritic conditions, whose joints are worn and are in painful conditions, by practicing several cycles of deep breathing, they find the pain disappear immediately, at least for an hour or so. Even as they progress from one round to the next – each round is 20 breaths, and a pause is done between each round to ensure respiratory alkalosis does not result in fainting – they begin to feel vibrations moving downward from the head towards the painful joints, and eventually the pain disappears. We explain this phenomenon as follows:
(a) Cause of the pain is because the muscles that pull the joints need to do more work for the joints to function effectively, since the smooth soft bone (cartilage) in the ends of the connecting bones are damaged, and smooth and easy gliding without friction is not possible. Without enough energy available for the muscles to move the joints easily, pain signals emerge.
(b) Pain disappears because the brain releases more oxygen (through blood supply) to those muscles to enable the joint mobility and healing process. This release of blood circulation to these muscles was not there previously.
(c) Question: Why did the brain not supply oxygen earlier if that was the solution? Reason is that the brain as the regulator of vitality utilization in each part of the body operates based on habitual conditioning of the neurons in the brain by past experiences of several years.
(d) How does the brain resolve the situation? Initially the brain gets confused when the passive breathing that it controls is overridden by the individual and too much oxygen becomes available. The brain is forced to reassess the energy needs of the various parts of the body. Then it realizes there is a need in these specific joints where there is pain and releases the oxygen by increasing blood circulation for those muscles.

SENSING OF THE SUBTLE BODY BY A TIBETAN DOCTOR

A DOCTOR'S TOUCH

This is the description of a western allopathic trained physician observing a Tibetan doctor, Yeshi Dhonden, the personal physician of Dalai Lama, using an approach that has some similarity to that described in this chapter to assess a patient. This was published by the Washington Post on October 27, 1998 in the ***Lifestyle and Wellness*** section. Web link is https://www.washingtonpost.com/archive/lifestyle/wellness/1998/10/27/a-doctors-touch/dc823337-fcee-4bb0-b453-a9b39887c17d/

It is an excerpt from Dr. Richard Selzer's book "Mortal Lessons: Notes on the Art of Surgery" (New York, Simon & Shuster, 1976). In 1998, when the Washington Post published this except, Dr. Richard Selzer was a retired physician who was on the faculty of the Yale School of Medicine. This incident, as described, occurred in the 1970s while Dr. Selzer was chief resident in surgery at Yale University.

Dr. Selzer describes the general skepticism of his colleagues, western trained allopathic physicians, towards spiritually inclined approach to health assessment. Further, the attire and appearance of a monk deviates from a scientific and white-coat approach to medicine. The patient examined is a woman who has congenital heart disease, a hole between the left and right ventricle of the heart. This has not been disclosed to the Tibetan doctor, and except for one senior doctor, none of the others observing know the diagnosis. The western trained doctors are watching the non-invasive examination and assessment of the Tibetan physician.

Dr. Selzer begins by describing the spiritual approach of the Tibetan doctor as follows: "We are further informed that for the past two hours Yeshi Dhonden has purified himself by bathing, fasting, and prayer."

Dr. Selzer describes three types of examination used by the Tibetan physician to diagnose the patient:

1. Intuitive sensing.

2. Pulse Examination as described in Figure 5.2.

3. Urine analysis – The Tibetan doctor's visual and olfactory examination of urine of the patient.

The approach of the Tibetan doctor in the sequential examination is described by Dr. Selzer as follows:

"Yeshi Dhonden steps to the bedside while the rest stand apart, watching. For a long time he gazes at the woman, favoring no part of her body with his eyes, but seeming to fix his glance at a place just above her supine form. I, too, study her. No physical sign nor obvious symptom gives a clue to the nature of her disease.

"At last he takes her hand, raising it in both of his own. Now he bends over the bed in a kind of crouching stance, his head drawn down in the collar of his robe. His eyes are closed as he feels for her pulse. In a moment he has found the spot, and for the next half hour he remains thus, suspended above the patient like some exotic golden bird with folded wings, holding the pulse of the woman beneath his fingers, cradling her hand in his. All the power of the man seems to have been drawn down into this one purpose. It is palpation of the pulse raised to the state of ritual. From the foot of the bed, where I stand, it is as though he and the patient have entered a special place of isolation, of apartness, about which a vacancy hovers, and across which no violation is possible."

The urine examination has been described as follows:

"The interpreter produces a small wooden bowl and two sticks. Yeshi Dhonden pours a portion of the urine specimen into the bowl, and proceeds to whip the liquid with the two sticks. This he does for several minutes until a foam is raised. Then, bowing above the bowl, he inhales the odor three times. He sets down the bowl and turns to leave."

After such examination, the Tibetan doctor and the western trained physicians in the hospital meet in a conference room to hear the Tibetan doctor's diagnosis which is described by Dr. Selzer as follows:

"Yeshi Dhonden speaks now for the first time, in soft Tibetan sounds that I have never heard before. He has barely begun when the young interpreter begins to translate, the two voices continuing in tandem -- a bilingual fugue, the one chasing the other. It is like the chanting of monks. He speaks of winds coursing through the body of the woman, currents that break against barriers, eddying. These vortices are in her blood, he says. The last spendings of an imperfect heart. Between the chambers of her heart, long, long before she was born, a wind had come and blown open a deep gate that must never be opened. Through it charge the full waters of her river, as the mountain stream cascades in the springtime, battering, knocking loose the land, and flooding her breath."

Then the senior doctor, the host of this event, who knew the diagnosis, answers, as described by Dr. Selzer:

"Congenital heart disease. Interventricular septal defect -- a hole in the wall between the left and right chambers of the heart -- with resultant heart failure."

As Dr. Selzer reflects: "A gateway in the heart, I think. That must not be opened. Through it charge the full waters that flood her breath. So! Here then is the doctor listening to the sounds of the body to which the rest of us are deaf. He is more than doctor. He is priest."

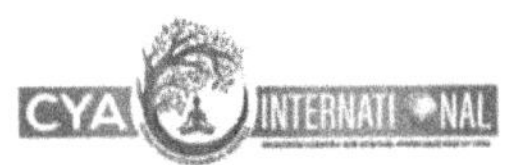

CHAPTER 6:

Yoga for Special Groups and Conditions

The previous chapters clearly note that yoga is about connecting into the cosmic intelligence, and real yoga practices are related to lifestyle and attitude of living that fulfill one's purpose of life with minimal reactivity that promotes *nādi* cleansing. However, in the common perception of yoga, the physical element has a predominant role, and cannot be avoided by anyone teaching yoga. In all situations, any yoga practice must be within the capacity of the individual focused on *nādi* cleansing.

While a general yoga session should be workable for a normally healthy person, people who are fragile or with injuries may require extra caution and modifications in practices. Such cases may be referred to an expert yoga teacher. Such conditions may include physical injuries, people in pain conditions, women who are pregnant, children, elderly who are fragile who may have difficulty in keeping balance or have limited mobility of joints.

In general, all these special circumstances are outside the domain of Instructor level training. Therefore, people who are not in a stable and healthy condition should not be in an instructor's class. Further, one should work with a disclaimer that if participants have doubts about their physical abilities, they should consult their physician, and their presence in an instructor's class assumes they agree to absorb any risk in participation.

Following are some notes on commonly encountered special groups with respect to approaches taken in yoga practice. In discussing them, the mechanism elements that point to *nādi* cleansing and the cosmic flow are instructive. It is important to note that this is only for information purposes to understand the depth of variation, and not for instructional application at the instructor level.

Role of Yoga for Children

From a traditional Yoga perspective, conventional *Haṭha Yoga* practices are not recommended for children before puberty. The yogic understanding is that the nature of being (natural programming) entering the *chakras* and *nādis* are not completed until puberty. Any technique that can have sustained physical pressure on the *nādi-chakra* system during the formative period before puberty can have undesirable impact.

However, the modern-day creation of children's yoga should be understood as a fun and games approach to physical and mental toning without the use of *Haṭha Yoga* techniques that can unwittingly create strain. Such an approach of fun and games should never impose rules or force children to do something they don't want to do.

UNDERSTANDING OF *CHAKRAS* AND *NĀDIS* FROM BIRTH TO PUBERTY

At birth only the *Ātma Chakra* (or the spiritual heart) is sensed. Then over the next few days the chakras emerge, but they remain like a cluster near the center of the body. As the baby grows, they move outward (towards the head and towards the perineum) and only between the ages of 5 and 7 the *chakras* realize their actual position. Even as the chakras are moving towards their actual position, *nādi* connections are forming. Soon after the *chakras* reach their final position the *nādi* connections become fully established.

While the natural programming of the child begins from birth (or even before), with the physical form being limited and the *chakras* and *nādis* not fully formed, the flow of the programs (*kleśha* and *karma*) are limited. Upon the *chakras* reaching their natural position and the *nādis* becoming fully formed, the descent of the programs become more accelerated. This heightened acceleration continues until puberty. Thus, we see an emergence of a new personality and physical being after puberty, that parents typically complain about the problem of adolescence.

At the time of accelerated descent of programs, any disruption caused by artificial pressure in the *nādis* can create lasting deficiencies in a person – like poor eyesight, poor digestion, etc. Therefore, before puberty, *Haṭha Yoga* practices are not recommended. However, after the *chakras* have attained their positions, and *nādi* connections are stable (between 5 and 7 years of age), transcendental meditative practices are considered suitable. Such meditative practices open the cosmic communication and allow for smoother reception of the accelerated downloads of the programs. Enough deep sleep is even more important during this period to enable better cosmic connectivity.

EFFECT ON CHILDREN FROM REGULAR MEDITATION PRACTICE

One of our regular practitioners and Life in Yoga instructor used to do daily morning and evening meditation for 20 minutes each time with his timer on. His infant daughter loved him and anytime he was home she would always be hovering around him constantly talking to him and engaging him to play with her. He would dote on his daughter and provide her good attention even as he stayed engaged in any household activity. However, the meditation time was special. He would tell her she had to be quiet while doing meditation. He would set the timer and sit for meditation, and his normally energetic daughter would become completely silent and would sit on his lap. For 20 minutes, she would not stir. Once the timer alarm went off, she would become her usual self, loudly demanding of her father's attention.

GUIDANCE FOR CHILDREN BY PARENTS HAPPENS NATURALLY

Swami Veda Bharati used to say that the very best way to learn meditation is wrapped in your mother's or father's meditation shawl. One adult initiate used to sit for his daily meditation every evening. Whenever he would sit down, soon his children would just gravitate to sit with him without being called. Meditation generates a field of peacefulness to which children and other creatures are naturally attracted.

Another friend and a senior teacher shared the following story from his childhood.

Every day in the late afternoon an atmosphere of peace and stillness would pervade the house so noticeably that he would go searching for the source. He would always find his father meditating. So, he would sit down, and in this way gradually learned to meditate from a young age. Years later he made his first visit to the ashram of his father's teacher in India. He sat down for the afternoon meditation and was amazed to find the very same feeling of stillness and silence in that room. Then he realized that this was the real source of the field of peacefulness he had always found in his father's meditation.

Yoga for Women during Menstrual Periods

Once we understand that yoga should be done in calmness and without strain, it is obvious how women during menstrual periods should follow their practice. Light practices, especially slow, deep breathing practices and meditation are recommended. Inversion practices should be avoided, so that the natural flow of the menstrual discharge is not affected.

Prenatal Yoga

Practicing Yoga during pregnancy has a wonderful ability to integrate and harmonize the woman's body, mind, and spirit. It creates a protected space for the growing baby and a positive, joyful experience for the mother to be. It also emphasizes specific poses, breathing, and relaxation techniques that help to:

- Improve physical strength - strengthens muscles used in labor & delivery, improve posture, improve circulation – heart & lung health – and increase endurance and build stamina,
- Relieve some physical discomforts of pregnancy (backache, heartburn, constipation, and leg cramps).
- Prepare a woman mentally and spiritually for the marathon of labor.

When can a pregnant woman start Prenatal Yoga?

Consultation with one's health care provider should be the first step before practicing physical elements of yoga to ensure one is in suitable health. Before the 12th week of pregnancy, miscarriages can happen without any external influence. Hence, care must be taken before starting the yoga sessions. Additional care must be taken in the cases of twin pregnancies, multiple pregnancies, or high-risk pregnancies. In general, most women do not start Prenatal Yoga in the first trimester because of the physical and physiological changes and adjustments going on in their body.

According to traditional wisdom, pregnancy is a manifestation of the presence of a new soul. Yoga practices strengthen the vitality and cosmic connectivity of the mother and the soul that she shelters. The key elements of these practices are maintaining good vitality, happy state of mind with good breathing, and meditative practices. Following is a broad description for the general needs and the type of practices divided by the trimesters.

First Trimester: (1st to 13th week of pregnancy)

It is a time of adaptation and has the highest risk of miscarriage. The possible causes are chromosomal abnormalities, problems with parental genes or anomalies in the uterus. This essentially points to improper cosmic programming affecting the fetal development, i.e., cosmic connectivity not being proper for the mother. It is also the period of morning sickness. During the first trimester, good deep sleep, stress-free living with nutritional diet is considered best for the mother for optimal fetal development. While in traditional societies the woman is taken care in a precious way with support from family members to take much rest and relax deeply, in modern societies with women engaged in the workforce, stress is more common. The yogic definition of stress is demands on the system being more than available energy as explained in Chapter 5. To counter stress, deep and slow breathing, relaxation, adequate good sleep, and meditation are the general recommendations of Prenatal Yoga at this time.

Second Trimester: (14th to 27th week of pregnancy)

It is a time of well-being. The body has successfully adapted itself to the pregnancy and usually this is a period when few problems occur. At this time gentle stretching, in sync with breath, can be added along with the deep breathing, relaxation, and meditation practices. Depending on the state of the person, conventional *āsanas* like the warrior pose and hip bending poses may also be added.

Third Trimester: (28th to 40th week of pregnancy)

It is often a time of discomfort and increased complaints due to the growth of the baby. Preserving the quality of respiration becomes the principal focus even as the other practices continue. The growing fetus tends to prevent diaphragmatic lower lung expansion. The continued meditative practice helps the woman to not only breath well with chest breathing, but also adds other yogic mechanisms of preserving energy.

This yoga teaching for a pregnant woman follows a holistic approach, which is done gradually with the evolution of the pregnancy and within the capacity of the woman.

Postnatal Yoga

Post-natal yoga begins 6 to 8 weeks after a normal delivery, and a couple of weeks later for those with C-section delivery. In either case, it is best to consult one's physician before beginning the practice. Post-natal practices are designed to help heal the body and mind after the strain of child delivery. These practices seek to repair the strained tissues back to their former glory, restore hormonal balance, ease pressure on the nervous system, help build up strength in the spine, minimize the effects of holding and feeding a baby, provide rest and instant relaxation, all of which aid emotional balance and relieve or avoid post-partum depression.

As always, every woman heals differently. The period to begin post-natal practices and the type of practices may vary from person to person. If one did prenatal yoga before delivery, the body may be ready sooner. The health care provider is in the best position to give personalized recommendations.

During the early postpartum weeks (before beginning post-natal yoga practices), walking is recommended for at least 10 minutes a day (assuming one did not have any complications). Resting is very important during this period.

Post-natal practices can be done for 6 to 9 months after the physician clears one for the practice. The practices generally include slow movement in sync with the breath, relaxing *Prāṇāyāma* practices, and meditation.

After the postnatal practices have balanced the system about 9 to 12 months after child delivery, normal yogic lifestyle may be renewed.

Yoga by Life Stages

While each person ages differently, in general, in the first half of life, when the person is free of disorders, yoga, particularly of the *Haṭha Yoga* variety need not be restricted, so long as one approaches in stages to build from the beginner's level to the advanced level. In later stages in life, mild or severe disorders such as weight-gain, inflexibility, arthritis, heart abnormalities, etc. may develop. Under these conditions physical elements of yoga (*āsanas*) need to be adapted to ensure they are gentle enough to avoid strain. Chair-based, slow movement in sync with the breath may be more appropriate. Such gentle practices, along with breathing and meditative practices, can serve a palliative and therapeutic role, in addition to helping to advance in spiritual awareness.

Yoga is about purification of the causal body, by working off our internal programs (*kleśha* and *karma*), that enables cosmic connectivity and heightened intuitive awareness.

As one ages, living life true to one's conscience, one naturally works off the internal programs (*kleśha* and *karma*). With already somewhat purified *nādis* by the aging process, there is no need for strong physical stimulations to advance in yoga. Mild stimulation of the spine, including neck and hips, and joints of the limbs are sufficient. With the inclusion of breathing techniques, vibration (mantra, music, etc.), power of intention, and training to be an observer, one can go a long way in yogic advancement. An example of chair-based gentle practices for physical mobilization, that is accessible to elders, is provided in Appendix 2.

Questions and Discussion Topics

1. Why is it important to treat special groups differently?
2. Children's yoga has become very popular. Is it appropriate from a yogic standpoint? Explain.
3. What is the importance of mental and physical balance for a woman at the time of pregnancy? Explore within your own cultural background how previous generations have dealt with pregnancy among the women in their families. Specifically, what were the pre and post-natal practices. Compare these against the lives of modern-day women and how it may affect pregnancy.
4. How will you approach beneficial practices for senior citizens? Consider both physical abilities and spiritual needs as you explain your answer.
5. Are *nādi* cleansing and purification of the causal body one and the same? If so, how. If not, what is the distinction?

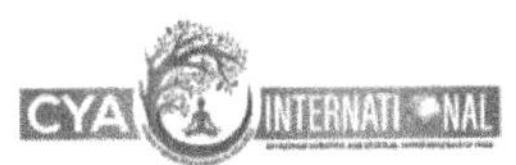

CHAPTER 7:

Growing Awareness by Yoga for An Instructor

As you begin your path as a yoga instructor, you should realize that it is only the building block towards becoming a yogi. A yogi is one who is well connected with the cosmic intelligence. The key to becoming a yogi is daily and regular practice of yoga. When we say yoga, we mean the meditative integration of gross, subtle, and causal levels of the body, that purifies the *nādis,* and in stages leads to connectivity with the cosmic intelligence. That connectivity along with inquiry within, in turn, leads to Self-Realization, which is the direct intuitive experience of the knowledge of all that exists. In any valid practice of yoga this must happen in gradual stages.

An inspiring story from the Upaniṣhads – third chapter, *Bhriguvalli*, of the *Taittriya Upaniṣhad* – describes the experience of a young man named Bhrigu, who is seeking to know wherefrom does all of existence come, how is it sustained and where does it all go.

Bhrigu's father, Varuna, asks him to do *tapas*. In common literature *tapas* is inappropriately translated as austerities. It has got to do with burning of programs (i.e., dissipation of *karma-kleśha*) in one's causal body by being a pure observer as the programs are activated by the *chitta*. *Tapa* means heat and heat is created in the body when the *chitta* activates and dissipates the programs. Thus, *tapas* is about purification. It is associated with meditation where one keeps the attitude of a pure observer. [By being unaffected by the activation of the *chitta*, with an attitude of inquiry and surrender to God, one is said to be practicing *Kriyā Yoga* in the language of the Yoga Sutras.]

After some *Tapas*, Bhrigu's initial experience is that food or matter is the source of creation and sustenance. The idea is very simple, like the explanation of Mufasa to Simba, in the Disney movie Lion King, where Mufasa explains that the lions eat the antelope, and when the lions die, they become part of the earth upon which grass grows which are consumed by the antelope – a material-based idea of cycle of life. This experience is called *annamaya* where *annam* means food.

Varuna, the father, tells Bhrigu to do more *tapas*. Bhrigu senses the vibration of energy – the *Prāṇa* that was explained earlier – and thinks that is the source of everything, by which everything grows and is sustained.

His father asks Bhrigu to do more *tapas*. Bhrigu discovers the power of the mind – energy flows where the mind goes. He thinks mind, called *manas* in Sanskṛit, is the source of everything.

Bhrigu is asked to continue his *tapas*. Then he understands the *karma* cycle that results in creation, existence, and dissolution. This is said to be *vijñyānam*. *Jñyāna* means knowledge and *vijñyāna* means special knowledge of cause and effect.

Father tells Bhrigu to continue his *Tapas*. Then he realizes *ānanda*, the joy of the highest intuitive realization, that happens in the state of cosmic connectivity, *Samādhi,* as we know from the Yoga Sutras. The highest realization is that the sentient being, perceived within, is connected to the source of creation (God), and the temporal body is the instrument of the sentient being to fulfill the purpose of the dynamics of creation. That realization is the source of ultimate joyfulness. This understanding is also the interrelationship of everything, the single cosmic program that manifests as many to fulfill the program of creation, existence, and dissolution. Thus, each entity that is created, does its cosmic role, and upon completion of its role it becomes free from rebirth.

Bhrigu's experience is personal and should be considered inspirational as one progresses in one's personal practice. This has been represented as the *Pancha-Kosha* system by some schools of yoga.

Questions and Discussion Topics

1. Consider where you are in your own yogic experience. Can you empathize in any way with Bhrigu's experience?
2. Can Bhrigu's experience be considered the universal standard?

As you finish the first section of this book, and get ready to advance further, if you ever thought yoga was a set of exercises, that impression must be permanently erased.

Now, fasten your seat belt and get ready to launch with real yoga practices!

Since breath connects the body to its higher functionalities, it can serve to stimulate higher awareness in yoga.

PART II – POWER OF BREATH IN YOGA

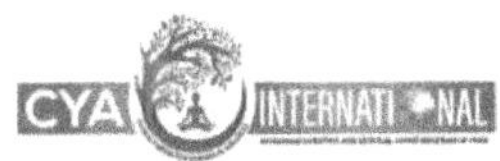

CHAPTER 8:

Introduction to the Power of Breath

Where energy flows, those functionalities become empowered and work with greater vigor. From a physiological perspective breath is the energy activator of the body. Breath supplies the oxygen, which mixing with the glucose produces energy in every cell of the body. Which cells or areas of the body will receive more oxygen (and glucose) with the brain directing the blood flow determines how our organs and faculties are physiologically energized. **The communication that regulates energy in the body is called *Prāṇa* and is closely related to how we breathe.**[34]

Following is an excerpt from Chapter 5 of the first part of the book:

> ***Prāṇa* refers to the vibrations that communicate to control energy regulation of the body that sustains life.** This view makes *Prāṇa* more than simple oxygen intake. From a medical sciences perspective, at a gross level, it relates to the activity of the Nervous System that controls passive respiratory rate, the heart rate, and hence the circulatory system. This results in the distribution of nutrients to different parts of the body for energy production in each cell of the body (cellular respiration), that supports all the organ systems. Thus, *Prāṇa* is considered the most important level of communication, without which none of the other *nādi* communications can function. At the instructor level, most yoga practices are designed to optimize the flow of this *Prāṇa*.
>
> Balancing the flow of *Prāṇa* to the left and right sides of the body is a concept unique to yoga and traditional medicine systems, where the left is considered our inner programmed entity and the right is considered the interaction and influence of the external environment. The left and right interacting together make us who

---

[34] From a physiological perspective the communication is through the nervous system. From a yogic perspective the underlying communication between the trillions of cells in the body and the cosmos (that the body is part of), results in the functioning of the nervous system. This can be appreciated only when one understands that cells of the body can be nourished with flow of oxygen and glucose keeping the body on life support systems (like ECMO – extracorporeal membrane oxygenation – heart-lung machine), but the person will never wake up and if the machine is stopped the body has no capability to breathe on its own. The failure of the system is that the underlying communication of the *nādis* connected with the cosmos and the trillions of cells of the body has stopped, and in modern physiology it is called 'brain dead', i.e. death.

we are at each living moment and serve us to fulfill our purpose of creation as an integrated element of the cosmos.

Where the mind goes, there the energy flows. Therefore, it is important to direct the mind in the right way . . . i.e., ensuring that it is in sync with the cosmic purpose of creation . . . failing which a systemic conflict arises that leads to physical or mental ill-health. ***Breath, in itself, can transform the mind. It can make sure the mind is in sync with the cosmic flow by targeting the zone of energy distribution.*** An important element of some breathing practices is the mental focus moving in and out of the lower part of the sternum or *Ātma Chakra* (noted in Chapter 5) that ensures the *Prāṇa* is in sync with the cosmic purpose.

Much has been written about the rhythm of breath on life and existence and is encapsulated in the term *Svara Yoga*.[35] ***In the yoga system, optimization of vitality and its distribution for various functions primarily through breath is called Prāṇāyāma.***

First Lesson in Breathing

The first lesson in breathing for most people is to recognize the difference between habitual breathing and natural breathing. If you observe a baby breathing while lying down, the rising and falling abdominal area is noticed prominently. This is enabled by the movement of the diaphragm. This is called natural breathing. In fact, the breathing is complete with slight expansion of the chest and shoulders even as the abdominal area bulges slightly in inhalation, and with contracting reverse movement in exhalation. However, because of stresses in life, people develop habitual breathing with only chest and shoulder that are referred as thoracic breathing and clavicular breathing respectively.

To overcome habitual sub-optimal breathing, two approaches may be considered.

- In a relaxed lying down supine position, one can make a conscious effort to observe the belly rise and expand with inhalation and collapse with exhalation. The sensitivity can be enhanced by using some weight like a sandbag, or the palm of the hands, over the abdomen. In time it will bring diaphragmatic sensitivity.

- Another practice called Sectional Breathing is used to develop resilience of each part of the lungs. First, the focus is on the diaphragmatic breathing using the lower part of the lung, then the chest and lastly the upper lobes of the lung. Practice details are provided in Appendix 1.

---

[35] *Svara Yoga* comes from an oral tradition of Tantra and while there are a few texts with the name, they do not adequately represent the meaning of *Svara Yoga*. Swami Rama discusses this in his book: Path of Fire and Light.

Anatomical and Physiological Nuances in Breathing

It is recognized that the average full lung capacity varies between 4 and 6 liters,[36] based on age, gender, and health of population. However, in normal unconscious breathing, air exchange in each breath (tidal volume) is only about 10% of the full capacity. In conscious deep breathing, one can utilize only about 30% to 40% of lung capacity,[37] because the anatomy is not built for full utilization of the lung space, perhaps to enable its other function which is getting rid of waste. The waste, besides carbon dioxide, includes potentially some 250 volatile substances including ketones, moisture (water is a by-product of cellular respiration), etc.[38] The capillaries flowing in the lungs also act as secondary filters of minute blood clots and other such unwanted particles. These are expelled through the exhaled air, and also as phlegm. Thus, for lung function, cleansing the waste may be considered as equal to or more important than oxygenation. Accordingly, the lung operates on negative pressure focusing on expulsion, so that it is always effortless to exhale while inhalation requires some mild effort. Therefore, exhalation is often said to be passive while inhalation is said to be active.

The lung is literally like a balloon ready to fill up. But it is a special type of balloon with millions of small balloons inside it – the air sacs or alveoli. As the alveoli expand, the lung also expands with the rib cage and chest, even as the diaphragm is pushed down and the belly comes out. The main function of the lungs is to permit air exchange – taking in oxygen and getting rid of carbon dioxide accumulated in the blood from energy production and any other waste substances. The real work is done by the alveoli within the lungs, specifically the inner surface of the alveoli where capillaries flow. There the exchange of air and other minute particles take place. There are between 300 million and 600 million alveoli in a person's lungs. The inner surface of the alveoli is very big in total capacity to permit maximum exchange of air and disposal of waste products. It is said that if the inner surface of the alveoli was spread out flat, it would cover the whole area of a tennis court.

When we use more parts of the lungs while breathing, greater is the efficiency of the air exchange and waste disposal. Better the breathing, better is the energy production in the body

---

[36] For a healthy 25-year-old adult the average lung capacity is thought to be 6 liters. See: Delgado BJ, Bajaj T. Physiology, Lung Capacity. [Updated 2021 Jul 26]. In: StatPearls [Internet]. Treasure Island (FL): StatPearls Publishing; 2022 Jan-. Available from: https://www.ncbi.nlm.nih.gov/books/NBK541029/ However, given the aging and health factors of a normal population, the average lung capacity is lesser than 6 liters.

[37] Vital capacity of the lungs, which is the maximum exhalation after full inhalation, is considered to be 80% of lung capacity. https://www.physio-pedia.com/Lung_Volumes#:~:text=Lung%20capacities,-Inspiratory%20capacity(IC&text=It%20is%20the%20maximum%20volume%20of%20air%20the%20lungs%20can,(4%E2%80%906%20L). However, the difference between the ability for gas exchange and the total air is called dead space which reduces the capacity utilization significantly. The dead space is the sitting air that never reaches the capillaries in the alveoli to enable gas exchange.

[38] Corradi M, Mutti A. Exhaled breath analysis: from occupational to respiratory medicine. Acta Biomed. 2005;76 Suppl 2(Suppl 2):20-9. PMID: 16353343; PMCID: PMC1455483. https://www.ncbi.nlm.nih.gov/pmc/articles/PMC1455483/

to maintain its functionalities. As noted in the previous section, in natural breathing the diaphragm also moves enabling all the lobes of the lungs to equally participate in air exchange and waste disposal. Because typically people breath with the upper lobes of the lungs due to stress, in yoga we pay special attention to the diaphragmatic movement, and there are special practices that focus on diaphragmatic breathing to stimulate the diaphragm and overcome years of bad breathing habits acquired because of stress.

Also, the COVID-19 pandemic brought to light the special role of prone positions. Because the lungs are more in the back and sides of the chest (with the heart and the esophagus using much of the space in the front part of the chest), those with breathing difficulties find it easier to breathe while lying down in a prone position (on the stomach) rather than a supine position (on the back). Of course, the seated position with the space for the chest to expand in all directions is the best for breathing practices. While for relaxation, in *Haṭha Yoga* practices, lying in a supine position is typically used (in *Śhavāsana* or corpse pose), prone position can also be used for relaxation (as in *Makarāsana* or Crocodile pose).

Furthermore, from an anatomical and physiological perspective modern medical science does not pay attention to the level of air flow from each nostril. In yoga it is considered very important to activate each hemisphere of the brain, and its consequent impact on unfolding of one's purpose in life as noted earlier.

PHYSIOLOGICAL VIEW OF SWAMI RAMA ON PRĀṆĀYĀMA
Path of Fire and Light, Vol 1 [pg27]

The first purpose in the art of *Prāṇāyāma* is to oxygenate the blood and not allow the energy that results from oxygenation to be dissipated. The second purpose is to eliminate as much waste material as one can. Therefore, one should inhale as much as possible and suspend the breath, so that there may be a more complete exchange of the gases. The third goal is to introduce pressure into the system, maintaining a proper balance between the outside and inside pressures. When this balance is not maintained, the nerves, and in turn the mind and muscles, are affected; the body trembles, and the mind fails to function normally. . . .The fourth purpose of *Prāṇāyāma* is the control of thoughts.

Overview of the Variety of Breathing Practices

There are four important objectives in breathing from a yogic perspective.

- ***Enabling waste disposal***
  - of carbon dioxide.
  - of blood clots and other wastes.
  - resulting in physiological cleansing.
- ***Ensuring optimal vitality and relaxation***
  - enabled by natural breathing, that is deeper. Without vitality nothing is possible, including higher yogic awareness.
- ***Ensuring the physical being is in sync with its cosmic/spiritual plan***
  - by balancing of left and right hemispheres of the brain.
  - by integration of some practices with the spiritual heart (*Ātma Chakra).*
- ***Allowing for internal and external air pressure balance***
  - lack of which results in 'decompression sickness' type of phenomenon. It is also known that for some people the coming of a thunderstorm caused by quick barometric changes in air pressure or sudden changes in temperature that affects pressure, can activate organisms and result in asthmatic attacks and even death.[39]

Nādi Śhodhana Prāṇāyāma (also referred as *Anuloma-Viloma Prāṇāyāma*) ensures that the mind is balanced by equally energizing the left and the right, i.e., one's internal program and the perception of the worldly situation that one encounters, and thus evoke the right response that is in sync with one's cosmic purpose.

Ujjayī Prāṇāyāma is a practice that stimulates the upper respiratory passage in the region of the vagus and glossopharyngeal nerves. The glossopharyngeal nerve is afferent in the pharyngeal region while the vagus nerve is mostly afferent below the pharyngeal region, ensuring the brain is better receptive of the energy needs of critical organs. Thus, the body's critical organs are appropriately nourished. In fact, the vagus nerve stimulates inflammatory reflexes and is known to help reduce inflammation in the body.[40] As described in the textual references, in *Ujjayī Prāṇāyāma*, the stimulation stretches from the throat to the spiritual heart (*Ātma Chakra)*, suggesting the link with one's spiritual purpose.

Bhastrikā Prāṇāyāma is a deep breathing technique that increases oxygen intake beyond what the brain naturally plans by regulating breath and heart rate. This creates a confusion in the brain, which finds something external (i.e., you) has usurped its control and forces it to review energy needs of organs in the body to use the excess oxygen. By dispersing more oxygen to low priority areas, the body's system is toned. In effect the brain resets its energy distribution

---

[39] https://www.lung.org/blog/can-a-thunderstorm-trigger-asthma

[40] Pavlov VA, Tracey KJ. The vagus nerve and the inflammatory reflex--linking immunity and metabolism. *Nat Rev Endocrinol*. 2012;8(12):743-754. doi:10.1038/nrendo.2012.189

pattern, often relieving pains in joints and muscles for those with weakness. This *Prāṇāyāma* is considered an energizer. However, removal of waste from the system in exhalation also makes it a cleanser. Textual references also suggest that both exhalation and inhalation must focus on the spiritual heart (*Ātma Chakra)* thus establishing the spiritual link with the flow of energy.

Deergha Śhvāsa is slow deep breathing with exhalation longer than inhalation that creates deep relaxation – effectively quietening the mind and resulting in lower demands on the system, and thus reducing stress.

Bhrāmarī is exhalation along with nasal humming. This results in vibrations that relax the organs in the head, thereby allowing for better balance of the jaws, sinuses, and the brain's hemispheres.

Certain *Prāṇāyāma* techniques from the *Haṭha Yoga* tradition where one inhales through the mouth and exhales through the nose are designed to move air into the GI tract and have interesting properties related to the enteric nervous system and the digestive process. Such practices are described as cooling for the body.

A breathing technique called ***Kapālabhāti*** that comes from the *Ṣhaṭkriyās* of *Haṭha Yoga* is considered a cleanser that creates heat in the upper back and head, while having impact on sympathetic, metabolic, and cognitive responses.[41] It is debatable whether it can be technically considered a *Prāṇāyāma* or just a cleansing practice.[42] In either case, it is a valuable breathing practice.

A trademarked practice called *Sudarśhana Kriyā* falls within a category of practices called ***Cyclical Rhythmic Breathing***. While it has significant beneficial properties, some people, whose *nādis* are not well-prepared, can have negative side-effects as well that may be transient. This is largely because this practice stretches a safety principle of yoga that requires all practices in yoga be done with minimal effort without strain.

An area that needs treading with care, is the role of suspension of breath, called ***Kumbhaka*** in yoga. In the traditional system of yoga, it is reserved for advanced practitioners whose internal purity is sufficient to withstand its impact. This is to avoid potential negative side-effects that may emerge for those whose purity of the *nādis* is not sufficient. Therefore, this segment is avoided in this instructor level presentation.

---

[41] Swathi PS, Raghavendra BR, Saoji AA. Health and therapeutic benefits of *Ṣhaṭkarma*: A narrative review of scientific studies. J Ayurveda Integr Med. 2021 Jan-Mar;12(1):206-212. doi: 10.1016/j.jaim.2020.11.008. Epub 2021 Jan 13. PMID: 33454186; PMCID: PMC8039332.

[42] *Haṭha Yoga* texts view *Kapālabhāti* as a cleansing practice as distinct and different from *Prāṇāyāma*.

Caution in Stimulating the Power of *Prāṇa* – A Safety Concern

Prāṇāyāma techniques can be very powerful. Because they are designed to regulate and channelize vitality, one should have the ability to withstand the impact. Therefore, these practices must be built up in slow stages.

Suspension of breath (*Kumbhaka*) creates pressure. If suspension of breath is done with the locks (*bandhas* described in the *Haṭha Yoga* section) it creates enormous pressure. If these practices are done by beginners whose *nādis* are not adequate to take the pressure, it can cause damage.

Strong visualization of the mind focusing on the path of the vitality flow – also creates pressure on the *nādis*. This too can create damage for beginners if the *nādis* are not adequate to take it.

The supreme guidance in yoga is that everything must be done with ease, with light effort, so that such practices can be mindfully meditative, and there can be no force in any such practice. If any practice feels forceful to the practitioner, it can forbode trouble.

The safest way to practice *Prāṇāyāma* techniques for a beginner is to keep the focus only on the breath without any visualization and without suspension of breath, and slowly develop the ability for inner awareness. As one advances, the inner awareness is enabled, and the practitioner can sense the path of vitality (the flow in the *nādis*). At that time, suspension of breath and visualization may be introduced. The ability to sense will then guide the practitioner to ensure that any suspension of breath or visualization does not create any undue pressure on the *nādis*. The ability to sense allows the practitioner to suspend breath and apply visualization slowly and carefully in stages.

The best way to understand the point is the following example.

If a person who has never exercised before, and whose muscles are stiff, tries to apply enormous force to lift something very heavy, it is likely that the person will inflict severe damage to the muscles and even could die of heart failure. One must realize that the average body has enough calories to lift a truck and throw it up 50 feet into the air. Practically this feat is impossible and if anyone were to try it, injuries or death may be the result. *Nādis* that regulate *Prāṇa* or vitality provide the communication to ensure production of energy as normally needed. If force is applied beyond one's normal usage, by willpower or compression during suspension of breath, it can result in serious damage.

HAṬHA YOGA PRADĪPIKĀ ON CAUTION AND RECOGNIZING PROGRESS

The Haṭha Yoga Pradīpikā's warning on any forceful practice is described as follows:

"Just as lions, elephants and tigers are controlled slowly by and by, in the same way breath is controlled by slow degrees; otherwise (i.e. by being hasty or using too much force) it kills the practiser." [Ch 2, Sutra 15]

The Pradīpikā distinguishes between doing breathing and regulating vitality which is the inner dimension of breathing as follows:

"When the whole system of *nādis* which is full of impurities, is cleaned, then the Yogi becomes able to control the *Prāṇa.*" [Ch 2, Sutra 5]

This is the idea of developing inner awareness, which comes along with a feeling of lightness in the body and the mind.

Interestingly the Haṭha Yoga Pradīpikā calls the *Nādi Śhodhana* as *Prāṇāyāma* and the eight other practices like *Ujjayī* and *Bhastrikā* as *Kumbhakas. Nādi Śhodhana* is suggested as more benign and beneficial. *Āsana* and *Nādi Śhodhana* are considered precursors to *Ṣhaṭkriyās* and *Kumbhakas* for safe practice.

Anchoring on the Yoga Sutras While Using *Haṭha Yoga* Texts

In the next few chapters, we extensively refer to traditional *Haṭha Yoga* texts to explain the methods of breathing practices. The use of the *Haṭha Yoga* texts is only for the description of selected practice methods, which must be applied adhering to the yogic principles enunciated in the Yoga Sutras, so that safety considerations for normal well-being are not compromised. *Haṭha Yoga* texts are chronologically more recent compared to the Yoga Sutras of Patanjali which is closer to the Vedic era. Hence, the *Haṭha Yoga* texts are possibly colored by later philosophies that emerged after the Vedic period. It is safer to stick to the Yoga Sutras for clear understanding of yoga and for safe application of practices.

Questions and Discussion Topics

1. Distinguish between *Prāṇa* and *Prāṇāyāma.*
2. Why do most people breathe with the upper lobes of the lungs?
3. Observe your breath and evaluate if you are breathing properly. Describe your breath and provide your recommendations for improvement.
4. Why does yoga think that proper breathing can help to unfold one's purpose in life?

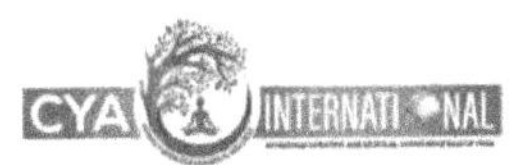

CHAPTER 9:

Nādi Śhodhana Prāṇāyāma

Nādi Śhodhana Prāṇāyāma (OR simply referred as *Prāṇāyāma* in the Haṭha Yoga Pradīpikā and *Nādi Śhuddhi Prāṇāyāma* in the Gheranḍa Samhitā) also popularly called *Anuloma-Viloma*[43] *Prāṇāyāma* is often simply described as Alternate Nostril Breathing, which is a great disservice to its importance. From an anatomical and physiological sense of modern medicine, it has no significance. However, from a yogic perspective, it is a very important practice. Let us examine this from the very Sanskṛit names of this practice.

The first name, *Nādi Śhodhana*, literally refers to purification (*Śhodhana*) of the channels of communication (*nādis*) through which life flow happens. In other words, it enables internal balance (of the *chitta*) through optimal communication.

The second name, *Anulom-Viloma*, is a little deeper in meaning. The prefix '*Anu*' indicates consistency in flow or in the system with some activity. The prefix '*Vi*' indicates either opposite (*Viparīta*) or special (*Viśheṣha*) which may be more appropriate in this case. *Anuloma* describes the flow of energy consistent with life circumstances. *Viloma* describes the flow related to special purpose of one's creation. In other words, *Anuloma-Viloma* balances the inner purpose of our spirit or soul with the external demands of temporal living. In doing so, one fulfills one's purpose of life (*Sva-dharma*) and in the process one purifies or burns off some of the programs (*karma* and *kleśha*) which is the cause of one's birth.

Purification happens when the program load reduces. Thus, breath itself can be a purifier that provides direction towards one's purpose of living, as one acts without reacting and thus preventing formation of new *karma*. This process of living consistently with one's purpose in life is also called *Kriyā Yoga* or *Karma Yoga*.

The Main Process

Haṭha Yoga Pradīpikā Chapter 2, Sutras 6-13 and Gheranḍa Samhitā Chapter 5, Sutras 39-57 describe the process as:

- beginning inhalation from the left nostril,

---

[43] We are not aware of an ancient textual reference of *Haṭha Yoga* for this name. We think it may come from an oral tradition of Tantra.

- exhalation from the right nostril,
- followed by inhalation from the right nostril, and
- completing the cycle by exhalation from the left nostril.

This process is followed by most yoga schools.

Both the texts also refer to suspension of breath upon inhalation and pay particular attention to slow exhalation. The Gheraṇḍa Samhitā specifically suggests exhalation should be twice as long as inhalation and suspension of the breath should be four times the inhalation.

The intent of these texts is clearly to optimize the communication of the *nādis* to permit higher meditative experience. Most yoga schools recognize that suspension of breath – *Kumbhaka* – should not be done before enough purification of the *nādis* has been accomplished. The general practice is to begin *Nādi Śhodhana Prāṇāyāma* without suspension of breath.

While the traditional texts talk of activating the *Suṣhumnā Nādi* by balancing the *Ida Nādi* on the left side of the body and *Piṅgalā Nādi* on the right side of the body, modern understanding of left and right hemispheres of the brain combined with experience of modern yogis have resulted in creative adaptation of this practice by different yoga schools.

Traditional texts do not provide details on number of cycles to be done. However, a count of 10 to 20 breaths is followed by many yoga schools. It can also be a time-based practice, which is better, since one should not hurry the breath. However, there is no limit on this practice, as it has no negative side-effects. Depending on the state of the person's mind, up to 20 minutes of this practice may be normally recommended, although for a regular practitioner, a couple of minutes itself may be transformative.

The flow of breath must be smooth and long, with flow in both nostrils similar in length and force, with exhalation longer than inhalation.

Logic of the Process – Role of Exhalation and Inhalation

From modern physiology we know some important facts that help to understand this practice.

- Lung function - The lung functions with negative pressure. It is always easier to exhale than to inhale. Thus, inhalation is active, and exhalation is passive in natural breathing.
- Hemispheres of the brain and body control – The left hemisphere of the brain, associated with logical thinking controls the right side of the body, and the right hemisphere of the brain associated with creative thinking controls the left side of the body.
- Brain, through the nervous system, controls natural respiration and heart rate to ensure adequate oxygen availability through circulation of blood for the functionality of organs.

When one begins breathing consciously, as opposed to natural unconscious breathing, the brain is impacted. Inhalation from one nostril activates the opposite hemisphere of the brain while exhalation relaxes. Understanding this provides the logic of the textual process of beginning with inhalation of the left nostril associated with the creative brain, which from a yogic perspective drives the soulful and cosmic (inner being) purpose of our lives in an intuitive way. Exhalation from the right nostril relaxes the left brain considered the logical brain, and from a yogic perspective the side that is influenced by external or worldly stimulations. The assumption, presumably, of the textual process is that most people are worldly focused and need to activate their right brain (through left nostril inhalation of *Ida Nādi*) while relaxing the left brain (through right nostril exhalation of the *Piṅgalā Nādi*) to bring internal balance between the left and right. After beginning thus, the process of alternating ensures that there is no overcompensation on either side, and to provide gradual balancing of the two hemispheres of the brain.

Realized Masters and advanced schools of yoga with deeper understanding of this process of respiration, *nādis*, and brain connection can adapt this practice as suitable for individual students. Following is an illustration.

Volume of air flow in each nostril reveals the state of balance between the left and right brain, or the *Piṅgalā* and *Ida Nādis* respectively. Whichever nostril has greater force in exhalation or inhalation, the opposite hemisphere of the brain is overactive relative to the other hemisphere. Exhalation relaxes the overactive side, and in inhalation from the opposite nostril activates the weaker side. This can be an accelerated way of balancing the two sides (of the brain or the two *nādis*), but must be used appropriately to ensure it does not overcompensate towards the weaker side. Presented on the next page is the protocol used by the Himalayan tradition.

Through the alternative nostril breathing process, both sides can be perfectly balanced given enough time of practice. However, there are methods to accelerate this balancing: role of the mind and *mudrās*.

Role of the Mind

Where the mind goes, there the energy flows. If one can visualize while inhaling from one nostril, the awareness crossing over to the opposite side behind the opposite eye and above the opposite ear and then going up towards the middle of the brain behind the upper part of the forehead when the inhalation is complete, and when exhaling from the other nostril visualize the mirror movement, the power of intention accelerates the balancing process of the two hemispheres of the brain. [See Figure 9.1 on the next page.] This should only be tried as an advancement to the next stage, and if there are any signs of discomfort, visualization should be avoided.

Role of *Mudrās*

Some schools pay great importance to the *mudrā* used, where the right-hand thumb is used to close the right nostril and the right-hand ring and little fingers are used to close the left nostril, while the index and middle fingers are folded into the palm. [See finger position of the lady in

Figure 9.1 below. This finger position is referred as the *Vişhnu Mudrā*.] Per se, there is no reasonable basis to conclude which hand or finger one uses has any significant impact.

Alternate Nostril Breathing of Himalayan Tradition

In this tradition, there are three steps that are repeated three times. The three steps are as follows:

STEP 1: Begin by exhaling from the nostril that has greater air flow; then inhale from the other nostril. Do the same breathing process two more times – exhale from the nostril with more air flow and inhale from the nostril with less air flow.

STEP 2: Reverse the breathing process. Exhale from the nostril with less air flow and inhale from the nostril with greater air flow. Do this three times.

STEP 3: Exhale and inhale from both nostrils – do this three times.

This 3-step process represents one round of the exercise. The usual recommendation is that you practice three rounds, alternating the starting nostril each time. Thus, the first and third rounds will be identical. However, the second round will have the breathing pattern of Step 2 (in the above description) in the first step followed by the breathing pattern of Step 1 in the second step.

When this pattern becomes familiar and natural, one may continue the pattern and complete three sets of three rounds. It takes between 30 and 45 minutes to complete and is a very good way to quickly reach a state of very profound mental and physical stillness. As the concentration improves, one may try changing the flow of breath mentally.

The exercise is usually performed after *āsanas* and relaxation and just prior to meditation. It should be done on an empty stomach, at least two hours after the last meal. It is best done before rather than after meals.

Figure 9.1:
ALTERNATE NOSTRIL BREATHING WITH VISUALIZATION

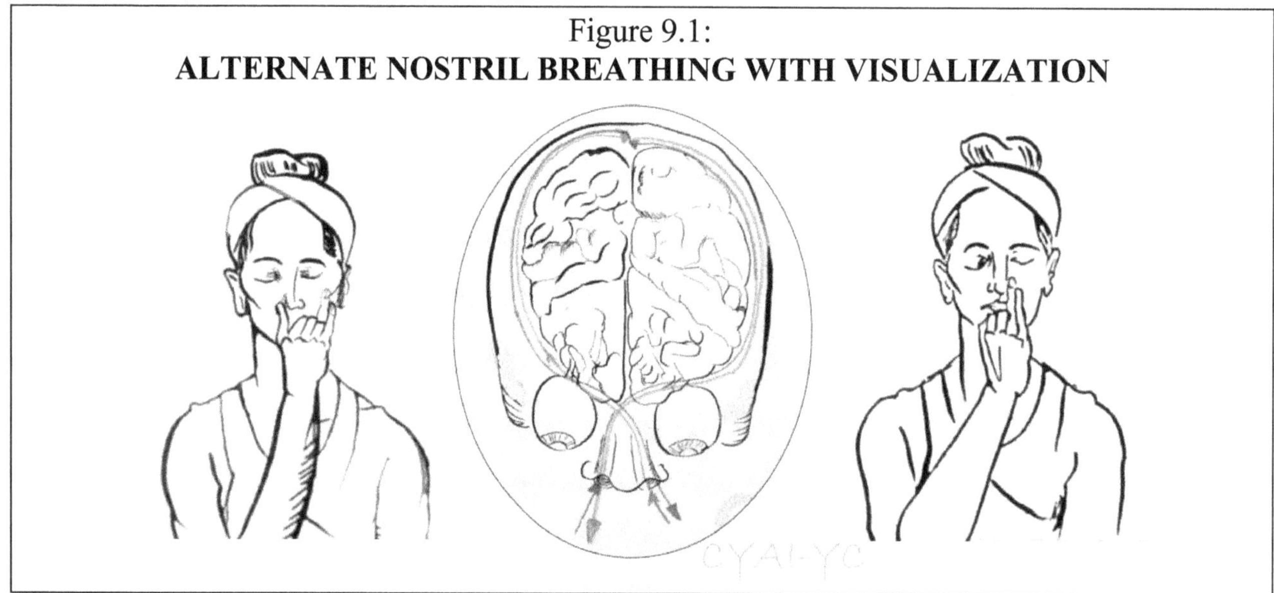

However, there are two interesting observations:

- Role of Elements Associated with Fingers – The thumb is associated with the space element and the ring and little fingers are respectively associated with the water and earth elements. Breathing through the right nostril pressing the left nostril with the ring and little finger focuses on the left brain, working through the *Piṅgalā Nādi* and our logical worldly existence which is mostly earth and water elements. Breathing through the left nostril pressing the right nostril with the thumb, which represents the space element, to connect through the Ida Nādi into the right brain for focus on our inner or cosmic purpose.
- Role of Index and Middle Fingers - Some schools of yoga extend out the index and middle finger and place it in the middle-upper part of the forehead. This serves subtly as the point of focus for the breath visualization – point of completion of the inhalation and point of beginning of the exhalation as explained in the visualization in the previous section. Also, these two fingers represent the air and fire elements that describe the role of the brain – air activating the oxygen intake for energy production, and fire directing the oxygen to where it needs to be utilized.

Nuances to Understand Effectiveness of this Practice

For an advanced practitioner, simply visualizing one's awareness in the middle-upper part of the forehead as one inhales with both nostrils, and visualizing the flow of exhalation downward towards the body's extremities can lead to the same effect. Here there is no focus on the breath in each individual nostril.

Advanced practitioners can also drive breath through each nostril without the aid of closing one nostril simply by intent.

In *Haṭha Yoga*, the connectivity of the left nostril to the right brain is called *Chandra* (moon) *Nādi*, and the connection of the right nostril to the left brain is called the *Sūrya* (sun) *Nādi*. *Chandra Nādi* stimulation is suggested for deeper relaxation by connecting with our inner being, while the *Sūrya Nādi* stimulation is suggested for increasing metabolic activity to deal with the external world. For people who are stressed *Chandra Nādi* stimulation is called for[44], while those who are depressed should stimulate *Sūrya Nādi*.[45] (See more details in Chapter 15.)

---

[44] This article speaks to *Chandra Nādi* stimulation reducing high blood pressure:

Bhavanani AB, Madanmohan, Sanjay Z. **Immediate effect of *chandra nādi Prāṇāyāma* (left unilateral forced nostril breathing) on cardiovascular parameters in hypertensive patients.** *Int J Yoga. 2012 Jul;5(2):108-11. doi: 10.4103/0973-6131.98221. PMID: 22869993; PMCID: PMC3410188.*

[45] See Chapter 5, in the first part of the book that notes: "In yoga, the path of flow of the left force is called *Ida Nādi* and the right flow is called *Piṅgala Nādi* and the interaction of the two are said to flow through the *Sushumna Nādi* which expresses the *Samāna*." These correspond to the *Chandra Nādi* and *Sūrya Nādi* which are *Haṭha Yoga* terms.

Therapeutic Benefit of this Practice

Nādi Śhodhana Prāṇāyāma is considered very effective for anxiety. From a spiritual perspective, anxiety begins when one is not consistent with one's cosmic plan. Balancing the two hemispheres of the brain is designed to bring one's temporal existence to be consistent with the cosmic purpose.

Questions and Discussion Topics

1. Try Alternate Nostril Breathing in three ways for 5 minutes in each mode: (a) without mindful focus (just mechanically); (b) with mindful focus on the breath going through each nostril; and (c) mindful journey of the breath between the nostrils and the middle of the top part of the forehead. Describe the difference in how you feel.
2. What is the spiritual significance of Alternate Nostril Breathing and mechanism of the spiritual intent?

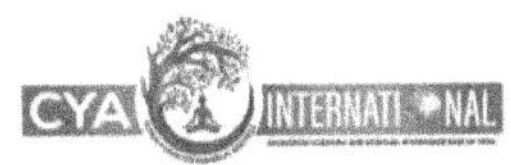

CHAPTER 10:

Ujjayī Prāṇāyāma

From a physiological perspective, *Ujjayī Prāṇāyāma* is often referred as vagal stimulation. Such a description shrouds the importance assigned to this practice in the yoga system. '*Ut*' in Sanskṛit means something that is hierarchically above, and '*Jayī*' means that which wins or is victorious. Combined by Sanskṛit rules it becomes *Ujjayī*, which means the highest, victorious *Prāṇāyāma*. This gives special insight into the spiritual importance of this *Prāṇāyāma* and some yoga schools keep this as the central element of their practice.

The Main Process

Haṭha Yoga Pradīpikā Chapter 2, Sutras 51-53 and Gheraṇḍa Samhitā Chapter 5, Sutras 69-72 describe the *Ujjayī* process. Both describe the inhalation as beginning with a firm mouth (lips closed) with breath being drawn with a sucking sensation with focus between the throat and spiritual heart (*Hṛidaya* or *Ātma Chakra* – see Chapter 5), i.e., the lowermost part of the sternum. Then both suggest suspension of the breath. The Haṭha Yoga Pradīpikā mentions that the exhalation should be through the left nostril, but the Gheraṇḍa Samhitā does not mention the nature of the exhalation. This creates a variety of different ways *Ujjayī* is practiced by different yoga schools.

The inhalation process creates a stimulation in the area from behind the nose (nasopharynx) all the way to the sternum. Different yoga schools approach it in different ways. Some focus on the back of the nose, while some focus on the sucking sensation that results in drawing in the glottis that is visible on the top of the trachea. Most importantly, it must be done with light effort that can be meditative with the focus on the stimulation between the pharynx and the sternum. Since suspension of breath – *Kumbhaka* – is considered a higher practice, it is not typically recommended. Some yoga schools exhale with both nostrils with the same constriction in the throat. Others use the left nostril exhalation.

As a way for easy instruction, Life in Yoga Institute suggests keeping the focus at the base of the mouth in the throat area and make a big smile. As the cheeks pull out in the smile, it creates a slight stretch in the throat area – specifically the vocal cords are stretched slightly. Slow deep breathing, that creates a mild sucking sensation while inhaling and a reverse sucking sensation while exhaling, stimulates the entire pharynx from behind the nose to the throat area, and the sensation extends all the way to the lower part of the sternum.

This practice can be done for a few minutes or for very long periods. There are no known negative side-effects.

Another yoga school does the *Ujjayī Kumbhaka*, i.e., suspension of breath, after inhalation, with the neck-chin lock (*Jālandhara Bandha*), and exhalation is done with a hissing sound between the teeth. This practice seems to have significant impact on the thyroid gland.

Anatomical and Physiological Assessment of this Practice

The primary stimulation of this practice as noted above is in the throat area – anatomically the pharynx, larynx, and the upper trachea. Two cranial nerves in this region are the vagus nerve and the glossopharyngeal nerve which may provide explanation for some of the physiological benefits of this practice. [Cranial nerves connect directly to the brain while other nerves connect through the spinal cord.] However, as noted in the beginning of this chapter, more often this practice is referred as vagal stimulation.

In the pharyngeal area the glossopharyngeal nerve is afferent, while the vagus nerve is efferent. In other areas, the vagus nerve, which is the longest nerve in the body, is primarily afferent. Afferent nerves carry information from the peripheral organs and tissues to the brain, as opposed to efferent nerves that carry instructions from the brain to the peripheral organs and tissues.

The vagus nerve has connection with the cardio-respiratory system and the digestive system. Being mostly afferent it has very interesting properties.

First, vagal stimulation is anti-inflammatory.[46] It is assumed that the increased efficiency of afferent communication results in the brain directing more blood flow and oxygen towards the areas of inflammation. Thus, *Ujjayī* can be effective for relieving asthmatic spasms and pains in different parts of the body where inflammation may be present.

Second, it increases nerve sensitivity. It is thought that lack of nerve sensitivity while sleeping causes the pharyngeal muscles to constrict or collapse and prevent efficient breathing. This results in snoring and sleep apnea. *Ujjayī*, working with the glossopharyngeal nerve and vagus nerve appear to relieve these problems in the pharyngeal area.

Third, it is supposed to balance the autonomic nervous system which controls the cardio-respiratory function. This creates a relaxing tone in the system, that reduces the heart rate and helps people to fall asleep. Also, many people can feel a meditative effect when they do *Ujjayī* for 10 to 15 minutes.

---

[46] Pavlov VA, Tracey KJ. The vagus nerve and the inflammatory reflex--linking immunity and metabolism. *Nat Rev Endocrinol*. 2012;8(12):743-754. doi:10.1038/nrendo.2012.189. https://www.ncbi.nlm.nih.gov/pmc/articles/PMC4082307/

Besides these benefits, Porges's Polyvagal theory explores deeper functionalities of vagal stimulation.[47]

Spiritual Insight of the *Ujjayī* Practice

There are two perspectives offered from practice experiences. First, it is thought that *Ujjayī* works through the *Suṣhumnā Nādi* balancing the *Samāna* and can be thought as combining the effects of the *Ida* (left) and *Piṅgalā* (right) *Nādis*. The balance of the two sides – the inner program and manifestation of external situations – is recognized as the fulfillment of one's purpose of life (*Dharma*). Thus, it is thought to lead to purification – depletion of the internal programs – preparing one for the higher experiences of yoga.

Second, the textual process of *Ujjayī* focuses between the throat and the spiritual heart. The spiritual heart, as noted earlier, is the area of the lower part of the sternum – referred as the *Ātma Chakra* (see Chapter 5). One can presume that anything connected with the spiritual heart or soul will have a higher impact on making one soulful.

The combined effect of the *Suṣhumnā* and *Ātma Nādi* (where the spiritual heart is located) can not only make the person *Dharmic*, but also less reactive. Therefore, it should help with rapid purification of the *nādis*. Perhaps that is the reason it is called *Ut-Jayī* – *Ujjayī* when the prefix is integrated – or the highest victorious *Prāṇāyāma*.

SPONTANEOUS *UJJAYĪ* EXPERIENCED BY SWAMI VEDA BHARATI

There are two types of *Ujjayī*. The first type is *Ujjayī* done as a conscious practice. The deeper practice occurs as a spontaneous *mudrā* in meditation. Late in life, in his afternoon meditations at Swami Rama Sādhaka Gram, Swami Veda Bharati used to sit down initially with a rather rounded posture because of the deterioration of vertebrae in his lower back. Within a few minutes of beginning the meditation, the *Prāṇa* would take over and his posture would straighten until it was perfectly erect. As the energy straightened the back of his neck and tucked his chin, he would begin an automatic *Ujjayī* breathing which had a rather different sound than when *Ujjayī* is done as a conscious practice. This is an example of how energy activations (*mudrās*) spontaneously manifest when one has sufficiently refined the practice of the fundamentals in yoga. Swami Veda used to refer to this approach humorously as "lazy man's yoga."

---

47 Porges, S. W. (2011). The polyvagal theory of emotion: Neurophysiological foundations of emotions, attachment, communication and self-regulation. New York, NY: Norton. ISBN: 978-0-393-70700-7

MEDITATIVE LIFE TRANSFORMATON WITH UJJAYĪ

Life in Yoga Institute's corporate program in Houston had the opportunity to witness the transformation of a 28-year-old with *Ujjayī* in 2018.

As part of the corporate wellness program employees could individually consult with a Life in Yoga yogi on-site during the yogi's monthly visit. This 28-year-old young employee walked in and said he would like to lose some weight. The yogi and the associate did not see him as overweight but humored him by taking his *nādi* reading. The peripheral nervous system was not in good balance. Hence, he was asked to do *Ujjayī* for 15 minutes. At the end of 15 minutes, the *nādi* reading indicated he had come back to normality. He also indicated he felt good after the practice. He was recommended to continue the practice twice a day – upon waking up in the morning and before going to sleep.

In the follow-up next month, he came to report he had good news. The yogi and his associate barely hid their amusement as he started by saying he had lost 2 lbs. Immediately thereafter he said his waist had reduced by 1 to 2 inches – likely the anti-inflammatory effect. Finally, he noted that the practice would take him into a meditative state where he could observe the follies of his own way of working that made him less effective at work. With regular practice, he had become stress-free and objective in his interaction with colleagues. He had become more confident and more receptive and could easily take criticism without feeling defensive. Second, his work had fewer mistakes and needed less rework. His colleagues noticed his improved interaction and work quality and appreciated it. This suggests the working in the *Suṣhumnā* and *Ātma Nādi* – performing one's role in sync with one's inner program and not being reactive.

Role of Mind and *Mudrās* for Accelerated Healing with *Ujjayī*

In the practice of *Ujjayī* the mind is entirely focused in the pharynx-throat area extending all the way to the lower part of the sternum. However, given its anti-inflammatory and pain-relieving nature, for those with specific joint pains stretching out the affected joints while doing *Ujjayī* brings accelerated relief.

Furthermore, pressing of the little finger, ring finger and middle finger (constituting the earth, water, and fire elements) with the thumb on the hand in the side of the body that is affected, pain or insensitivity can be more rapidly relieved.

The extension of *Ujjayī* described in these two paragraphs above should be treated as advancement and applied only when the practitioner is ready and there is no discomfort in the practice.

Avoiding Ineffective Practices

Some schools of yoga do *Ujjayī* with a loud sucking sensation and focus on the loud sound. The effort put in the process causes strain for most people and can tire the person very quickly. Such an approach is violation of the yogic principle of light effort without strain that can be meditative which is a standard for all yoga exercises. Any strain in the practice of Ujjayī must be avoided.

Questions and Discussion Topics

1. Reflect on why *Ujjayī* is considered the highest *Prāṇāyāma*. Provide your considered thoughts on this view.
2. Since *Ujjayī* is practiced differently by different schools of yoga, what would you say is the common denominator that makes it effective?

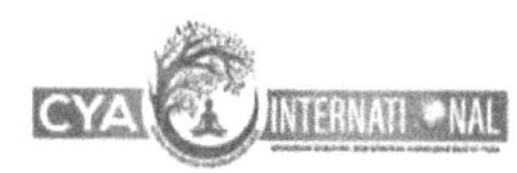

CHAPTER 11:

Bhastrikā

Bhastrikā means "like a *bhastrā*," where *bhastrā* means bellows of a blacksmith. Bellows are used by blacksmiths to increase heat (energy) in the fire by pumping in more air – specifically the oxygen component of the air that further heats the fire. Filling the bellows can be relatively quick but blowing the air out into the fire is done smoothly and slowly so that the fire's heat is increased. Air is never blown too fast as it may disturb and make the flame unstable.

In effect, *Bhastrikā* is deep breathing done with focused effort where exhalation is slower than inhalation. One can have about three times more air exchange than normal in this practice. The practice has variations across yoga schools, and any practice that is done without strain and with smoothness will be considered yogic.

Textual Process

Haṭha Yoga Pradīpikā chapter 2, sutras 59 to 67 and Gheranḍa Samhitā chapter 5, sutras 75-77 describe Bhastrikā as follows.

Haṭha Yoga Pradīpikā points to *Padmāsana* (Lotus pose) as the seated position to begin *Bhastrikā*. It may be assumed that this refers to aligned and vertical spine. From this seated position one exhales with effort that is focused from the *Ātma Chakra*[48] to the throat and then the forehead. Then, one inhales rapidly feeling the fullness in the *Ātma Chakra*. And thereafter, one continues the same exhalation and inhalation as noted in the first exhalation and inhalation. When one feels worked out (mild fatigue) then one should inhale from the right nostril (*Sūrya Nādi*) and hold the breath in *Kumbhaka* for a short period. Thereafter exhalation is done with the left nostril.

The Gheranḍa Samhitā uses the term *Bhastrikā Kumbhaka* and suggests that it should be done like the motion of a blacksmith's bellows. It should be done slowly, and upon completion of twenty breaths, one should hold the breath in *Kumbhaka* for a short period. It recommends that three rounds of twenty breaths each, followed by *Kumbhaka* has positive impact on health.

---

[48] *Ātma Chakra* is located just behind the sternum as described in Chapter 5 of Part 1 and is often referred as the spiritual heart and in these ancient texts the word "*hṛit*" or hidden is used.

Variety of Practice Approaches

For beginners, getting the rhythm of the breath flow without creating strain in the system is very important. Simply focused on deep breathing without visualization is a good beginning.

Swami Veda Bharati of the Himalayan tradition used to train beginners in slower breath first to ensure that they do not strain before making the speed faster.

TEACHING OF BHASTRIKĀ BY SWAMI VEDA BHARATI

Swami Veda Bharati taught the practices of *Kapālabhāti* and *Bhastrikā Prāṇāyāma* in a similar systematic manner. Even though, in the way these practices are taught in the tradition of the Himalayan sages, involve vigorous breathing, Swami Veda always taught newcomers to begin with a much slower pace, less effort, and a smaller number of repetitions, in order to give enough time to allow the body to prepare for more vigorous and intense repetitions. The main aspect of his teaching to promote smooth progress for students was that the speed and intensity of the practice should always allow the body to remain stable and that the vigorous breathing should not create jerks, involuntary movements or physical tension in the body.

Kaivalyadhāma uses the textual process of twenty quick breaths followed by inhalation from the right nostril, holding the breath and exhalation from the left nostril.

For beginners, Life in Yoga uses deep inhalation followed by slower exhalation as a starting practice where each cycle of inhalation and exhalation combined may take 7 to 9 seconds – about 2 to 2.5 seconds for inhalation, 4 to 5 seconds for exhalation, and brief pauses in-between inhalation and exhalation. Each round has twenty breaths, and three or more rounds are practiced until fatigue in the muscles and joints are eliminated. Once the practice is mastered, the textual process of focusing on the *Ātma Chakra*, throat, and forehead, as one begins in exhalation, is introduced. Inhalation follows with focus on the *Ātma Chakra*. This becomes the visualization in all the breaths in each round of twenty breaths each. The slow breathing is taken from the Gheraṇḍa Samhitā that notes the word "*shannaih*" (meaning slowly) to indicate the quality of the breath.

To be in sync with the expansion of the lower, middle, and upper parts of the lungs for full breathing, some schools of yoga use movement of the hand along with the movement of the abdomen, shoulders, and chest in deep breathing. One starts with a loose fist by the side of the shoulders with elbows by the side of the chest when fully exhaled with the contraction of the belly and chest, and the shoulder pulled down. Then as one inhales one lifts the elbows a little, stretching the shoulders and opening the palms as the chest and belly expand. There is no such mention in the textual references, but it seems to help people to breathe deeply. Life in Yoga promotes this approach, although with a caution that breathing must be slow, and the movement of the hands smooth and limited only to promote expansion of the chest and lungs. It should not result in full stretching out of the hands or be converted into a hand exercise that can strain the shoulder.

Figure 11.1
BHASTRIKĀ WITH HAND MOVEMENTS

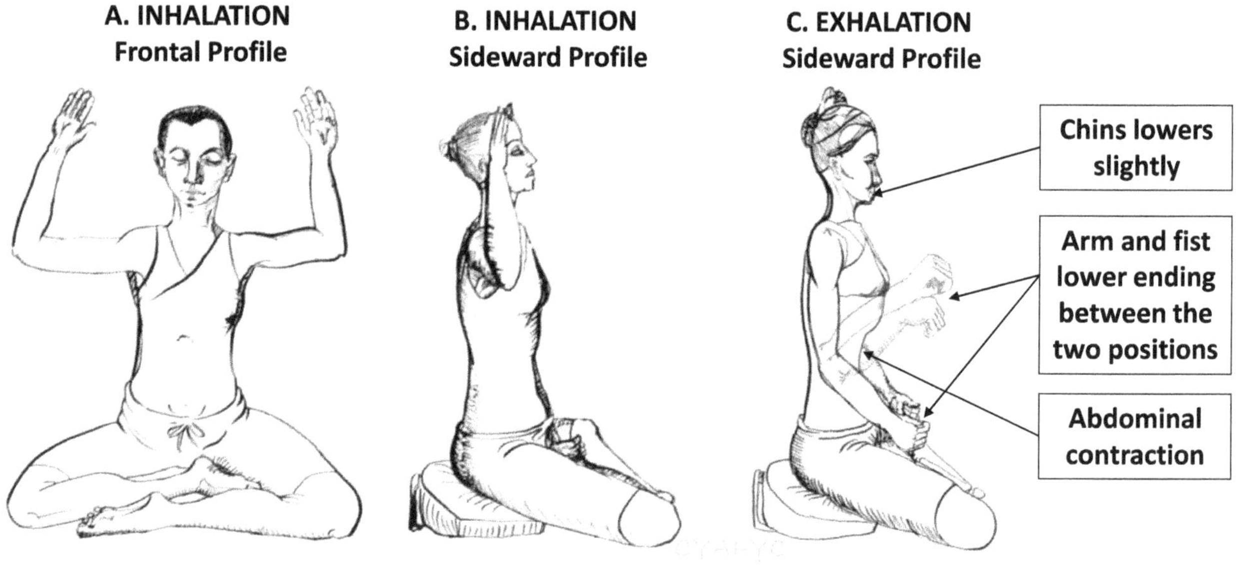

A. INHALATION Frontal Profile

B. INHALATION Sideward Profile

C. EXHALATION Sideward Profile

Chins lowers slightly

Arm and fist lower ending between the two positions

Abdominal contraction

Physiological Process

From a physiological standpoint, *Bhastrikā's* focus is to ensure we use more of the lungs than the typical 10% of the capacity used in normal unconscious breathing. Therefore, it does not matter whether one begins with relaxed long exhalation or active deep inhalation, since the cycle will eventually ensure maximum air exchange. The key to best practice is to use all the five lobes of the lungs – the two lobes of the left lung and the three lobes of the right lung.

Diaphragmatic insensitivity, COPD, or other respiratory disorders, for some people may result in poor usage of the lobes of the lungs. When one does not feel the deep breath, to breath better and make better usage of the lobes, one should not strain. It is more important that this practice be done with ease rather than trying to do with strained effort to get all the lobes to breath. In time, with regular practice, deficiencies can be improved, especially diaphragmatic resilience.

The physiological view of breathing relates to the role of the brain and the blood chemistry as part of cellular respiration in the energy production of the body. Energy is produced locally in every part of the body to maintain its functionality. However, the brain decides how much of oxygen from our breathing will be distributed to each part of the body through the blood supply. Thus, in a passive state when one is not focused on the breath, the brain controls the respiration and heart rate to optimize what the brain considers as the needs of the body. From a biochemical process, this revolves around the oxygen and carbon-dioxide content in the blood. Oxygen from the fresh inhalation makes the blood more alkaline and carbon-dioxide produced from the energy production of our cells makes the blood more acidic. The body's varied functionalities with all the ionic exchanges are designed to be optimized when the pH level is 7.4 for the blood and fluids in the system. The oxygen buffering system in the blood cells allows the body to normally maintain this pH level within a small variation between 7.35 and 7.45.

From a physiological perspective, there is a maximum buffering capacity within the system. Rapid or deep breathing (like in *Bhastrikā*), overriding the passive control of the brain, increases air exchange much beyond normal levels, resulting in increased oxygen in the blood supply. Initially the buffering system stores the excess oxygen to ensure that the pH level in the blood does not increase substantially. As one continues to breath and the pH level increases with more oxygen, the brain gets confused resulting in a person passing out from respiratory alkalosis. Therefore, to avoid risk of passing out, *Bhastrikā* is never done for more than 20 breaths at a time, after which one observes the sensations in the head. Only after the sensations subside does one go onto the next round of 20 breaths.

When rounds of 20 breaths are repeated in many rounds, something extraordinary happens. It starts with vibrations or sensations in parts of the body with weak muscles or joints. After enough rounds, usually between 3 to 10 rounds, any joint pain or muscle pain fully disappears. We think of this as resetting the brain, where the brain begins to direct more blood flow to the areas of pain or weakness. This allows for release of the excess oxygen that cannot be stored since the buffering system is maxed out. Thus, the energy starved cells which are the source of the pain and weakness are enabled to produce more energy to resolve the pain.

Pain in the system is a nerve response to indicate that an area needs attention. As a result of wear and tear or damage from an accident to joints, the connective tissues and muscles that move a specific joint need more energy to move the joint effectively. Without more energy available, pain comes as the signal. *Bhastrikā* done in several rounds, overcoming the pain, suggests that the blood carrying more oxygen becomes available to these connective tissues and muscles, to relieve pain.

OVERCOMING PAIN IN JOINTS AND MUSCLES WITH *BHASTRIKĀ*

On October 1, 2016, a 45-year-old female in Tampa, Florida approached us at Life in Yoga Institute with complaint of right hip and left shoulder pain, and occasional migraine headache. She also complained of a lot of tiredness in the muscles of the lower and upper limbs. We did 10 rounds of *Bhastrikā Prāṇāyāma*, with 20 breaths in each round, and at the end of which all her pains were gone.

This is something we see all the time with older people with arthritic join pain.

Yoga Views of the Process and Impact

While the yoga process is designed to revitalize the body and mind, there is also a spiritual component in the textual process. This is suggested by the focus on the *Ātma Chakra* (lotus of the spiritual heart - soul) while inhaling, as if directing the intention of the breath to the *Ātma Chakra*. While exhaling the focus begins from the *Ātma Chakra*, moving up the throat and forehead, as if the *Ātma Chakra* is directing the brain to suitably use the vitality of the breath.

Revitalizing without the anchor in the *Ātma Chakra* only leads to balance in the energy, without necessarily being in sync with the soul's plan. Inhaling into the *Ātma Chakra* evokes the soul's intent in applying the energy. Exhaling from the *Ātma Chakra* to the throat (*Viśhuddhi Chakra*) suggests that the throat where *Kūrma Nādi* is stimulated ensures supreme balance within (Yoga Sutras 3:32). Moving from the throat to the forehead suggests the association with the *Ājñyā Chakra*. The *Ājñyā Chakra* is considered to be the controller of the lower *chakras* through which the functions of the body and mind execute. Thus, the visualization suggests the empowerment of the *Ājñyā Chakra* to execute the soul's intent.

For an advanced practitioner, a single round of 20 breaths of *Bhastrikā* done with focus on these points can create a strong meditative silence and eliminate all discomfort in the body. Done for three rounds creates a state of meditative stillness that is difficult to describe.

DISTINCTION BETWEEN BREATHING AND DIRECTING VITALITY

When Swami Veda Bharati taught special sessions on the refinement of *Prāṇāyāma* practices to a selected group of long-term students at his ashram in Rishikesh, one of the students repeatedly asked questions related to the physical methods of performing the practices of *Bhastrika Prāṇāyāma*: what is the movement of the diaphragm, what happens with the chest area, the abdomen, the facial muscles, the phases of inhalation and exhalations? Swami Veda's reply was: "what is your intent, are you trying to do *Prāṇāyāma* or *śhvāsāyāma* (breathing exercise)?" His humoristic reply was to bring the students back to the essence of the practice and not just to emphasize the physiological breathing happening in the gross body.

Caution in this Practice

Bhastrikā should be done after attaining left and right balance in the system, failing which the increased energy can increase any imbalance. Such balance can be attained in a variety of ways: by calm observation, by spinal stimulation practices, alternate nostril breathing, etc.

Questions and Discussion Topics

1. The textual approach requires *Bhastrikā* to be done in *Padmāsana* (lotus pose). What is the significance of this requirement? Does that mean that those who cannot do *Padmāsana* cannot do *Bhastrikā*?

2. Since the *Bhastrikā* practice is done differently by different schools of yoga, what is or are the common denominator/s of all practices that produce/s the net effect of *Bhastrikā*?

3. Start meditative practices in two different ways. Start with regular *āsanas* to bring alignment in the body and go into meditation after a minute or two of Alternate Nostril Breathing. In a second modality, sitting with erect spine, immediately after a minute or two of Alternate Nostril Breathing do 3 to 5 rounds of *Bhastrikā* and then begin meditation. Describe the difference and postulate a spiritual hypothesis for the difference.

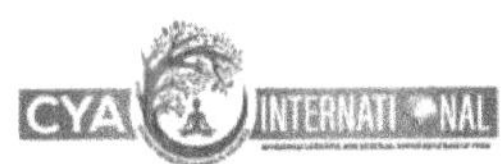

CHAPTER 12:

Deergha Śhvāsa – Long Deep Breath

While Haṭha Yoga texts don't refer to *Deergha Śhvāsa* (long deep breath), the more authoritative Yoga Sutras in the second *pāda*, Sutra 50 states *Prāṇāyāma* is done with long, subtle, and quiet breath. Because this is such a simple and powerful technique for deep relaxation and inward awareness, it is used by almost all schools of yoga. Long deep breathing, with exhalation longer than inhalation reducing normal breath rate of 15 per minute to 6 breaths per minute, has shown to be every effective in reducing systolic blood pressure along with deep relaxation.[49]

As a beginning practice, this is helpful for practitioners to observe and build diaphragmatic sensitivity.

The Process

It really does not matter whether one begins with exhalation or inhalation, since the cycle of several breaths bring the necessary rhythm. However, if we were to exercise a choice, it is always preferable to begin with exhalation, since it is passive and relaxing.

However, the first step in relaxation is to have a comfortably seated or lying-down posture where the spine is aligned and straight.

Exhalation begins in a natural slow pace with a sense of letting go unwanted stuff. Inhalation that is deep and slow follows thereafter. Typical inhalation takes 2 to 4 seconds while exhalation takes twice as long with natural pauses between inhalation and exhalation. Such practice is done with full mindfulness.

Modified Process with Greater Benefits

This same slow breathing done with lifting of the shoulders as one inhales to stretch the spine and rotating backward and relaxing the shoulders as one exhales, seems to enhance the effect of

---

[49] Russo MA, Santarelli DM, O'Rourke D. The physiological effects of slow breathing in the healthy human. Breathe (Sheff). 2017;13(4):298-309. doi:10.1183/20734735.009817

the relaxation in the central nervous system. However, care should be taken that this does not create unnecessary stress.

Questions and Discussion Topics

1. What is the benefit of this slow, deep breathing?
2. Why is it suitable for most beginners?

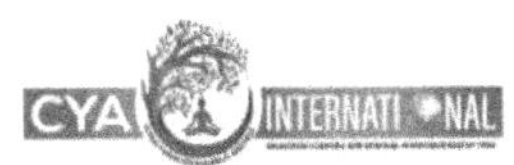

CHAPTER 13:

Bhrāmarī

"*Bhrāmarī* " refers to the buzz of a bee and derives from the Sanskṛit word "*Bhramaraka*". "*Bhramaraka*" means "bumble bee."

Like all *Prāṇāyāma* it is practiced by keeping the head, neck, and trunk in the same alignment. It could be performed with or without the hands according to traditions. The practice focuses on nasal sound with breath that resonate upward into the head.

Depending on the tradition, this may be practiced for a few breaths or for a few minutes.

Textual Process

This practice is referred in the Haṭha Yoga Pradīpikā Chapter 2, Sutra 68, and in the Gheranḍa Samhitā, Chapter 5, Sutras 79-82.

The Haṭha Yoga Pradīpikā states that when yogis practice filling up in rapid inhalation with the sound of a male bumble bee, and while exhaling make a sound like a female bumble bee, they experience a sensory joy within their consciousness. This is *Bhrāmarī Prāṇāyāma.*

The Gheranḍa Samhitā states a practice with a similar name called *Bhrāmarī Kumbhaka* differently. The practice is to shut the ears with one's hands in the middle of the night when everything is quiet, after taking inhalation and holding the breath. In this state different sounds will be heard within and after all have gone, the *anāhata* sound is heard. Within that resonance there will be light, and the mind when immersed in that light, one reaches the awareness of the cosmos.

In effect, according to these texts this practice gives high level of inner happiness and can lead to a deep meditative experience. The common element in both is that there is some sound involved whether actively created by breath or experienced within. While the Gheranḍa Samhitā speaks to closing the ear, the Haṭha Yoga Pradīpikā focuses on the sound of exhalation.

Thus, *Bhrāmarī* is a *Prāṇāyāma* whose practice and technique vary depending on the traditions.

Mudrā used with *Bhrāmarī*

The gestural position of the hands, "*hasta mudrā*," used along with the *Bhrāmarī* breathing by many yoga schools is the *Ṣhaṇmukhī Mudrā*. The term "*Ṣhaṇmukhī*" comes from the Sanskṛit word "six" ("*Ṣhat*"), and "*Mukhi*" refers to the face or openings.

The position of the hands should be over both eyes, both ears, the mouth, and partial constriction of the nostrils. Hence its name, "*Ṣhaṇmukhī*", which means "six-faced" implying restricting the functionality of the six openings.

Neither the Haṭha Yoga Pradīpikā or the Gheranḍa Samhitā mention this *mudrā* in the context of *Bhrāmarī.*

Figure 13.1: ***ṢHAṆMUKHĪ MUDRĀ***

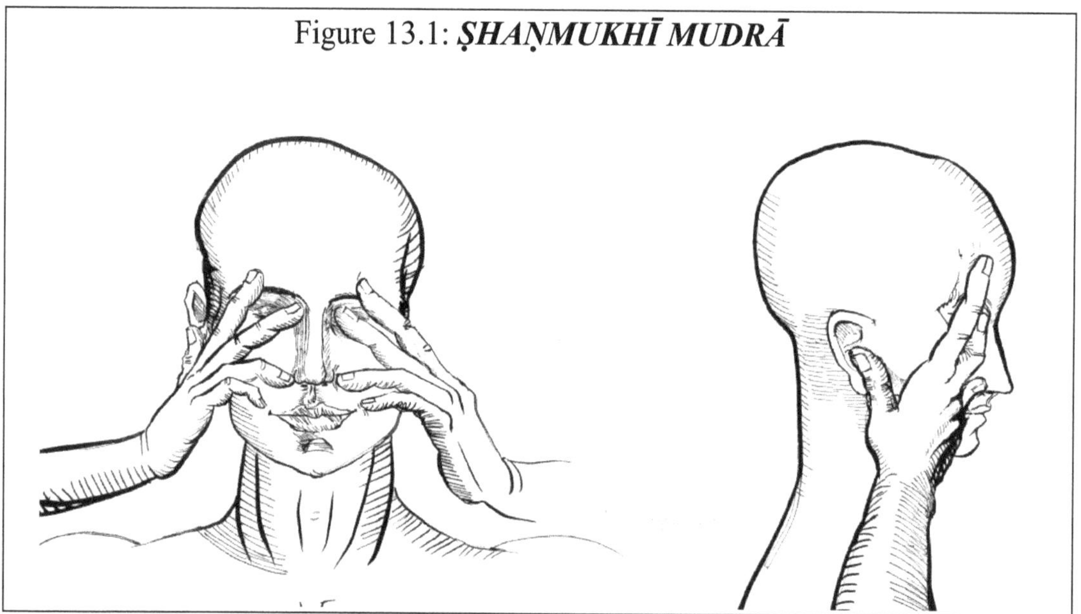

Variety of Practice Approaches

Most yoga traditions focus on taking a deep breath and making a nasal humming sound while exhaling. The *Ṣhaṇmukhī Mudrā* is used by most of these traditions. In this type of humming, the resonating sound comes from the throat area moving upward.

The Himalayan tradition of Swami Rama adheres to the Haṭha Yoga Pradīpikā. Humming is done in both rapid inhalation and slow exhalation with the focus of the resonating sound in the nasal and pharyngeal areas. The difference in the sound in inhalation and exhalation is thought to be the difference between a male and female bee.

SWAMI RAMA'S TIPS FOR SINGERS AND SPEAKERS

When *Bhrāmarī* is practiced back and forth imitating the hum of the male and female bees as taught by Swami Rama of the Himalayas, it helps to refine the voice and prolong the ability to manage the breath. This is the basic practice of the Himalayan tradition and is recommended for singers and speakers.

The Assessed Psychosomatic Impact

Following suggestions have been made regarding the vibrations of *Bhrāmarī* by yogic practitioners:

- It promotes deep mental relaxation that also has a somatic impact. The mental impact can result in cessation of intrusive, negative thoughts that result in better mental balance. On the somatic side, perhaps with the slower breathing and through the mechanism of the vagus nerve and the parasympathetic tone, the deep physical relaxation can reduce the allostatic load and result in lowering the systolic blood pressure.
- Such psychosomatic impact may be helpful for improving sleep quality.
- The impact of the vibrations in the throat and head areas may help to relieve any issues in the region, like sinus pressure, nasal congestion, health of jaws, thyroid, etc.

An area that merits further inquiry is the mechanism of the benefits from *Bhrāmarī.* The resonance of the sound affecting other sinuses in the body, like the Valsalva sinus, may be worth investigating. Whether the impact on the Valsalva sinus can affect the performance of the heart muscles is an interesting question. We have seen this correlation from *nādi* reading in two cases.

Questions and Discussion Topics

1. The description of *Bhrāmarī Kumbhaka* from the Gheraṇḍa Samhitā is very different from what is generally practiced by most schools of yoga? How would you justify significant variations from the description in a traditional text.

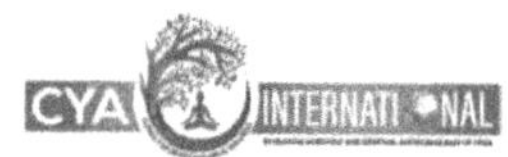

CHAPTER 14:

Kapālabhāti

Kapāla refers to the head or forehead and *bhāti* refers to lustre. Thus, *Kapālabhāti* is known to induce heat in the system, particularly in the upper back and neck, and the forehead. In the Tibetan Buddhist system, a similar practice is called *Tumo* breath.

Kapālabhāti, although a breathing practice, may not be considered a *Prāṇāyāma*. As suggested by the Haṭha Yoga Pradīpikā it is viewed as a cleanser that precedes *Prāṇāyāma*. It is referred to as one of the six cleansing practices called *Ṣhaṭkarma or Ṣhaṭkriyā*.

The practice involves short exhalations from the belly, done without strain (light effort in a smooth manner). It begins from a position of a drawn in belly after full inhalation. The pressure of the full breath with belly drawn in results in forced exhalation with the belly drawing in further. The recoil motion automatically ensures inhalation. Thus, in this practice exhalation is active and inhalation is passive. This practice is also often referred as diaphragmatic breathing with the diaphragm lifting-up in exhalation and relaxing in inhalation. Upon exhalation, one may also experience a slight pelvic floor lift. Figure 14.1 below shows the lifting diaphragm and contracting belly in the side view of exhalation (C) in contrast to A and B views.

Figure 14.1: **DIAPHRAGM AND BELLY MOVEMENT IN KAPĀLABHĀTI**

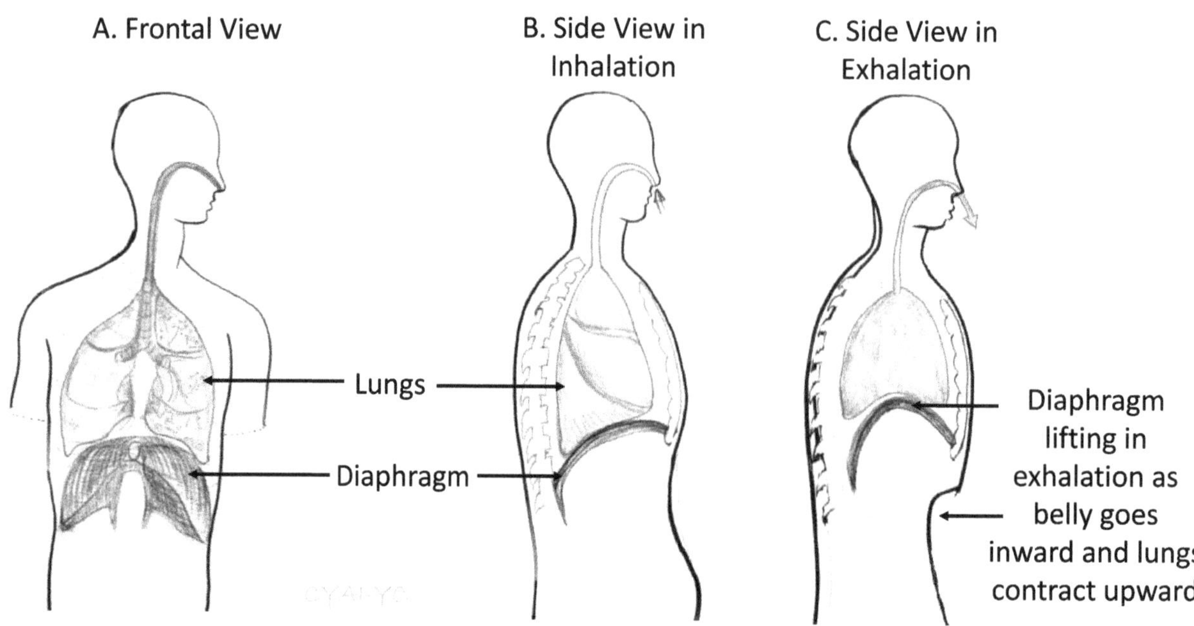

One way for beginners to train themselves is to sit erect and pronounce the syllable "HA" with an open mouth. This approximates the correct motion of the abdomen and diaphragm while doing *Kapālabhāti*. However, once the sensitivity of the abdomen and diaphragm is recognized, the practice should be continued with a closed mouth.

Textual Process

This practice is referred in the Haṭha Yoga Pradīpikā Chapter 2, Sutras 35-37 and is described as follows.

> When one does exhalation and inhalation like the bellows in complete absorption, it is called *Kapālabhāti*, and it removes all *kapha* (phlegm congestion) from the system. (Thus), similar to completing the (other elements of) *Ṣhaṭkarma* [see *Haṭha Yoga* section] that remove the faults of *kapha* and impurities, one becomes ready for *Prāṇāyāma*.

The text does not recommend the specific duration of the practice. When done without strain, a person can do it for a long time, even 15 minutes or longer. In some schools of yoga, they do three rounds of 20 breaths each with relaxation in-between each round.

It should be noted that the description of *Kapālabhāti* in the Gheranḍa Samhitā (1:55-60) is substantially different and is actually nasal cleansing with air (like alternate nostril breathing) or water (*Jala Neti*).[50]

Physiological and Psychosomatic Benefits of the Practice

Diaphragmatic breathing activates the air exchange in the lower lobes of the lungs while also serving as a cardio-respiratory exercise. For those with breathing disorders where activating the lower lobes of the lungs is beneficial, *Kapālabhāti* is particularly useful.

In the Yoga-Ayurveda tradition it is said to improve the digestive fire. Therefore, it is considered as toning for the gastro-intestinal tract and beneficial for those with metabolic syndrome. There have been cases of type-2 diabetes who have pancreatic insufficiency[51] who have been able to get off insulin with this practice.

Also, from an Ayurvedic perspective, it is consistent with the view expressed in the Haṭha Yoga Pradīpikā, where *Kapālabhāti* is described as a cleanser. In the Ayurvedic expression, the digestive fire of *Kapālabhāti* is supposed to digest, dissolve, and expel toxins.

---

[50] *Jala Neti* is described in Appendix 3 and is also referred in Chapter 19, *Ṣhaṭkarma* in the *Haṭha Yoga* segment of the book.

[51] It is important to note pancreatic insufficiency is a small subset of cases of type-2 diabetes. The more common variety is insulin resistance for which this practice may not be relevant.

It is said in Ayurveda that one should have the capacity to digest and expel the unwanted stuff of whatever we take from the environment – which can be whatever we take through the mouth, nose, skin, or mind. This can also be expressed from a spiritual process of clearing out the unwanted stuff so that the *nādis* are prepared for higher spiritual activity.

Extension of *Kapālabhāti* Practice

Once a person has been trained sufficiently in *Kapālabhāti*, some schools of yoga alternate the exhalation of *Kapālabhāti* from one nostril to the other in each subsequent breath. It is usually done to cleanse the nostrils and sinus channels more effectively.

Caution in *Kapālabhāti* Practice

Expert practitioners of *Kapālabhāti* can do it smoothly with much vigor. When others who are not so accomplished try it with the same vigor, they end up creating strain in the system. We have known a number of people, who have practiced *Kapālabāti* with strenuous vigor, finding themselves requiring surgery for hernia, after many months of regular practice. It is very important that this practice must be done with smoothness and ease, without strain.

Because many schools of yoga have tended to teach *Kapālabhāti* with much vigor, it is commonly suggested that those with high blood pressure should avoid doing this practice. When done without strain, it has not been found to increase blood pressure.

Since *Kapālabhāti* increases heat in the face, it is known to help eyesight, but for those with glaucoma caution is recommended. Consistent with the basic rule of yoga that no part of the body may be strained, those with recent abdominal surgery or any abdominal pain should avoid doing this practice to avoid strain in the healing wounds.

Questions and Discussion Topics

1. What are common mistakes that can happen in the practice of *Kapālabhāti*?
2. Practice *Kapālabhāti* without strain for 15 minutes (with breaks if needed) and observe any sensation of heat in any part of the body. Describe your experience.

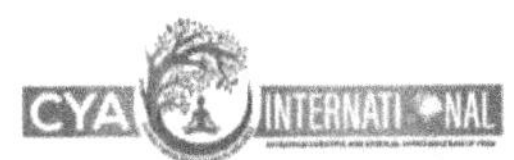

CHAPTER 15:

Other Breathing Practices

Haṭha Yoga Pradīpikā and Gheranḍa Samhitā discuss many more breathing practices. In addition, other traditions have developed innovative techniques beyond the textual methods. We make a brief reference here to make sure an instructor is aware of these practices, but these are not meant for teaching at the instructor level.

Practices of Inhaling through the Mouth

There are two traditional practices of inhaling through the mouth and exhaling through the nostrils that come from *Haṭha Yoga* texts. They are called *Śheetalī* and *Seetkārī.* Mouth inhalations like these are thought to direct more of the air into the GI tract and help with reduction in acidity, while cooling the body. The purpose is intended to balance the heating and cooling of the body. It is typically suggested for practice during the hot summer months or anytime the body feels excessive heat.

However, there are other methods to balance the heating and cooling in the yogic tradition. The balance comes from the balancing of the processing of the *chitta* by limiting reactivity and being true to one's conscience (following one's *Sva-dharma*). It is important to bear in mind yoga is about spiritual awareness at a much higher level as stressed in the Yoga Sutras. These practices coming from the *Haṭha Yoga* tradition, that are more in the physical dimension, may not be necessary for daily practice.

One should also be mindful that the nostrils have filters to limit the entry of unwanted substances from entering the lower respiratory tract. Such filters are not there in the mouth, and part of the air inhaled through the mouth also goes into the lungs. Hence mouth breathing should be generally avoided, and only when absolutely required exercised carefully in a clean environment.

Practices of Varied Inhalation through the Nostrils

Different yoga schools have developed techniques of varied breathing that have significant impact in cleansing the *nādis*, even though some of these practices may not be smooth with light effort as recommended by general yoga principles. ***These practices need to be approached with extreme caution, since for those with significant imbalances, it can be destabilizing. These practices may be practiced only under the supervision of an experienced teacher.*** Two such practices are described here.

Breathing Discretely – This is a practice where each inhalation is done by three discrete sniffing or sucking motions through the nostrils and each exhalation is done in the same way.

Cyclical Rhythmic Varied Speed Breathing – This practice involves multiple cycles of breathing where breathing speed goes from relaxed slow breathing to very fast breathing in stages. Typically, four or five stages are involved where each stage is about 20 to 40 seconds. Throughout this practice, eyes are fully and firmly closed. Following is a step-by-step description:

1. Slowest breathing - In the first stage, breath is slow and relaxed.
2. Slightly increased speed of breathing - In the second stage, the speed is slightly increased and focused.
3. Continued increment in stages - Speed is thus increased in one or two more stages until in the final stage the breath is very fast and obviously strained. This rapid breathing is done for about 20 to 25 seconds.
4. Going back to slowest breathing - Then it goes back to the slow and relaxed breathing, as in Step 1, at the beginning of the next cycle.
5. Repetition of cycles – Steps 1 to 3 are repeated 3 to 5 times.
6. Final slow breathing - After the last cycle of rapid breathing, there is a long stretch of slow and relaxed breathing.
7. Lying Down – After the final relaxing breathing, the practitioner lies down for deep relaxation observing the senses for about 15 minutes.
8. Final Opening of Eyes – Only after the deep relaxation, like emerging from deep meditation, the practitioner sits up and slowly opens the eyes looking straight into the palm of the hands.

The two practices described above involve jerky or irregular breaths. Inherently they create sporadic pressure on the *nādis* during the irregular, forceful motion of the breath as it tries to clear the *nādis*. Such force can accelerate *nādi* cleansing, but at the same time it is not completely free of the potential of the force to go the wrong way and create unwanted disturbance in the psychosomatic system. When done with mantras or sounds this unwanted potential is mitigated to some extent. When visualization involves connecting into cosmic intelligence for guidance, such risks can be completely avoided.

Variations of Alternate Nostril Breathing

Alternate Nostril breathing when done according to the previously explained textual process (See Chapter 9) is safe and works to balance the system in a slow and methodical way. However, recognizing its impact on the hemispheres of the brain and the yogic notion of left and right, four different kinds of breathing practices can be applied, but not at the instructor level. This is because any excessive or inappropriate use of these techniques can result in imbalances.

- *Sūrya Prāṇāyāma* is inhaling and exhaling through the right nostril only.
- *Sūrya Bhedana Prāṇāyāma* is inhaling from the right nostril and exhaling from the left.
- *Chandra Prāṇāyāma* is inhaling and exhaling through the left nostril only.
- *Chandra Bhedana Prāṇāyāma* is inhaling through the left nostril and exhaling through the right.

Practice of Breath Suspension

Practice of breath suspension, in the traditional system of yoga, is reserved for higher practices of yoga and not recommended at the instructor level. The practice of suspension of breath is more powerful and if done inappropriately it can lead to negative consequences. The forms of breath suspension are the following:

- *Bāhya Kumbhaka* or holding out the breath after full exhalation,
- *Antar Kumbhaka* or holding in the breath after full inhalation.

Both of these types of breath suspensions can be done with or without compression.

Antar Kumbhaka creates more pressure in the system than *Bāhya Kumbhaka.* Accordingly, *Antar Kumbhaka* should be approached with extra caution since the held breath creates pressure on the *nādis*. *Bāhya Kumbhaka* can be relatively safe if the exhalation before the *Kumbhaka* and inhalation after the *Kumbhaka* are done very slowly and smoothly, while holding out the breath is done without compression. Slow motion avoids jerky pressure and holding out the breath without compression avoids pressure in the holding phase.

Compression, in these two *Kumbhakas,* is created with *bandhas* or locks, that are described in the *Haṭha Yoga* section. Their application must be approached with even greater caution because of the added pressure on the *nādis*. Again, done with *Bāhya Kumbhaka* with very slow and smooth exhalation before the compression and very slow and smooth inhalation when compression is released is relatively safer. Therefore, in modern day yoga practices, *Bāhya Kumbhaka* has become more prevalent in general use.

Esoteric Practices

Murchchhā, *Plāvinī*, and *Kevala Kumbhaka* are described in Haṭha Yoga Pradīpikā Chapter 2, Sutras 69-75, and in the Gheranḍa Samhitā, Chapter 5, Sutras 83-89.

Murchchhā Prāṇāyāma refers to a practice of breath that creates a peaceful feeling arising from a swooning sensation.

Plāvinī is a technique of breathing to fill the belly with air that enables floating in water.

Kevala Kumbhaka is a state when one is neither inhaling nor exhaling. This is an advanced state that can be reached because the *nādis* are cleansed to a point where it is able to absorb *Prāṇa* from the environment, without depending on breath.

In traditional *Prāṇāyāma*, the word *Sahita* refers to Prāṇāyāma with inhalation and exhalation, while *Kumbhaka* refers to *Prāṇāyāma* with suspension of breath.

A Final Caution on These Practices

These practices emerge from the *Haṭha Yoga* and *Tantra Yoga* traditions that tend to force *nādi* cleansing towards building higher awareness beyond the physical body by physical force. This speaks to the history of these traditions and their non-Vedic influences. The safest approach is the Yoga Sutras approach of gradual *nādi* cleansing by living life true to one's conscience without reactivity to situations that don't involve one's duty. Use of gentle practices described in chapters 9 to 14 should be more than sufficient for safe and effective spiritual advancement.

Questions and Discussion Topics

1. The *Haṭha Yoga* system considers *Prāṇāyāma* techniques to be approached with care after adequate purification with *āsanas* and Alternate Nostril Breathing. Can you suggest why this caution has been stated?

2. Some schools of yoga suggest that *Prāṇāyāma* alone can lead a person to the highest level of awareness. Can you discuss the arguments to justify this statement and arguments to oppose this statement?

3. Should we assume that the eight breathing practices from the Haṭha Yoga texts should be the only ones considered valid? Or is it acceptable to adopt other practices and if so with what caution?

4. Should one ever consider any practice that involves inhalation by mouth? If so, what should be the precaution? If not, why? Present your justification for both positions.

In all breathing practices, realizing the power of breath, it is important to recognize that it can cut both ways.

Correct practices can give significant benefits, while inappropriate practices can have detrimental effects.

Therefore, these should be done with caution and under the guidance of a good teacher.

PART III – *HAṬHA YOGA*

16. Understanding Anatomy and Physiology for Safe Instruction
    - Physiological Energy Production and Distribution System
    - Understanding the Nervous System
    - Cardio-Respiratory System
    - *Chakras*, Glands, and Hormones
    - Digestive and Excretory System
    - Immune System
    - Anatomical and Physiological Safety Parameters
17. Introduction to *Haṭha Yoga*
    - Progression and Study of *Haṭha Yoga*
    - Historical Development of *Haṭha Yoga*
    - Perspectives in Mode of Practice
18. *Āsanas*
    - Method to Perform *Āsanas*
    - Distinguishing Between Yoga *Āsana* and Gym Exercises
    - Dyanamic and Static Yoga *Āsanas*
    - Progression in Yoga *Āsanas*
    - Physical and Metaphysical Perspectives of Yoga *Āsanas*
19. *Ṣhaṭkriyās* or *Ṣhaṭkarma*
20. *Prāṇāyāma* Overview
    - Terminology and Sequence in *Haṭha Yoga*
    - Correlation Between Metabolic Rate and Breathing Rate
    - Yogic Adage on Longevity
    - Physiology of Breath Holding
21. *Mudrās* and *Bandhas* – An Overview
    - Application of Hand-Finger (Hasta) *Mudrās*

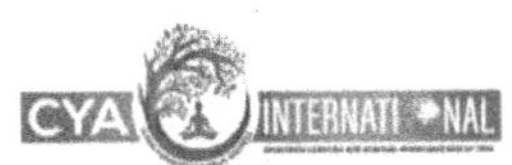

CHAPTER 16:

Understanding Anatomy and Physiology for Safe Instruction

For safe instruction there is no need for extensive understanding of anatomy and physiology like that of a physician.

Some Yoga schools that emphasize *āsanas* may focus on the anatomy of the gross body to the degree of mapping the 600 or so muscles and 206 bones and ensuring their alignment in every practice. Such focus takes one away from the real dimension of safe yoga practice.

The second *pāda* (chapter) of the Yoga Sutras, Sutras 46-47, state an important safety principle of yoga. If there is peaceful, pain-free, happy state in any yoga practice, where one can be in meditative engrossment infinitely, there can be no violation of safety. A peaceful face and slow rhythmic breathing are indicators of this. Anytime the breath is irregular or fast, or the face is cringing, one can know something is wrong. These external indicators of potential violation of safety are easy to notice and an instructor can take immediate action to stop the practice for the practitioner.

Underlying the breath and facial expression are the energy production and distribution system of the body, that is captured in the cardio-respiratory and the neuro-muscular systems. Understanding these is all that is required for an instructor who is dealing with normally healthy people to lead a practice protocol in which the instructor has significant mastery. While it is not essential to know the endocrine system that underlies the observed impact on the cardio-respiratory and neuro-muscular systems, in the field of *Haṭha Yoga* some yogis in the last century have associated the *chakras* with glands. Also, since yoga provides stress release, knowing something about stress hormones is useful. To empathize with those who may not be normally healthy, some understanding of the aging, digestive and excretory processes, as well as the immune system may be helpful.

Physiological Energy Production and Distribution System

Energy in the body is produced in every cell of the body by taking oxygen and glucose from the blood. The body's system maintains the glucose level in the blood at a suitable level all the time releasing from its storage[52] as needed, while the oxygen comes continuously from our regular breathing of the lungs. The pumping of the heart and the circulatory system ensures that the blood, carrying the glucose and oxygen, reaches all the cells in all parts of the body.

Several cells together form tissues and organs which have specialized functions. The energy of the cells of each tissue or organ helps to perform its function: whether it be functioning of the brain with energy produced by the brain cells; or pumping of the heart with the energy of the cells of the heart; or bending your finger by the extension and contraction of the muscles in the finger joints facilitated by the energy in the muscle cells; or even the production of hormones in the glands like for example insulin in the Islets of Langerhans in the pancreas.

The decision to send more blood (with glucose and oxygen) to some parts of the body and less to other parts of the body, or even how much of glucose and oxygen is needed for the body's systems is made by the brain and communicated through the nervous system.[53] Thus, the nervous system controls your heart rate and passive respiration rate (when you are not focused on your breath) to ensure adequate oxygen (and glucose) in blood circulation. In essence, the nervous system is the communicator and default decision maker of the energy production and distribution in our body system, unless you seek to disrupt it by seeking to control some of its functions through yogic practices. Examples of such practices and how they affect the nervous system were ample in the previous section on the breathing power of yoga.

Understanding the Nervous System

The nervous system is viewed relative to location and functionality of the nerves in the following ways:

- Central Nervous System (CNS) and Peripheral Nervous System (PNS)
- Autonomic Nervous System (ANS) and Voluntary Nervous System
- Parasympathetic and Sympathetic Nervous Response
- Motor Nerves and Sensory Nerves, also referred as Efferent and Afferent Nerves respectively.

The CNS consists of the brain and the spine. The PNS is the network of nerves going into the rest of the body from the brain and spine. While most of the PNS connects through the spine, there are twelve nerves called the cranial nerves that directly connect into the brain. These

---

[52] Excess glucose after digestion of consumed food is converted into glycogen by insulin and stored in the liver and muscle/adipose tissues to ensure that glucose level in the blood does not go too high. These are released by conversion of the glycogen, fat like substance, into glucose by glucagon when blood glucose goes too low in the blood.

[53] "The regulation of blood glucose is generally stated to be under the control of the endocrine system. But the endocrine secretion is itself regulated by the central nervous system, especially the hypothalamus." Kumar VM. Neural regulation of glucose homeostasis. Indian J Physiol Pharmacol. 1999 Oct;43(4):415-24. PMID: 10776456.

cranial nerves mostly control the functionalities of the face/head and neck. However, the tenth cranial nerve, called the vagus nerve, goes further down to connect into the cardio-respiratory and the gastro-intestinal (GI) systems.

When we are not actively focused on breathing or any activity, some automatic functions continue as default activity. Examples are breathing, pumping of the heart and digestion of food. All these automatic controls are exercised by that side of the system that is called the Autonomic Nervous System (ANS). But when you choose to lift your hand or move your leg, or talk, it is the Voluntary Nervous System in operation. Both the Autonomic and Voluntary Nervous Systems are part of the PNS.

The ANS is divided into three kinds of functionalities:

- Parasympathetic when the body and mind are in a peaceful state and not affected by any stress,
- Sympathetic when the stress hormones kick up, and the breathing rate and heart rate typically go up,
- Enteric that controls the GI (gastrointestinal) tract that seems to have an independent brain-like control on its local energy utilization.

Figure 16.1: **NERVOUS SYSTEM STRUCTURE**

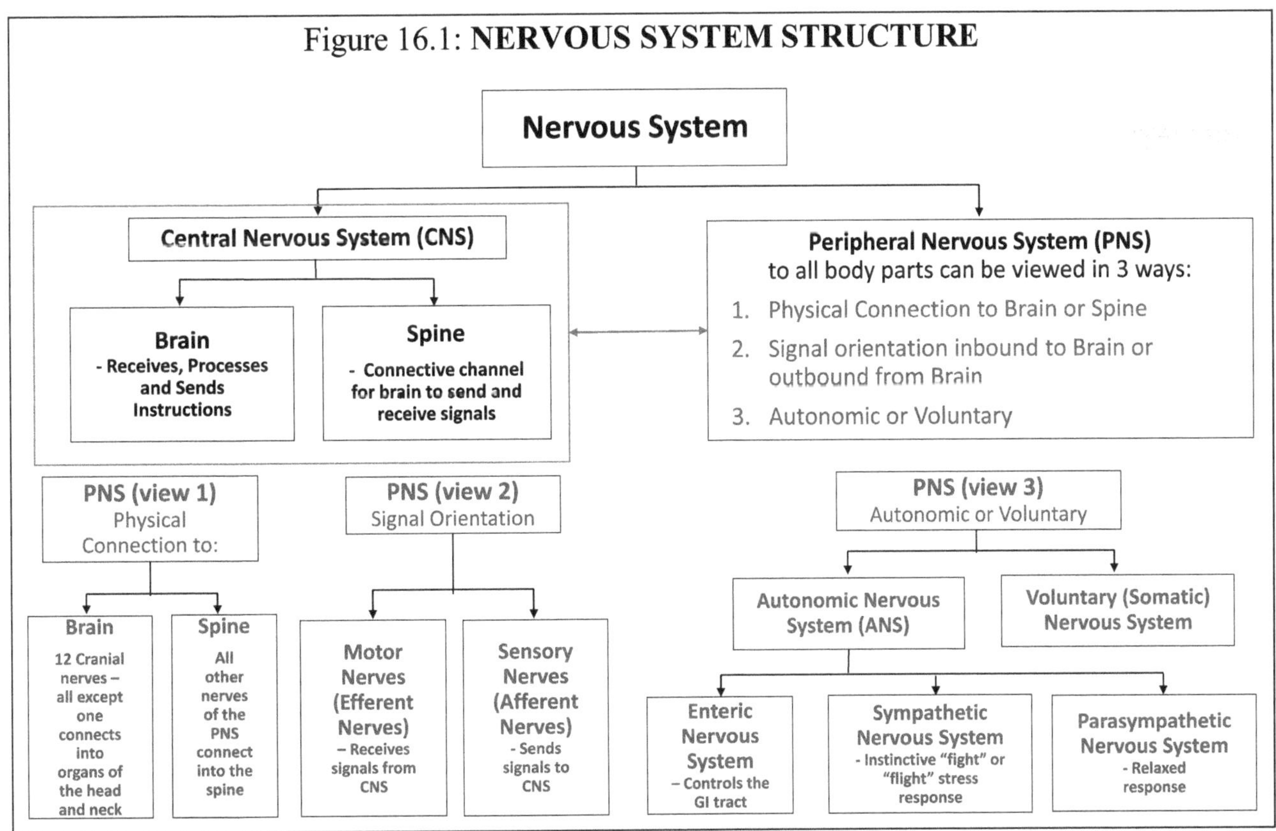

Motor Nerves carry messages to different parts of the body from the CNS, while the Sensory nerves send messages to the CNS from different parts of the body that communicate their energy requirement and utilization status. Another way to say the same thing is that efferent nerve functionality communicates from the brain to the rest of the body, whereas afferent nerve functionality communicates from the various body parts to the brain.

The mechanics and responsiveness of the nervous system, particularly the ANS, to stress and relaxation provides the insight needed to ensure compliance with the requirements of yoga.

Cardio-Respiratory System

It is clear from the discussion of the nervous system and energy production in the body that if the overall nervous system fails, breathing and pumping of the heart stops. Then the person is said to be brain dead and essentially a dead person. However, even if the nervous system is operational, failure of the respiratory system or the cardiovascular system would result in the same death of the nervous system, because the brain cells will not be able to receive its oxygen and glucose to produce its energy to do its function. Thus, the cardio-respiratory system has its own importance.

In fact, in any practice, the cardio-respiratory system should not be overloaded to the point of break-down. Accordingly, the safety requirement in yoga is to ensure breath always stays normal during any practice or quickly returns to normal after mild stimulation. In the *Haṭha Yoga* system, between *āsanas*, resting after stretching is designed to regain normal slow breathing. But as noted in the Yoga Sutras, even the stretching in any part of the body should be with mild effort so that there is no pain. Pain in any part of the body while doing yoga practices is a signal that this part of the body is not getting enough blood flow (glucose and oxygen) to produce enough energy to do the yoga practice.

Following is an overview of the components and functionalities of the cardio-respiratory system.

- ***Heart***, which is located about the middle of the chest with a slight leftward tilt of the lower end. It has four chambers. The two upper chambers (atria) receive blood. And when they contract, they send the blood to the two lower chambers (ventricles) which pump the blood out of the heart. The left side receives oxygenated blood from the lungs, and it sends the blood to all parts of the body. The right side receives the deoxygenated blood after circulation in the body, and it pumps the blood into the lungs to get oxygenated before sending it to the left side of the heart.
- ***Lungs*** are two in number and sit in the chest cage behind the heart. The right lung has three lobes (superior, middle, and inferior), while the left lung has two lobes (superior and inferior). [Some of the space on the left chest is taken by the heart which on the right side is available for the division of three lobes in the right lung.] The key gas exchange component of the lungs are the tiny air sacs called alveoli, that are in millions in each lobe. The deoxygenated blood pumped from the right side of the heart through the pulmonary artery distributes into smaller blood vessels with the tiniest ones being the capillaries which are thinner than a hair. These capillaries run through the gossamer

like web of the alveoli where air exchange takes place. Oxygen is taken from the fresh air coming through the breath into the lungs, and carbon dioxide, produced as a by-product of energy production (along with moisture and other waste), is released.

- ***Respiratory channels*** from the nose-mouth area continue into the trachea in the throat area that goes down and split into the right bronchus and left bronchus which divide further until it goes into all the lobes of the lungs.
- ***Circulation*** of oxygenated blood begins through the aorta at the mouth of the left ventricle of the heart. The aorta segment just outside the heart has the opening for the blood vessels, called the right main and left main coronary arteries, that take the oxygenated blood to the walls of the heart to help produce energy for the heart cells to keep the heart pumping. Further along, the aorta divides into other vessels to take blood upward towards the head and upper body organs, and downward towards the legs and lower body organs.
- ***Capillaries*** coming out of the arteries provide the gateway for cells to take oxygen and glucose from the blood and release the carbon dioxide (and water) coming from the energy production of every cell. The deoxygenated blood ends up in the vessels called veins which return the blood to the right atrium of the heart through the superior vena cava from the upper parts of the body, and the inferior vena cava from the lower parts of the body.

Figure 16.2:

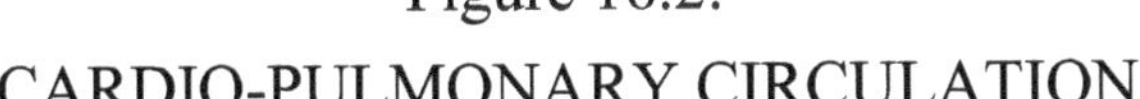

CARDIO-PULMONARY CIRCULATION

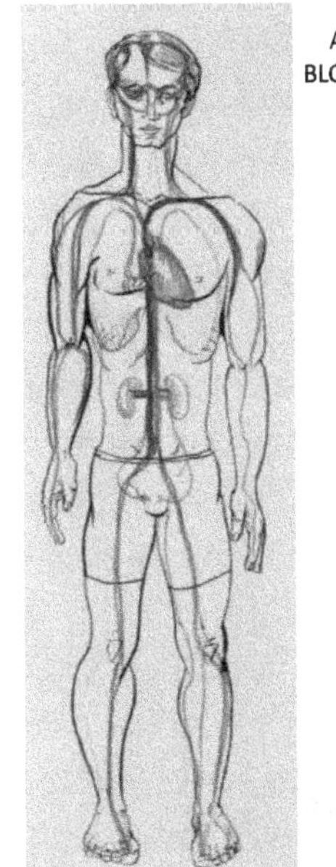

A. CIRCULATION OF THE BLOOD THROUGH THE BODY

B. HEART-LUNG CIRCULATION FOR OXYGENATION

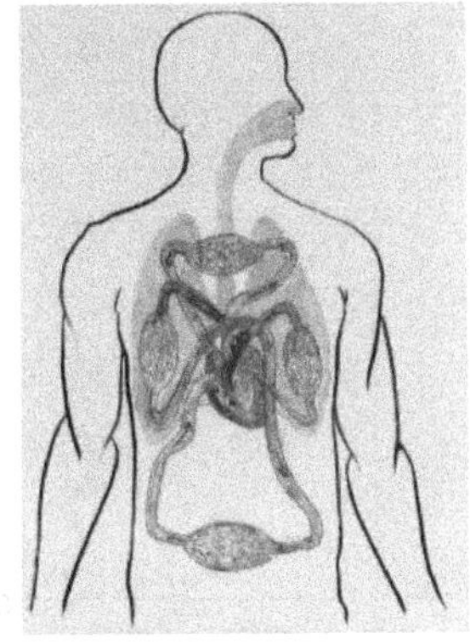

The blue indicates the veins carrying deoxygenated blood while the red indicates oxygenated blood in the arteries.

- ***About 15% of the fluids of the blood leak*** out into the areas outside the cells while going through the capillaries before reaching the veins. These are reabsorbed by separate channels called the lymphatic vessels that carry the fluid all the way to the upper chest (clavicle area) and drain into the subclavian vein which empties into the superior vena cava that brings the deoxygenated blood back to the right atrium of the heart to carry on the circulation.

Any disruption in this entire cardio-respiratory function will be registered in the nervous system, and it will result in irregular breathing and a facial expression that deviates from a peaceful demeanor. If a practitioner, even with little effort exhibits any of these undesirable signals, that is in the province of a physician. The yoga instructor is only responsible to warn practitioners to avoid strain in any practice. Capacity for individuals vary. What is strenuous for one person may be a smooth effortless flow for another.

Chakras, Glands, and Hormones

In yoga, some yogis and physiologists have speculated a relationship between *chakras* and glands, and the hormones secreted by these glands. From an instructor level perspective, the real focus is on stress hormones that are expected to be tamed by relaxing yoga practices that bring balance to the body. The hypothalamus, pituitary and adrenals are considered the critical glands for stress management. Other important glands are the thyroid and pancreas, which have metabolic impact. The functioning of the body's system through genes, neurotransmitters and hormones is complex and is reserved for higher level learning. Figure 16.3 below depicts specific glands/organs associated with each *chakra*.

Figure 16.3:
ORGANS ASSOCIATED WITH EACH *CHAKRA*

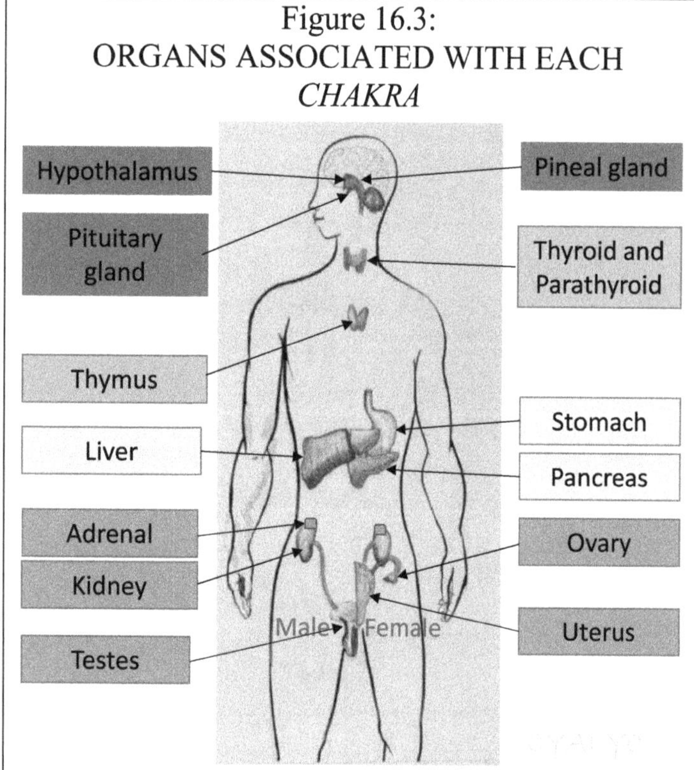

The color coding above corresponds to each *chakra*. Organs that produce hormones related to five *chakras* are noted above with the bottom-most *chakra* and the top-most *chakra* (refer to figure 5.3 in chapter 5) not having any hormone producing organ associated.

Each of these glands produce one or more hormones that impact the functionality of the body. The glands are divided into endocrine and exocrine glands. Those glands whose hormones directly come into the blood system are called endocrine, while those that enter other parts of the body are called exocrine. Enzymes produced by the walls of the stomach, liver, and intestines (and saliva produced by the salivary glands or sweat from the sweat glands) are exocrine examples. Stress hormones, like cortisol and adrenaline, enter the blood directly from the adrenal glands, and are therefore part of the endocrine system. On the metabolic side, our focus will be on insulin and glucagon produced by the pancreas and thyroxine levels related to the thyroid. Accordingly, most of the health-related focus of yoga will be on the endocrine system rather than the exocrine.

Digestive and Excretory System

The digestive system comprises of many parts from the mouth through the entire alimentary canal as shown in the diagram below (Figure 16.4: left panel). Of greatest interest is the liver.

Liver filters out the toxins produced or ingested in the body. If the liver fails, the accumulated toxins enter the brain which kills the person. Stress hormones are toxins in the system and the liver needs to remove them from the system. Many medications, especially steroids, create excessive load on the liver and over a long term can weaken the liver.

In a conventional sense, the excretory system consists of the urinary system (Figure 16.4: right panel) and the fecal excretion through the anus after the digestive process. However, from a yogic perspective we also stress on exhalation and sweat.

Figure 16.4

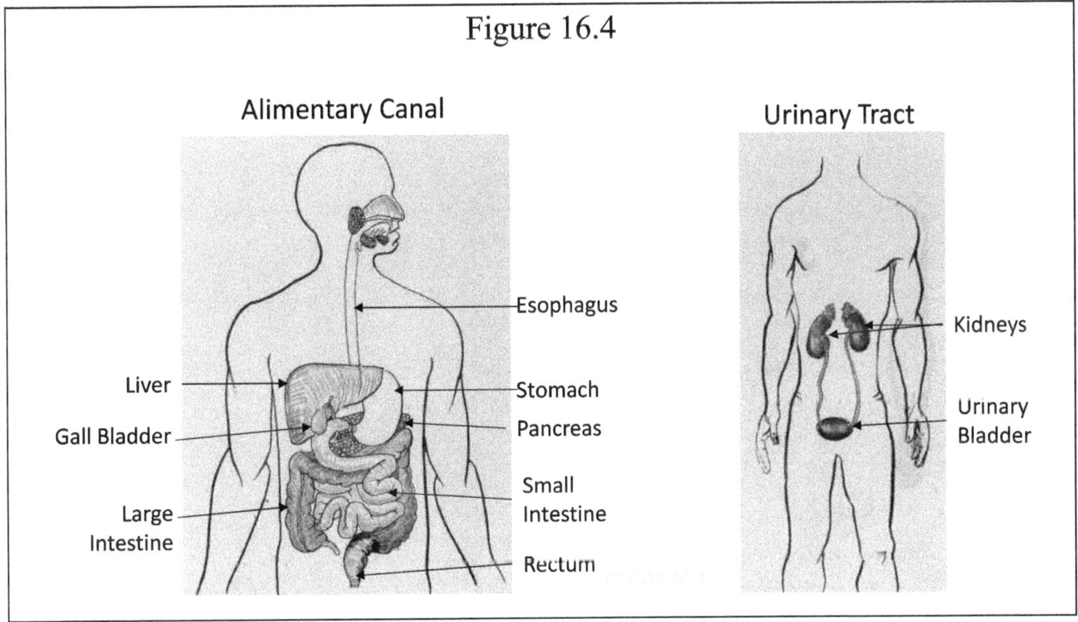

Immune System

From a conventional medicine perspective, the immune system is primarily meant to recognize and fight off any invading organisms that can damage the body. The system is divided into two classes: innate immunity and adaptive immunity.

Innate immunity comes from the memory of infection whether from an earlier infection or inherited memory. This memory is stored in the white blood cells: granulocytes (neutrophils, eosinophils, and basophils), monocytes, and lymphocytes (T cells and B cells). [White blood cells are also called leukocytes.] Chief method of immune system activation is through the circulatory system, particularly the lymphatic system where lymphocytes in the lymph nodes constantly review the overflow from the blood circulation (15% of the blood flow). They are ready to act from their memory. The spleen, tonsils and certain mucous membranes in the body also act as filter mechanisms to ward off infections. The leukocytes are produced in the bone marrow.

Adaptive immune system relates to new memory created from an infection or vaccine, as understood in modern medicine. Modern medicine does not fully understand the source and mechanism of building adaptive immunity but finds a strong correlation with good sleep.

From a yogic standpoint, adaptive immunity comes from the cosmic intelligence into which we are all connected. Also, yoga does not view the immune system simply as the fighting mechanism of the body to ward off invaders, but also thinks of it as the intelligence to repair the body. This secondary aspect of the immune system is being slowly recognized in allopathic medicine.

Anatomical and Physiological Safety Parameters

While observing breath and facial expression is a good way to assess safety of practices, there are additional parameters that are helpful.

All yoga practices should be done with aligned spine. From a conventional medicine perspective, the spine is part of the central nervous system (CNS). If the communication of the CNS is impeded because of a distorted spine, the body will not have the interconnectivity to supply the energy needs to many organ systems. Energy optimization is an important goal of yoga practices. It helps to create balance and prepares the body for higher awareness in meditation. A practitioner may use back support to keep an aligned spine in meditation.

All motions should be slow, smooth, and easy. Whether through degeneration from aging or injuries, many people develop weakness in joints and muscles. Slow motion prevents overstretching and unwanted injuries. Easy joint mobility exercises, done in sync with breath, serve as a good precursor to additional yoga practices.

Āsanas are thought to stimulate *nādis* possibly through *Marma* points (and even perhaps acupuncture points). *Marma* points are present in many parts of the body with concentrations in the neck area, back, hips and near the joints of the limbs.

Haṭha Yoga practices, that are suited to be within the capacity of the individual, should aim to provide the following physiological parameters, while observing the safety precautions:

- Spinal alignment
- Pelvic flexibility
- Joint Mobility
- Muscle strengthening
- Cardio-respiratory strengthening

Questions and Discussion Topics

1. What is the physiological basis (in terms of blood flow, nervous system response and energy production) of understanding injuries while engaged in physical elements (*āsanas*) of yoga practices? After explaining the physiological basis of injuries, justify in your own words how to avoid injuries.

2. Yoga seeks to bring supreme balance in the body-mind (and spirit) system. Examine the role of the nervous system with respect to the body-mind balance. Explore all aspects of the central and peripheral nervous systems that contribute to the body-mind balance.

3. Conventional medical understanding is that for an average adult in a resting state the brain consumes about 20% of the oxygen available in the body. Consider the role of the brain and the nervous system, and explain why this may be the case, and how it affects the cardiovascular system over the lifetime.

4. It is sometimes said that the enteric nervous system has a brain of its own. "Even while it communicates with the CNS, it is capable of operating on its own." In the context of this statement examine the usual prescription that yoga exercises are not recommended immediately after a meal. Rather yoga practices are recommended when the stomach is light.

5. Some dedicated yoga practitioners will often wake up early in the morning, even when they have not had adequate sleep, to pursue their daily yoga practice. Do you think this is right yogic behavior? What is the implication for the physiological system?

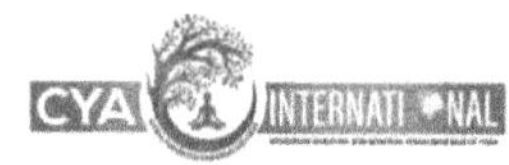

CHAPTER 17:

Introduction to *Haṭha Yoga*

The tradition of *Haṭha Yoga* is embedded in the knowledge that goes back several centuries (while the Yoga Sutras go back a few millennia). However, from a traditional textual perspective on *Haṭha Yoga* practices, Gheranḍa Samhitā and Svātmarama's Haṭha Yoga Pradīpikā are generally considered as principal references, while Śhiva Samhitā and Gorakśha Śhataka serve as additional references. However, these texts cannot be considered authoritative on yoga principles and philosophy. The word written ***haṭha*** means force in Sanskrit. [54] The idea of force is inherent in many of the practices in the original texts and the approach of *Haṭha Yoga* has a strong focus on physical elements. Even though Svātmarama's Haṭha Yoga Pradīpikā clearly speaks to a spiritual objective, the approach of ***haṭha*** may not be fully consistent with the principles of the Yoga Sutras. Therefore, *Haṭha Yoga* cannot be safely practiced without anchoring in the principles of yoga expounded by Patanjali in the Yoga Sutras. Accordingly, modern application of *Haṭha Yoga* practices, by schools that focus on the Yoga Sutras of Patanjali, is somewhat selective and modified to the capacity of the practitioner to avoid forceful and intrusive methods.

Haṭha Yoga, unlike other approaches to yoga, begins with the grossest aspect of the human awareness, the physical body, which for most people is a natural point of self-identification, and hence the popularity of *Haṭha Yoga* worldwide. In stages, when one begins to identify with the inner vibrations of the physical body, it not only allows for enhanced physical control in the somatic domain, but it also allows for control of the psyche in the realm of emotions and states of the mind. This brings balance and harmony within the body-mind system of thoughts, words, and deeds, which prepares one to seek a higher transcendental awareness.

---

[54] *Haṭha* is also described by some scholars to be made up of two words, ***ha*** and ***ṭha***. Associated with sun and moon, heat and cold, male and female principles, *Haṭha* is thought to be the balancer. We are not aware of any ancient textual reference to this meaning.

Progression and Study of *Haṭha Yoga*

The progression and study of *Haṭha Yoga*, as expressed in current times,[55] can be summarized as follows.

- *Āsanas* (postures) are meant to align the *nādis*.
- *Ṣhaṭkriyās*, also called *Ṣhaṭkarma*, are internal cleansing techniques designed to purify the *nādis*.
- *Prāṇāyāma* practices are designed to improve the vitality flow even as it further purifies the *nādis*.
- *Bandhas* (locks) are intended to improve the functioning of the *nādis* with gentle nudges;
- *Mudrās* are positionings with hands and body for channeling energy.
- Meditation (called *Laya Yoga* in the *Haṭha Yoga* tradition) is to settle the mind and to become a pure (non-reactive) observer.
- From this state, one advances to experience the vibrations of existence – *nāda-anusandhāna*.

It is important to find the appropriate yoga practices suited for each person according to their capacity and need over the lifespan. It is generally associated with their personality and programmed nature (*karma-kleśha*) which is expected to be changing over the lifespan.

Historical Development of *Haṭha Yoga*

Haṭha Yoga texts are relatively recent – between 500 to 1,000 years old – compared to the Yoga Sutras and Vedic understanding of yoga which are much older. Within the *Haṭha Yoga* approach *Ṣhaṭkarma* arc considered the older practices dealing with internal physical cleansing, and the *āsanas* as later developments that came with the written texts. It is also likely that the *mudrā* elements came from the *Tantra Yoga* system.

Given the recency of the *Haṭha Yoga* texts (relative to the Yoga Sutras) and their approach focused more on the physical elements of the body in the practices, it appears that they may have been influenced by the *Sānkya-Yoga* philosophy and Buddhism. The Tantra elements can also be associated with Mahāyāna Buddhism, and the *Ṣhanmata* system (six forms of worship) designed by Shankaracharya.

---

[55] The organization of these practices is somewhat different in the Haṭha Yoga Pradīpikā. *Āsanas* are followed by *Prāṇāyāma*, which is considered as Alternate Nostril Breathing (*Nādi Śhodhana*). Thereafter the Ṣhatkriyas are considered for further purification. Then eight breathing practices are introduced thereafter, and are called *Kumbhakas*, which these days are called the eight *Prāṇāyāmas* of Haṭha Yoga. Also, *bandhas* and *mudrās* are integrated as one single concept in the traditional texts.

Perspectives in Mode of Practice

In the last century there has been a tendency to portray *Haṭha Yoga* as physical culture, given the physical orientation of *Haṭha Yoga*. Yogic practices give direct health benefits to everyone regardless of their spiritual objectives. Physical and mental health benefits are well recognized by physiological research.

Most practitioners of yoga usually begin with the physical aspects with a focus on either sports or physical health. While the benefits of the physical postures (*āsanas*) are to energize and remove the stiffness and stagnancy accumulated either in sleep or during the day (e.g., at the office sitting in a chair, hunched over a desk), the deeper stress reduction from mindfulness happens concurrently without specific intent. The energization of the body and mindfulness naturally pave the way for higher meditative practices.

Finally, all approaches to yoga are essentially experiential rather than theoretical knowledge or intellectual exercise. It can be adapted to individual needs through practice and experience.

Questions and Discussion Topics

1. *Haṭha Yoga* appears to be the most popular form of yoga in the world today. Examine the reasons for this popularity.

2. Why do we insist on adherence to the principles from the Yoga Sutras while using *Haṭha Yoga* approaches?

3. What would you say are the commonalities and differences between the Yoga Sutras of Patanjali and the *Haṭha Yoga* texts, and how would you parse them in your application as a yoga instructor? [Hint: Examine the emphasis or views on learning to be a pure observer with less reactivity and the concept of *Sva-dharma* (purpose of birth) and historical philosophical influences.]

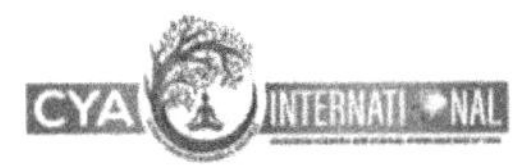

CHAPTER 18:

Āsanas

Hathasya Prathama-angatvāda-Āsanam poorvam-uchyate.
Kuryātta-āsanam sthairyam-ārogyam cha-angalāghavam. [In Sanskṛit]

हठस्य अङ्गत्वात् आसनं पूर्वं उच्यते
कुर्यात् तत् आसनं स्थैर्यं आरोग्यं च अङ्ग-लाघवम्

Āsana is explained as the earlier (or first) part of Hatha. Having done *āsana* one attains steadiness, health and lightness of the body parts. **[Haṭha Yoga Pradīpikā (1:17)]**

Implication: *Āsanas'* impact on health and vitality helps to pave the way for furthering in yoga.

Āsana means physical posture or position in Sanskṛit.

In the Yoga Sutras of Patanjali there is a concise definition of yoga *āsanas* and how they should be done:

- **स्थिरम् सुखं आसनं** "*Sthiram sukham āsanam*"[2:46] Steadiness and comfort-giving is *Āsana.*
- **प्रयत्न शैथिल्य अनन्त समापत्तिभ्याम्** "*Prayatna śhaitilya ananta samāpattibhyām*" [2:47] – Effort must be light along with infinite engrossment (in the *āsana*).

This implies that the *āsana* position should be steady and comfortable. It should be done with light effort and must lead to meditative engrossment. Thus, we can see that yoga *āsana* are practiced for development of the practitioner's ability to remain comfortable in a position for an extended length of time, as is necessary during meditation. There is no place in *āsana* practice for force or staying in a posture that is uncomfortable or painful.

Method to Perform *Āsanas*

The Haṭha Yoga tradition pays particular attention to attaining a posture, maintaining it and its release. All of this is done in sync with the breath. After taking a full breath, during slow and gradual exhalation a posture is attained. The gradual movement ensures that one does not overstretch and hurt the muscles. And while maintaining the posture, one continues to observe the breath and sensations. Typically, the sensations vary with expansion in inhalation and relaxation in exhalation. The posture is typically maintained for at least a couple of minutes.[56] It is thought that physiologically a minimum of 90 seconds is required for neuro-vascular stimulation for sufficient blood flow to be directed into the stretched muscles to provide significant relaxation upon release of the posture. Like the gradual motion of attaining the posture, release of the posture is done while exhaling after taking a last deep breath in the posture.

The *Haṭha Yoga* method of attaining, maintaining and release of *āsanas* relieves the stiffness of the body. The body becomes resilient, postures which seemed impossible become easy to perform, and steadiness and grace of movement develop. When the flow of *Prāṇa* is increased through purification of the *nādis*, the body may also move into certain postures by itself, and *āsanas*, *mudrās*, and *Prāṇāyāma* occur spontaneously. This results in a greater awareness of the vibrations within and better control of the senses (*Pratyāhāra* of the eight-fold yoga of Patanjali).

Haṭha Yoga, therefore, not only strengthens the body and improves health, but also enhances inner awareness. The mind and body are not separate entities although there is a tendency to think and act as though they are. Every mental distortion or imbalance has a corresponding imbalance in the physical being. The gross form of the mind is the body, and the subtle form of the body is the mind. Haṭha Yoga, through the physical body processes of *āsana* and *nādi* cleansing practices, seeks to impact the mind and correct any imbalance.

Thus, the body becomes full of vitality and strength, the mind becomes light, creative, joyful, and balanced, manifesting as confidence in all areas of life.

Distinguishing between Yoga *Āsana* and Gym Exercises

Yoga *āsanas* have often been thought of as a form of physical exercising. However, they are not exercises in the conventional sense, but rather techniques which place the physical body in positions that cultivate relaxation, and internal awareness. Part of this process is the development of good physical health by stretching, massaging, and stimulating the *Prāṇa* channels (*nādis*) and internal organs. The key difference is that yoga is without strain that leads to physical and mental relaxation preparing for spiritual awareness. Whereas in exercising, strain is involved in the work-out, and while there are some physical and mental benefits, they are not as deep, and the effect is not as conducive for spiritual awareness. Following is a more detailed review of the differences between *āsana* and conventional gym exercising, ranging from the physical to mental effects.

---

[56] Caliskan E, Akkoc O, Bayramoglu Z, Gozubuyuk OB, Kural D, Azamat S, Adaletli I. Effects of static stretching duration on muscle stiffness and blood flow in the rectus femoris in adolescents. Med Ultrason. 2019 May 2;21(2):136-143. doi: 10.11152/mu-1859. PMID: 31063516.

YOGA *ĀSANAS* AND EXERCISES

	Subject	*Āsanas*	Physical Exercises
1	Speed of Execution	Done very slowly and smoothly with awareness and focus on breath, without strain.	Done vigorously with some speed involving strain. It often tends to be rapid and jerky.
2	Effect on Muscles and Formation of Lactic Acid	Stretches and relaxes muscles while neutralizing lactic acids because of practice without strain and with regular breathing.	Builds muscles by making them shorter and bulkier; may produce lactic acid due to anerobic activation from excessive strain.
3	Relaxation Impact	Makes one feel refreshed immediately after practice. Eliminates fatigue and rejuvenates.	Strenuous exercises may make one feel tired and exhausted immediately after practice.
4	Energy Levels	Conserves and enhances energy.	Consumes energy and may cause exhaustion.
5	Cardio-respiratory Impact	Optimizes lung capacity and heart rate variability.	Has similar impact but may be limited.
6	Effect on Brain Centers	Activate awareness, attention, and parasympathetic tone (relaxation), while stimulating balance in the two hemispheres of the brain.	Stimulate sympathetic tone initially before relaxation, and not designed to balance the two hemispheres of the brain.
7	Flexibility & Mobility of Joints	Improves Substantially.	Not as effective.
8	Development of awareness	Builds awareness of body and mind – psychosomatic integration – leading towards spiritual awareness.	Focuses on body awareness – limited impact on psychosomatic integration; body is viewed as a mechanical process.
9	Integration of personality	Develops and integrates all aspects of our personality – physical, mental, emotional, and spiritual; contributes to emotional intelligence.	Focuses mostly on the physical aspects of personality; has some impact at the mental and emotional level.

Dynamic and Static Yoga *Āsanas*

As noted earlier, holding of a posture at least for a couple of minutes is the traditional approach of Haṭha Yoga. However, motion-based *āsanas* practices have crept into modern day Haṭha Yoga for the following reasons.

- **Warm-up Needs** – For most normal people there is a need to warm-up for loosening of body tightness and stimulating *nādi* flows especially in cold weather. For warming up purposes, *Sūryanamaskar* and *Chandranamaskar* are common yoga practices before beginning regular *āsanas*, although other approaches to loosening joints and increasing energy flow may also be used. These are best done smoothly with awareness, synchronized with the natural flow of breath for effective loosening of the body and stimulation of *nādi* flows. Dynamic movements that are forceful or jerky, not only violate the principles of yoga as referred in the Yoga Sutras 2:46-48, but also negate the purpose of warm-up which is to avoid injuries from excessive stretching. Therefore, forceful, or jerky practices even in warm-up is inappropriate.

- **Need for Gentle approach for Some Groups -** For beginners and the fragile or elderly population motion-based practices are much gentler and better suited. For such groups, a complete session can be done just seated in a chair, with suitable motions in sync with the breath that helps to stimulate the *nādis*. [See Example in Appendix 2.]
- **Integration of *Tantra* approaches in *Haṭha Yoga*** – Some yoga systems in the last few decades have started using motion with breath awareness as part of *āsana* practices. This approach called *Prāṇakriyā* has been a traditional part of the *Tantra Yoga* system. Its appearance in *Haṭha Yoga* in recent times with the name of *Vinyasa* appears to have been the discovery of its value.

It is worthwhile to note that static practices have a more subtle and powerful effect on the *nādis* and have a faster cleansing impact on the *nādis* than dynamic practices. However, the ability of the practitioner and the level of cleansing needed will govern the appropriate application of these approaches.

Progression in Yoga *Āsanas*

The guidance of yoga sutra 2:47 on *āsanas* is clear. Practices are to be done with light effort, in one's zone of comfort. Therefore, in common practice, *āsanas* are planned at three levels, from beginners (and those with disabilities) to intermediate to advanced.

The beginner's regimen should be performed by those who have never practiced yoga *āsanas* before, who are infirm in any way and who are therefore unable to perform the more advanced practices. This regimen consists of mindful gentle movements in sync with regular and relaxed breathing – movements that seek to ease the muscles supporting the spine from the neck to the tailbone, and mobilizing joints of the shoulders, hands, hips, and legs that result in deep relaxation for the body and mind. While this may be the building block towards more advanced *Āsana* practices for most beginners, for some people, especially the elderly population, this alone may be sufficient preparation for the higher meditative aspects of yoga. This is because, as one lives over several decades, typically the *karma* and *kleśha* get fulfilled by meeting the various challenges of living. As a result, natural *nādi* purification of some significant degree may have already happened. [Appendix 2 describes a typical beginner's regimen.]

The intermediate regimen practices consist of *āsanas* that require greater flexibility and a reasonable level of muscular strength. Common *āsanas* in this category are spine stretching practices like *Bhujangāsana* (Cobra pose), *Dhanurāsana* (Bow pose), *Śhalabhāsana* (Locust pose), *Uṣhtrāsna* (Camel pose), *Setubandhāsana* (Bridge pose), etc. done within the capacity of the individual. Sideward stretching practices include *Trikonāsana*, *Vakrāsana*, *Ardhamatsyendra*, etc. Balancing poses include variations of *Veerabhadrāsana* (warrior pose) and *Vṛikśhāsana* (tree pose). With good balance and flexibility, in this category, practices like *Halāsana* (plough pose), *Sarvangāsana* (Shoulder stand) and *Matsyāsana* (fish pose) may also be included. The stretching and stimulation introduce the mind to the subtler aspects of the posture that in stages lead to greater inner awareness.

The advanced regimen practices require a higher level of muscular strength and stronger sense of balance allowing for extensive control over the musculoskeletal system. Common Āsanas in this category include *Śhirasāsana* (head stand), *Kākāsana* (crow pose), *Mayurāsana* (Peacock pose) and variations of them. This is for those who have already mastered the intermediate regimen of *āsanas* and no longer feel the stretch and stimulation from them. Thus, an instructor and student of yoga must understand attainment of a posture is not the goal, but rather stimulation of the *nādis* without strain that enables higher inward focus. Therefore, it is best to plan the progression of practices under the guidance of a yoga expert.

Āsanas for deep relaxation are common to all levels of practices. Common relaxation practices include *Śhavāsana* (corpse pose), *Makarāsana* (crocodile pose), *Bālāsana* (child pose), etc. Haṭha Yoga tradition requires relaxation after each *āsana* for short durations, and a long relaxation at the end of the practice. It is recognized that it is in relaxation that the *nādis*' communication is enhanced, while during the *āsana* practice *nādis* are stretched.

Physical and Metaphysical Perspectives of Yoga *Āsanas*

The Yoga Sutras of Patanjali (2:27) notes that intuitive wisdom (*Prajñā*) which comes from connectivity with the cosmic intelligence (in *Samādhi*) is attained after crossing seven boundaries, obviously referring to the first seven of the eight aspects of *Aṣhṭānga* yoga, where the eighth is *Samādhi*. While this may create an impression that these are seven sequential attainments, it is well recognized that each of the seven aspects reinforce the others and can be considered as seven legs supporting one system. In fact, Patanjali himself in sutra 2:45 notes that the last of the *Niyamas* leads to *Samādhi*. In this context, progression in *āsanas* along with greater purification, affects all the other seven aspects of yoga, and can have an integrative effect on the three levels of the body (gross, subtle, and causal, as referred in Chapter 5).

However, the physical dimensions of *āsanas* that influence the psychic dimensions should be appreciated separately for deeper understanding. The linkage can be attributed as follows: physical health leads to optimized vitality, leading to balanced frame of mind, which in turn prepares one for the metaphysical experience.

Physical health aspects of *āsana* can be noted as follows. From a yogic standpoint, the improved communication of the *nādis* stimulates the body's own corrective mechanism and restores health. It begins by rectifying hyperactivity on one end, or sluggishness on the other end. It has been noted among high school and college level population that *āsanas* begin to correct restlessness of the body and mind, while counteracting the sluggishness of depressive tendencies. In older populations with chronic health conditions, *āsanas* have the impact of better management of the conditions. The key elements that enable this is the better flow of vitality and a mind that develops the ability to be calm and less reactive. In effect, in the progression of *āsana*, breathing becomes normalized. In other words, *Prāṇāyāma* element that controls vitality gravitates towards optimization. That is the reason a yoga instructor pays attention to the nature of the breath as indicative of stress or relaxation. With the calming of the breath in *āsana*, inner awareness builds (*Pratyāhāra*). As we know from the Yoga Sutras (2:55), *Pratyāhāra* leads to complete control of the sense organs, and hence its restorative effect on the physical body.

Mental health aspects of *asanas* are now well-recognized. [57] They immediately flow from the optimized vitality and control of the sense organs. In fact, deep relaxation comes from good vitality and calmness of the mind. This goes back to our yogic view of stress – when demands on the system exceed the available supply of vitality to fulfill the demands. [See Chapter 5.] With strong vitality and demands on the system reduced by a calm mind, relaxation is achieved. One can empathize by reflection that temper is lost when the body-mind composition's vitality resources are strained.

Thus, *āsanas*, also stimulating the other aspects of *Ashṭānga* yoga can lead to internal transformation in stages. It is a feeling of well-being with a sense of internal joy and peace. It allows one to sleep better and adapt to environmental demands more easily. This sense of well-being is attained by regular practice that reprograms our nature.

OBSERVANCES OF FOOD & WATER WHILE DOING YOGA PRACTICE

Yoga is done with light stomach so that the energy of cleansing the *nādis* is not focused on digestion. Therefore, yoga done early in the morning before breakfast is considered best. For later in the day practices, it is suggested that two to four hours should elapse after a meal, depending on the heaviness of the meal.

Also, unlike the popular image of those working out in a gym having a bottle of cold water next to them and sipping as they sweat, in yoga, drinking water during a practice session is not recommended. Cold water is considered worse than hot water. Water consumption during yoga practice diverts the energy of *nādi* cleansing to absorption of the water in the digestive tract. Further if cold water is consumed, warming it to body temperature is additional energy loss. If a person cannot avoid thirst while doing yoga practice, it is recommended that they sip water that is beverage hot. This way the heat, more than the body temperature, also provides some energy for absorption so as to negate the impact of significant energy withdrawal from *nādi* cleansing.

---

[57] Mehta UM, Gangadhar BN. Yoga: Balancing the excitation-inhibition equilibrium in psychiatric disorders. Prog Brain Res. 2019;244:387-413. doi: 10.1016/bs.pbr.2018.10.024. Epub 2019 Jan 3. PMID: 30732846. https://pubmed.ncbi.nlm.nih.gov/30732846/

Streeter CC, Gerbarg PL, Saper RB, Ciraulo DA, Brown RP. Effects of yoga on the autonomic nervous system, gamma-aminobutyric-acid, and allostasis in epilepsy, depression, and post-traumatic stress disorder. Med Hypotheses. 2012 May;78(5):571-9. doi: 10.1016/j.mehy.2012.01.021. Epub 2012 Feb 24. PMID: 22365651. https://pubmed.ncbi.nlm.nih.gov/22365651/

Streeter CC, Whitfield TH, Owen L, Rein T, Karri SK, Yakhkind A, Perlmutter R, Prescot A, Renshaw PF, Ciraulo DA, Jensen JE. Effects of yoga versus walking on mood, anxiety, and brain GABA levels: a randomized controlled MRS study. J Altern Complement Med. 2010 Nov;16(11):1145-52. doi: 10.1089/acm.2010.0007. Epub 2010 Aug 19. PMID: 20722471; PMCID: PMC3111147. https://pubmed.ncbi.nlm.nih.gov/20722471/

Questions and Discussion Topics

1. This chapter discusses the differences between gym/sports exercises and yoga. Is it possible to transform some gym/sport exercises into yoga by slight modification in attitude or method of performance? Explain with examples.

2. What is the essential difference in the psychosomatic impact of static versus dynamic *āsanas*?

3. Why is it sufficient for many seniors (people of advanced age) to work with mild and easy practices of *āsanas* to advance in yoga?

4. Is it appropriate to state that the highest advancement in *āsana* leads to *Pratyāhāra*? Explain.

5. If a person is feeling very thirsty while doing yoga, and is unable to focus within, what would you suggest?

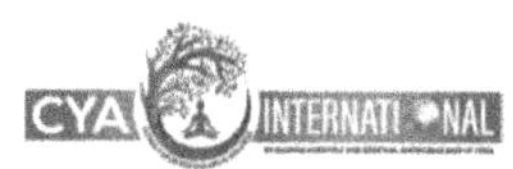

CHAPTER 19:

Ṣhaṭkriyās or *Ṣhaṭkarma*

Haṭha Yoga system, focused on physical cleansing, pays particular attention to certain practices that are referred as *Ṣhaṭkarma* or *Ṣhaṭkriyās*. *Ṣhat* means 'six' and *karma* (or *kriyā*) means 'action,' 'process,' or 'practice.' These are referred in the Haṭha Yoga Pradīpikā (2:22-35) and the Gheranḍa Samhitā (1:12-60).

These actions are meant for deeper physical cleansing of the internal body-parts beyond the stretching of the muscles in *āsanas*. Both the *āsanas* and the *kriyās* are designed to open the *nādis* for better communication. This is explained in the Haṭha Yoga Pradīpikā (2:21) as follows:

> *Meda-shleshma-adhikaha poorvam Ṣhaṭkarmāni samācharet.*
> *Anyastu nā-charettāni doshānām samabhāvataha.*
>
> मेद-श्लेष्म-अधिकः पूर्वं षट्-कर्माणि समाचरेत्
> अन्यस्तु नाचरेत्-तानि दोषाणाम् समभावतः
>
> When fat or phlegm is excessive, the *Ṣhaṭkarma* (or six cleansing techniques) should be practiced before (higher-level practices). Others, in whom the doshas are balanced, need not do them.

Ṣhaṭkarma practices are used before *Prāṇāyāma*[58] and other higher yoga practices, as needed, for eliminating the imbalances. These techniques should be learned from experienced yoga practitioners to avoid inappropriate application or wrong methods of practice that may negatively affect the practitioner.

These set of practices consist of six groups in the following order as stated in these two texts:

- Haṭha Yoga Pradīpikā (2:22) – *Dhauti*, *Basti*, *Neti*, *Trataka*, *Nauli* and *Kapālabhāti*.
- Gheranḍa Samhitā (1:12) – *Dhauti*, *Basti*, *Neti*, *Laukiki*, *Trataka* and *Kapālabhāti*.

---

[58] While commonly the eight breathing practices (*Sūrya Bhedana*, *Ujjayī*, *Seetkāri*, *Śheetalī*, *Bhastrikā*, *Bhrāmari*, *Murchchha*, *Plāvini*) of *Haṭha Yoga* are referred as *Prāṇāyāma*, in the Haṭha Yoga Pradīpika (2:44) they are called *Kumbhakas*. The Alternate Nostril Breathing is referred as *Prāṇāyāma* in the Haṭha Yoga Pradīpika and can be done even before the *Ṣhatkriyās*.

Nauli and *Laukiki* are the same practice but described with different names by the two authors. Also, there is some variation in the description of some of these practices between the two authors.

DOṢHAS OF AYURVEDA EXPLAINED IN BRIEF

As explained in Ayurveda, the three essential elements of body composition are *kapha*, *pitta*, and *vāta*. *Kapha* consists of earth and water elements and is associated with steadiness and calmness. *Pitta* consists essentially of fire element with a component of the air element and is associated with energetic dynamism. And *vāta* consists of the air and space element, associated with an imaginative nature. In Ayurveda, each person's innate nature as a composite of *kapha*, *pitta* and *vāta* is called *Prakṛiti*.[59] When the mind cultivates desires and reacts excessively to what the senses perceive, it can take one away from one's innate nature. The changed nature is called *Vikṛiti*. The gap between *Prakṛiti* and *Vikṛiti* is an imbalance, called *doṣha* (or fault) in Sanskṛit. [According to both Ayurveda and *Haṭha Yoga*, the presence of imbalance (*doṣha*) will eventually result in illness.]

When *kapha* becomes excessive, it usually manifests as phlegm in the throat and respiratory tract along with inflammation, and the body becomes excessively sluggish. When *pitta* becomes excessive it causes acidity and excessive heat in the body while creating phlegm in the GI tract along with inflammation, and the person typically becomes angry and fastidious. When *vāta* is excessive it results in a flitting mind that is unable to remain focused with gas building in the system (especially the colon) along with inflammation in the joints. The person may come across as an unsteady or nervous personality. Excess of one is actually deficiency of another. Thus, deficiency and excess are two sides of the same coin that manifest in the way described above. Thus, balance may be restored by reducing the excess or increasing the deficiency or by both.[60]

The first focus in *Haṭha Yoga* is to bring balance in the system. Hence, each of these *kriyās* are targeted to relieve phlegm and inflammation in specific areas that are affected.[61]

---

[59] The use of the word *Prakṛiti* here for an individual (the microcosm) should not be confused with the cosmic context of *Prakṛiti* (macrocosm) as the initial program of creation.

[60] For instance, the practice of *Kapālabhāti*, one of the *kriyās*, removes phlegm from the respiratory tract while increasing digestive fire in the belly. Thus, it is used to reduce *kapha* and increase *pitta* to restore the balance of the two.

[61] The mind that strays from its innate nature resulting in imbalance in the physical system is sought to be corrected by the physical techniques of *Haṭha Yoga*. While this approach forces one to become internally aware of the physical state and thus with greater concentration develops less reactivity of the mind, other yoga approaches seek to impact the mind more directly. Examples of psychosomatic cleansing include Alternate Nostril Breathing and *chakra* cleansing (see chapter 26).

The cleansing focus of these practices are summarized in the following table:

ṢHAṬKARMA PRACTICE	INTENT OF PRACTICE
Dhauti	Stomach and esophagus cleansing as described in HP (2:24); Alimentary canal cleansing as described in GS (1:13-44)
Basti	Colon and rectum cleansing (HP 2:26, GS 1:46,48)
Neti	Nasal tract cleansing (HP 2:29, GS 1:50)
Nauli or *Laukiki*	Abdominal stimulation (small intestine, liver, pancreas, spleen) (HP 2:33, GS 1:52)
Trāṭaka	Eye stimulation (HP 2:31, GS 1:53)
Kapālabhāti	Cleansing of phlegm from the system overall, mostly focused on the respiratory tract and nasal-head area (HP 2:35, GS 1:55-60)

A logical view of *Ṣhaṭkarma* cleansing or stimulation can be viewed from the top of the body to the bottom as follows:

- *Trāṭaka* – eyes
- *Neti* – nasal tract
- *Dhauti* – esophagus and stomach
- *Nauli* – abdomen
- *Basti* – colon and rectum
- *Kapālabhati* – overall and integrative cleansing

Many of these practices, as described in these texts, would be considered intrusive and would not be recommended by modern day health care providers. Yoga masters, with vast experience accumulated over many years, have modified some of these practices that are accessible to most people.

Accordingly, for the beginner level, only two practices are recommended:

- *Jala Neti*[62] – Nasal tract cleansing with water (see Appendix 3)
- *Kapālabhāti* – as described in the Haṭha Yoga Pradīpikā and in Chapter 14 of this book.

The other practices mentioned here are only for the purpose of information.

---

[62] Neti described in the texts is actually called Sutra Neti. The Jala Neti is a simplification that has come from practice traditions. Sutra Neti is the process of using a string (normally a rubber catheter is used in current times) to cleanse out the posterior nasal passages. It is not recommended at the introductory level.

Questions and Discussion Topics

1. What is the yogic purpose of the *Ṣhaṭkriyās* (*Ṣhaṭkarma*)? Review the mechanism of yoga and explain in those terms.

2. Examine the cleansing effect on the *doshas* of the six types of practices noted (*Ṣhaṭkriyās*). Consider which of the three *doshas* (as noted in Ayurveda) are addressed by each one of these six practices:
   - *Trātaka* focused on eyes but having impact beyond the eyes on which *doshas*?
   - *Neti* focused on the nasal tract but having impact beyond the nasal tract on which *doshas*?
   - *Dhauti* focused on the esophagus and stomach impact on which *doshas*?
   - *Nauli* focused on the abdomen impact on which *doshas*?
   - *Basti* focused on the colon and rectum impact on which *doshas*?
   - *Kapālabhati* focused on the abdomen and the lower respiratory tract impact on which *doshas*?

   [Consider the *Pratyāhāra* effect from each practice, if relevant.]

3. If each of these six practices in question 2, examine the effect of the five types of communications (*Pancha Prāṇā*: *Prāṇā*, *Apāna*, *Vyāna*, *Udāna* and *Samāna*).

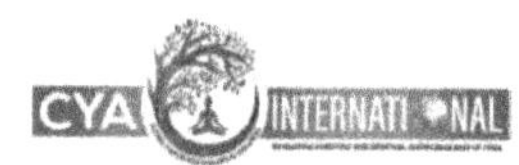

CHAPTER 20:

Prāṇāyāma Overview

Prāṇāyāma, as practiced by most yoga schools, is discussed comprehensively in Part II of the book (The Power of Breath in Yoga). In this chapter, we discuss a few *Haṭha Yoga* perspectives.

- First, Terminology and Sequence in *Haṭha Yoga*
- Second, Correlation between Metabolic Rate and Breathing Rate
- Third, *Haṭha* Yogic Adage on Longevity
- Lastly, Physiology of Breath Holding

Terminology and Sequence in *Haṭha Yoga*

The Haṭha Yoga Pradīpikā calls the Alternate Nostril Breathing as *Prānāyāma* with the name of *Nādi Śhodhana.* This comes early in the second chapter which focuses on *nādi* cleansing. Thereafter, it presents the *Ṣhaṭkarmas.* Then, it unfolds the eight breathing practices that are associated with *Haṭha Yoga* under the name *Kumbhaka*: *Sūrya Bhedana*, *Ujjayī*, *Seetkārī*, *Śheetalī*, *Bhastrikā*, *Bhrāmarī* , *Murchchhā*, *Plāvinī.* In common practice, most schools refer to these as *Prānāyāma.*

The *Haṭha Yoga* perspective of *Ṣhaṭkarma* preceding these eight *Kumbhaka* practices should not be confused with *Nādi Śhodhana* which can be done before the *Ṣhaṭkarma* even according to *Haṭha Yoga.* Thus, from a common usage perspective of *Prānāyāma* the Haṭha Yoga Pradīpikā speaks about nine practices, not eight.

Correlation Between Metabolic Rate and Breathing Rate

It is recognized that the normal breathing rate for people range from 10 to 20 breaths per minute. The rate of breathing appears to be largely related to the oxygen need in the body which corresponds to the metabolic or energy production rate. In babies the breathing rate is on the higher side of the spectrum to feed the energy production rate for the child's growth. For adults the breathing rate depends on their level of stress. As noted in Chapter 5 (The Underlying Mechanism of All Yoga Approaches), the yogic definition of stress is demands on the system being higher than the supply of available energy. [In physiology it is called allostatic overload.] Increased stress increases the breathing rate and metabolic rate and has immediate collateral impact on the nervous and cardiovascular systems. As one ages the metabolic rate naturally comes down, but the breathing rate may or may not depending on the dead space of breath. The dead space of breath is the sum of two parts related to ventilation efficiency. First, when people have shallow and quick breathing, most of the air in the breath never reach the alveoli to exchange the oxygen and carbon dioxide. This is one part of the dead space in breath. Second, through disuse and/or damage to alveoli, the blood perfusion in some capillaries may have ceased. In such non-functional alveoli any contact with fresh air does not allow for exchange of oxygen and carbon dioxide. This is the second part of the dead space in breath.

Thus, breath driven by metabolic need works according to the stress level, ventilation efficiency and growth needs of the body, and it works through the nervous and cardiovascular systems. The impact of stress on the nervous and cardiovascular system has been well studied. It is recognized that slower and deeper breathing of about 6 breaths per minute has a deep relaxing and restoring impact on the body-mind systems.

Yogic Adage on Longevity

Accordingly, there is an often-repeated *Haṭha Yoga* adage:

> "Life is a period between one breath and the next. A person who only breathes half, lives only half his life. He who breathes correctly, acquires control of the whole being."

It is often said: "If one breathes deeply and slowly then one lives longer; if s/he breathes rapidly, it leads to a shorter lifespan." The faster breathing rate is associated with tension, fear, anxiety, etc. A person who is breathing slowly is relaxed, calm and happy, which is conducive to longevity. Thus, it is popularly said in *Haṭha Yoga* tradition that longevity in measured in the number of breaths. Of course, from the spiritual understanding of the Yoga Sutras, one is born to fulfill one's purpose in life for the cosmic flow. Therefore, longevity is not an absolute number of years for everyone. Proper breathing leads to completion of one's full life with greater awareness and less reactivity. Often the correlation between age of animals and their breathing rate is quoted in the context of making this point.[63] This *Haṭha Yoga* view is contextual to the physical awareness rather than the deeper purpose of life as understood in the Yoga Sutras.

Physiology of Breath Holding

Besides the rate of breath, the holding in or holding out of the breath has profound impact on the ventilation and the rebuilding of the body. Holding of breath after inhalation appears to improve air exchange in the alveoli and reduce dead space. Holding out the breath, causing

---

[63] The Curious Connection Between Breath Rate and Longevity. https://drherbz.wordpress.com/2016/04/28/the-curious-connection-between-breath-rate-and-longevity/

intermittent hypoxia and hypercapnia, appears to have impact on stem cell production and body's rebuilding mechanism.[64]

It is important to note that holding the breath without creating pressure within the system is one thing, while the use of *bandhas* (compressed locks) is another matter. Inducing pressure with *bandhas* can create negative impact for a person whose *nādis* are not purified enough. Therefore, *bandhas* are not recommended for beginners. It is also important to note that when holding the breath without pressure, it should be done without discomfort or strain, and should be held only for as long as there is no discomfort. The capacity will differ from person to person.

Questions and Discussion Topics

1. The Haṭha Yoga Pradīpikā is specific that the eight *Kumbhakas* (*Prāṇāyāma* techniques) mentioned in the text should be done only after cleansing with *āsanas* and *kriyās*. However, the Yoga Sutras are not so specific. Examine the physiological and metaphysical aspects of *Prāṇāyāma* and address the following questions:
   (a) Is there a difference in what constitutes *Prāṇāyāma* as understood from the Yoga Sutras and the Haṭha Yoga Pradīpikā?
   (b) If there is a difference, please explain. If there is no difference, how do you explain the approaches of the Yoga Sutras and the Haṭha Yoga Pradīpikā?

2. Discuss the methods and the pros and cons of breath holding.

---

[64] Ma T, Grayson WL, Fröhlich M, Vunjak-Novakovic G. Hypoxia and stem cell-based engineering of mesenchymal tissues. Biotechnol Prog. 2009 Jan-Feb;25(1):32-42. doi: 10.1002/btpr.128. PMID: 19198002; PMCID: PMC2771546. https://pubmed.ncbi.nlm.nih.gov/19198002/

Malshe PC. Nisshesha rechaka Prānāyāma offers benefits through brief intermittent hypoxia. Ayu. 2011;32(4):451-457. doi:10.4103/0974-8520.96114 https://www.ncbi.nlm.nih.gov/pmc/articles/PMC3361916/

Lepicovská V, Dostálek C, Kovárová M. Hathayogic exercise jalandharabandha in its effect on cardiovascular response to apnoea. Act Nerv Super (Praha). 1990 Jun;32(2):99-114. PMID: 2399805. https://pubmed.ncbi.nlm.nih.gov/2399805/

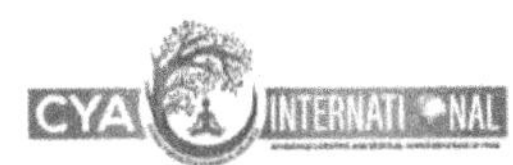

CHAPTER 21:

Mudrās and *Bandhas* – An Overview

Mudrās and *bandhas* are discussed in the main *Haṭha Yoga* texts like the Haṭha Yoga Pradīpikā, Gheraṇḍa Samhitā, Gorakśha Ṣhataka, and in the Śhiva Samhitā. In these ancient texts, *mudrās* and *bandhas* are combined as one unit in their functionality. These are stimulations of certain parts of the body that create a profound sense of inner balance for spiritual stimulation.[65] In modern day verbiage they are often described as psycho-neurotransmitters. They may be considered comparable to bio-meridians of the acupuncture system. However, unlike acupuncture that uses needles, stimulations of *mudrās* and *bandhas* are done by voluntary muscle pressure alone.

MUDRĀS-BANDHAS DESCRIBED IN TRADITIONAL HAṬHA YOGA TEXTS

The traditional Haṭha Yoga texts list the *mudrās* and *bandhas* as follows, none of which involve finger positions:

Haṭha Yoga Pradīpikā (Ch 3): *Mahāmudrā, Mahābandha, Mahāvedha, Khechari, Uddiyāna Bandha, Mūla Bandha, Jālandhara Bandha, Viparita Karani, Vajroli* and *Śhaktī-chālana.*

Gheraṇḍa Samhitā (Ch 3): *Mahāmudrā, Nabhomudrā, Uddiyāna Bandha, Jalandharam Bandha, Mūla Bandha, Mahābandha, Mahāvedha, Khechari, Viparita Kari, Yoni, Vajroli, Śhaktī-chālani, Tādāgi, Mānduki, Shāmbhavi, Ashvini, Pāshini, Kāki, Mātangi, Bhujangi* and the five *Dhāraṇās (Adho, Ambhasi, Vaiśhvānari, Vāyavi, Nabho*)

Gorakśha-Ṣhataka (32-37): *Mahāmudrā, Nabhomudrā, Uddiyāna Bandha, Jalandharam Bandha, Mūla Bandha, Khechari*

Śhiva Samhitā (Ch 4): *Yoni Mudrā, Mahāmudrā, Mahābandha, Mahāvedha, Khechari, Uddiyāna Bandha, Mūla Bandha, Jālandhara Bandha, Viparita Kriti, Vajroli* and *Śhaktī-chālana*

The *mudrās* and *bandhas* of traditional Haṭha Yoga are not relevant at the introductory or instructor level. However, the 33 ancient religions of India used many hand and finger positions to evoke the *mudrā* type of stimulation.[66] These became part of the Tantra system of yoga and the *Nātya Śhāstra* of *Bharata-Nātyam* dance form. Swami Satyananda Saraswati of the Bihar

---

[65] The language in these texts refer to Kundalini and the *nādi* system which is left for general discussion in the Tantra segment of this book.

[66] The traditional description of *mudrās* and *bandhas* don't use hands. Very likely they became integrated with the yoga system from the Tantric system of *Nyāsa*.

School of Yoga in his scholarly book ***Āsana Prāṇāyāma Mudrā Bandha*** presents his own five group classification as follows (an integration of the types of Mudrās and Bandhas from various systems):

- *Hasta Mudrās* – hand and finger positions
- *Mana Mudrās* – head *mudrās*
- *Kāya Mudrās* – body positions
- *Bandhas* or locking of *mudrās*
- *Adhara Mudrās* – related to the perineum

The ease of hand and finger positions have made some hand *mudrās* very popular for therapy and meditation.[67] In this introductory level, we will limit our discussion to principles and application of hand and finger *mudrās* for meditations purposes only.

Application of Hand-Finger (*Hasta*) *Mudrās*

Mudrās involving the fingers and hands can be very useful for meditative practices. Conscious awareness of this process rapidly leads to introspection and internalization. The *mudrā* principle for hands and fingers is associated with the five-element representation in the five fingers[68] as follows:

- Thumb is associated with space,
- Index finger is associated with air,
- Middle finger is associated with fire,
- Ring finger is associated with water,
- Little finger is associated with earth.

As discussed in Chapter 5 (The Underlying Mechanism of All Yoga Approaches) communication with each functionality of the body – *Prāṇā, Apāna, Vyāna, Udāna* and *Samāna* – is associated with each of these elements. Since *Udāna* associated with the space element (connecting into the cosmic consciousness) is the re-programmer of functionalities, the thumb is involved in all the hand *mudrās* with or without the combination of one or more of the other fingers to stimulate the necessary communication.

For meditation purposes, three hand-finger positions may be used. The appropriate one is selected based on what feels best – feeling of lightness that helps meditation – for the practitioner:

---

[67] The fields of acupressure and even reflexology (including the feet) may have some relationship to this simplistic use of the hands and feet. Finger tapping of different parts of the body in the Emotional Freedom Technique may be similar. [Crenshaw, Carol. (2017). EFT for Meditation. Fultom, CA: Energy Psychology Press. Stapleton, P. (2022). The Science Behind Tapping: A Proven Stress Management Technique for the Mind and Body. Carlsbad, CA: Hay House Publishing.]

[68] Some texts in the last century have proposed a different schematic of matching elements to fingers, which has been widely propagated on the internet.

- ***Dhyāna Mudrā*** – One palm over the other, both facing upward, with the thumbs touching each other resting on the lap is the position of the *mudrā*. Which palm comes of the top is specific to each person and should be tested for what feels best. The thumbs pressing each other allows for stimulating *Udāna*.
- ***Chit or Chin Mudrā*** – Palms open (facing upward) and separated, resting on the knees comfortably, with each thumb touching the respective index finger is the position of this *mudrā*. This stimulates the *Prāṇa* and *Udāna* together to energize meditation. It may not feel as light as the previous *mudrā* but is used by many people.
- ***Open Palms*** – Keeping both palms open (facing upward) and loose, resting on the knees is another option to consider for meditation.

Figure 21: MEDITATION MUDRĀS

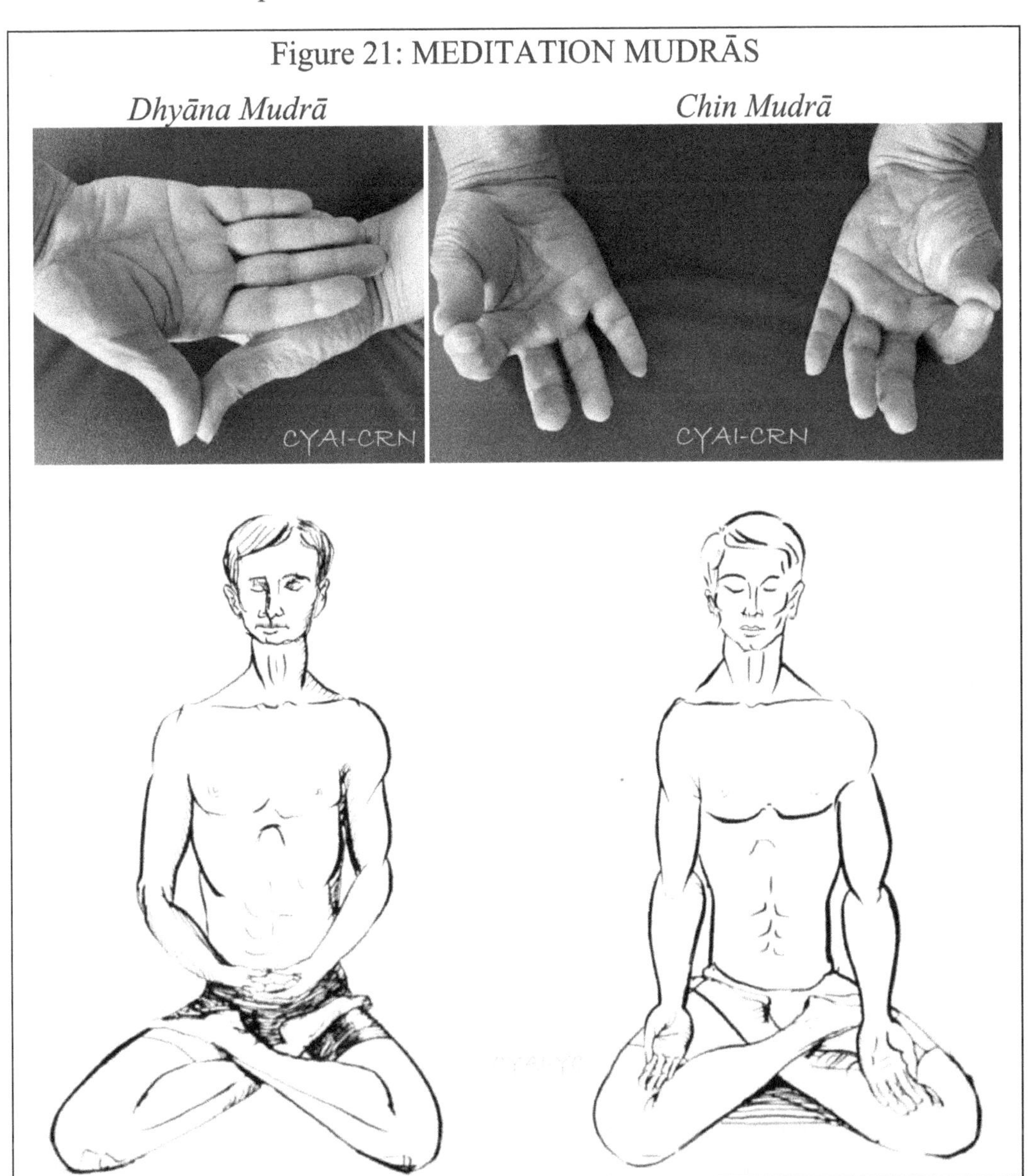

The *mudrā* of choice should be left to the practitioner since previous use of any of these *mudrās* will gravitate one towards that as their comfort zone. Finally, the mind-belief system is more powerful than any *mudrā*.

The common *bandhas* used by many schools in conjunction with *Kumbhaka* are *Mūla Bandha*, *Uddiyāna Bandha*, *Jālandhara Bandha* and *Mahābandha* (commonly also called *Tribandha*). These are reserved for discussion in the higher level.

CAUTION IN *KUMBHAKAS* DONE WITH *BANDHAS*

Swami Rama taught that breath suspension (*Kumbhaka*) should not be practiced until a substantial amount of emotional purification of the *chitta* has been accomplished. His explanation, which cannot be verified by physiological research, is that *Kumbhaka* strengthens all of one's karmic impressions (*samskāras*) across the board. Premature practice of *Kumbhaka*, then, guarantees a more difficult process of accomplishing the purification and stabilization of the *chitta* (*chitta-prasādana* in Yoga Sutras 1.33) in preparation for deeper practices of meditation. Signs and symptoms of readiness for *Kumbhaka* are described in the Haṭha Yoga Pradīpikā (2:19). Swami Veda Bharati also added that the spontaneous occurrence of *Kevala Kumbhaka* in meditation is also a sign of readiness.

Questions and Discussion Topics

1. There is a distinction between the *mudrās* and *bandhas* of the Haṭha Yoga texts and the *mudrās* of the fingers/hands that have come from other traditions. Understanding this distinction, in your opinion are the *mudrās* and *bandhas* of Haṭha Yoga texts useful for conducting a yoga class by an instructor? Explain.

2. Are the finger *mudrās* useful for any purpose? Explain

The predominance of the physical focus of the *Haṭha Yoga* approach and its impact on physical and mental health can make one less receptive to the spiritual potential.

Tantra is the means for the higher realization of yoga.

PART IV – TANTRA APPROACH TO YOGA

22. Concept of Tantra and its Application
    - The Basis: Science, Yoga Philosophy and Tantra
    - Common Applications
    - Religious Applications
    - Applications in Yoga
    - Yoga's Requirement of *Dharma*
    - The Special Place of Kashmir Shaivism in Tantra

23. *Kuṇdalinī Yoga* System
    - Understanding the Awareness of *Kuṇdalinī*
    - Non-Validated Conceptions
    - Conclusive Understanding of the Value of the Kuṇdalinī System

24. Tantra as Integral to Yoga – Integration of Gross, Subtle and Causal Body
    - *Samyama* of Yoga Sutras is Tantra
    - Yoga Concept of Three Bodies and Role of *Dharma* Assumes Tantra
    - Tantra is Apparent in Certain Yoga Practices

25. *Prāṇakriyā*

26. *Chakra* Vibration Practice
    - Vibrations for each *Chakra*
    - Repetitions in each *Chakra*
    - Use of *Mudrās* in each *Chakra*
    - Application of *Chakra* Vibrations

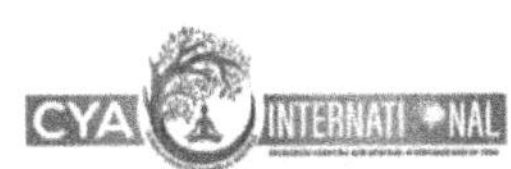

CHAPTER 22:

Concept of Tantra and its Application

Tanu Trayete Iti Tantraha (तनू त्रायते इति तन्त्रः) is the Sanskṛit grammar and root meaning statement that effectively says ability to go beyond the physical body is *tantra*. Typically, it refers to vibrational connection that can go beyond the body. Its relevance is widespread in many aspects of living – in religious contexts, in power of sound vibrations and intention, and it has scientific relevance to the nature of wireless communication and even phenomena related to weather, climate, earth, solar system and the universe. Of course, it also has application in yoga, which applies to all aspects of creation.

The Basis: Science, Yoga Philosophy and *Tantra*

Physical sciences understand creation – viewed as the universe of galaxies – as a vibrating entity. Vibration is caused by oscillating minute particles that result in propagative waves. The phenomena of electrical power generation and distribution through copper wires, or wireless communication (like our common mobile phones) have in common the principle of electromagnetic propagation. Light is considered both a wave and a particle and visible light fits in the middle of the electromagnetic spectrum. We find it completely acceptable for such an electromagnetic communication, triggered from a remote button or an app on our smart mobile phones, to remotely unlock our cars, turn on our lights or other electrical appliances. At the same time, it would seem somewhat farfetched to think the power of the mind can create waves (telepathically) to trigger actions remotely.

However, such forms of telepathic communication have been demonstrated by the physicist Michio Kaku with special eyeglasses that capture thought and wirelessly send the waves to induce action.[69] Artificial limbs these days are being prepared by Dustin Tyler at Case Western Reserve University for those who have lost a limb in a war or accident that take instructions from the brain and move almost like normal limbs.[70]

All these in the scientific world are real life *tantra*, where we use mechanical devices as the intermediary to enable vibratory communication.

---

[69] Michio Kaku: Future of the Mind. https://mkaku.org/home/articles/excerpt-from-the-future-of-the-mind/

[70] https://www.cleveland.com/news/2021/02/cwrus-human-fusions-institute-melds-man-and-machine-with-high-tech-prosthetics.html

Beyond the mechanical devices, scientists recognize today that motion of planets and stars, and even climatic conditions and weather are governed by the four forces of nature.[71] Effectively all of creation is *tantra* dynamics.

Within the physical world electromagnetic frequency is considered the basis of wireless communication. When it comes to live beings like us, the element of *tantra* can be subtler transcending beyond the electromagnetic spectrum. While we exist within the communication potential of audio and electromagnetic frequencies in the temporal world,[72] the subtle being that existed before we were born and may exist after we leave the body exists outside this communication spectrum. Until there is further development in quantum physics beyond Higgs boson, our scientific understanding of it is limited.

Yoga, as a theistic philosophy, explains the first creation of God (*Īśhvara*), called *Prakṛiti* or Cosmic Consciousness (the One *Chitta*), as simply dynamically programmed energy that unleashes creation.[73] *Prakṛiti*, in Sanskṛit parsed as *Prakṛishṭa Kṛiti* (प्रकृष्ट कृति) literally means composition (*Kṛiti*) divinely connected in its core (*Prakṛishṭa*). Thus, with the innumerable number of entities in creation that includes each one of us, all of creation is considered a distributed computing system wirelessly connected into the cosmic dynamics of the One Cosmic Consciousness. Each one of us, as cosmically programmed entities with some degree of free will, do activities that roll into the cosmic flow by our thoughts, words, and deeds. Meditative connectivity that provides intuitive guidance, sometimes called voice of the conscience in religious parlance, guides us towards keeping us in track with the cosmic plan. [And when the mind goes astray and we deviate from the cosmic plan, resulting in ill-health, is another matter for which remedy is yoga.]

Now, connecting into the Cosmic Consciousness or even at a lower level[74] that is beyond our physical bodies, that help us intuitively sense and influence people and things around us, is the

---

[71] The four forces of nature recognized by the Standard Model of physics are, gravitation, weak force, electromagnetism, and strong force. While there has been some success in showing the underlying unity between some of the forces, the holy grail in physics that remains is to find a unified theory of all the four forces. https://www.space.com/four-fundamental-forces.html and https://nautil.us/a-brief-history-of-the-grand-unified-theory-of-physics-236493/ provide detailed insights for those seeking further details.

[72] Our mobile phones are examples of transcendence from audio to electromagnetic frequencies (EMF) when we talk on the phone, and conversion from EMF to audio when we hear. The transcendence process beyond into the subtler dimension that yogis experience is yet to be scientifically discovered.

[73] In *Sāṅkhya* philosophy, the Yoga concepts of *Prakṛiti* and the One Cosmic *Chitta* are parsed further. The Cosmic *Chitta* is considered a processor with no intent of its own. *Prakṛiti* processes its intention through the Cosmic *Chitta*. The innumerable individual *chittas* or processors are part of *Prakṛiti*'s processing of its intent, where each individual *chitta* processes some of the intent of *Prakṛiti* to be governed and integrated within the processing of the Cosmic *Chitta*.

[74] Cosmic connectivity is understood to be at different levels. Ability to intuitively anticipate events is considered a low level of connectivity. Abilities like controlling the weather, aspects of nature, is considered a very high level of ability.

zone of *tantra* in Yoga. The connecting ingredient is vibrations.[75] ***There are two sides of vibration: the waves that connect and the messages or instructions that they carry.***

A SCIENTIFIC AND PHILOSOPHIC PERSPECTIVE ON TRANSCENDENCE

One hypothesis is that transcendence beyond the electromagnetic spectrum is facilitated by 'scalar waves', and the messages or instructions that they carry, that spin around the scalar waves, are called 'torsion field.'

The best way to understand scalar waves is to understand what happens in Transcendental Meditation. It is said in yoga that a person's composition of internal programs (*karma* and *kleśha*) when activated by energy flow emanates a composite vibration by which the person acts and reacts as part of daily living. An equal and opposite vibration is called the personal mantra of the person, which scientifically would be called 'harmonic vibration.' In transcendental meditation, it silences the vibrations of the internal programs that emanate in all directions. The outcome is a feeling of lightness and a single line of awareness lifting upward, experienced like a column above the head. Since the vibrations of the internal programs have energy, and the harmonic vibration also has energy, the energy cannot be lost, but it manifests as scalar waves felt like a column above the head. Intentions travel upward spinning around the scalar waves as torsion field, and intuition or result of the intention is also conveyed in a downward flowing torsion field.

While vibrations are in the electromagnetic spectrum, scalar waves appear to go outside the electromagnetic spectrum, possibly permeating into a fourth dimension or beyond. The philosophical sense coming from Vedic understanding is the concept of *dahar-ākāsha* or the space between the smallest particle through which the higher reality and God can be accessed. In our model we consider the subtle being of anyone (consciousness) existing in the fourth dimension – the place from which everything comes before birth, and where it goes when the body is dead. That individual consciousness integrates with the cosmic consciousness as part of the cosmic flow. The cosmic flow is in the control of *Prakṛiti*, and *Īśhvara* is the unmanifest beyond that.

Common Applications

There are many common applications of *tantra* in daily life that go beyond remote appliance connection that we accept on faith and don't think much about it. There are two aspects to these *tantra* applications: role of power of intention, and induction of connection by stimulants.

[75] While the examples given relate to the electromagnetic spectrum, much of Quantum Theory of physics is still unexplored and unknown. The type of oscillations that carry connectivity and information may be beyond the electromagnetic spectrum. We can speculate that even neutrinos whose function is unknown do oscillate. So, there is much yet to be discovered from a conventional scientific perspective.

Often called, the '**power of positive thinking**', or simply put '**power of intention**', works differently for different people.[76] We observe this in such phenomena as praying for someone's health, seeking blessings, faith healing, placebo effect, etc. None of these are equal for everyone. Some people can fulfill their intent most of the times, while others are unsuccessful. Placebo effect does not happen for all even if they have faith. Also, if you observe healers (like Reiki, Prānic, Shamanic and Voodoo healers) not every healer is equally effective. This is because power of intention is only the message or instruction, but without the waves that connect effectively adequate success is not evidenced. Further, even a successful healer meets failure every now and then – why? The target of the intention may have a block to receive, and that may be the cosmic intent. In yoga, the one with the highest connectivity who can overcome any obstacle in connecting with the power of intention is called *Pradhāna Jayī* (Yoga Sutras 3:49) or the one who has control over the Cosmic Consciousness enabling one to do anything with mere thought.[77] From a yogic perspective that is not necessarily good. Anyone with such power diverting the natural dynamics of the Cosmic Consciousness is considered one who has not fully realized the nature of existence.

The second aspect of common *tantra* applications is the **connectivity by stimulants**. Such stimulants include psychedelic drugs, use of mantras and *mudrās*, invocation of an elevated spirit, places with induced cosmic connection like pyramids, temples and such sacred places, and gems, stones, metallic body adornments and insignia. Places and objects that act as stimulants are called *yantra* in the yogic system. In Sanskṛit, *yantra* means an (inanimate) object which pervades beyond itself. These can be thought as vibration transmitting hubs that can help you transcend. The common aspect of all these types of stimulants is that they open the pathways of connection, and thereby enabling the power of intention to work.

As a yogi, the focus is on cleansing the *nādis* by living a life consistent with the cosmic flow without being excessively reactive. That opens the channels of communications beyond the body without being dependent on external stimulants, although in initial stages help with stimulants like sacred places and mantras are useful.[78] The realized yogi, understanding oneself as only an instrument of the cosmic flow, is always cautious about using the power of intention.

---

[76] Bengston WF. Crossing disciplinary boundaries: going beyond even meta-analysis of distant intention. J Altern Complement Med. 2012 Jun;18(6):525-6. doi: 10.1089/acm.2012.0443. PMID: 22784337.

[77] This ability to do anything with mere thought is only within what has been created by *Prakṛiti* through the Cosmic flow. *Īshvara* or God is considered beyond *Prakṛiti and* is the Supreme source of everything. That is the reason from a yogic perspective this ability to do anything with mere thought is not considered the highest level of realization.

[78] Cleansing of the *nādis* by gradual purification with yoga practices induces the connectivity beyond the body. In this case no external stimulants are required. It is important to note that external stimulants provide temporary opening of the *nādis* within a person to experience beyond the body, but purification through yoga results in having the *nādis* open all the time – called *Nirbeeja Samādhi* in yoga.

PURE *SAṄKALPA*

The power of intention is called *Saṅkalpa* in *tantra* literature. This can be thought of as similar to the *Dhāraṇā* component of *Ashṭānga* Yoga. However, in the higher spiritual domain, intuition that guides one towards an intention is considered as revealing the purpose of the person's life (one's *Sva-dharma*). This is of a higher order than *Dhāraṇā*, and of a higher order than the common understanding of *Saṅkalpa* as only solemn affirmation. Therefore, it is referred as *pure Saṅkalpa.*

The AHYMSIN tradition describes *Saṅkalpa* as follows:

One of the powers of the purest part of *chitta*, which is called *buddhi*, is the formation of intentions, or *Saṅkalpas*. These intentions, from this relatively subtle layer of *chitta*, can be quite powerful even though they are generally not forceful. Commonly people speak of "will power" as if the exertion of will requires a substantial effort. Unfortunately, that is the zone of "I, as the doer" instead of the yogic attitude of one being an instrument of the cosmic flow that "lets things happen through this body as the instrument." In truth, the more gently a *Saṅkalpa* is expressed, it is intent of the cosmos expressed through the instrument of the person. Thus, greater is the power and effectiveness of such *Saṅkalpa*. It is much more like the "still, small voice" of conscience that guides the cosmic intent through a person. Swami Veda Bharati often described it as "gentle as the decision to give oneself in love."

This view of *Saṅkalpa* assumes a significant level of cosmic connectivity with purification of the *chitta* that enables one to sense and affirm one's purpose of life.

Religious Applications

Every religion has some form of *tantra* practice in its rituals. At the superficial level they are limited to the power of intention. At the deeper level they also open the channels of communication through three approaches:

- ***Places of group worship*** – where through years of meditative practices and perhaps other rituals there is established connectivity, which often people feel as lightness or joyful feeling while in those places.
- ***Priest as the conduit in religion*** – priests, through daily meditative and other ritualistic practices are expected to have clear *nādis* to communicate beyond the physical body and convey the requests of the believer.
- ***Individual cleansing practices*** – through mantras, *yantras*, *mudrās* and other yoga-type practices.

All over the world we see people flocking to places of religious worship, no matter what religion. This role of pilgrimage is to foster deeper connectivity with the higher consciousness.

Priest serving as a conduit is present in many religions and is used for many purposes. Some examples are the following. Warding off evil and bringing blessings is used for births, marriages, and major acquisitions like houses and automobiles. Even some governments use such approaches to build new installations or even to launch new aircrafts and ships used for protection of the country. Priests also serve for spiritual initiation for the faithful. They also serve to convey the spirit of the dead to its final destination. Perhaps the highest role for priests serving as conduits of spiritual connectivity is in the consecration of places of worship, where they bring the connectivity into the place or object of worship.

Individual practices within religion are ritual practices that may include prayers and observances. While the ritual is done individually it can be done alone or in groups. These are like daily meditation, prayers, etc. and annual observances.

All of these are inherently *tantra* practices.

Applications in Yoga

Now that you understand *tantra* it is easy to see that a key element of yoga is *tantra* – the ability to experience beyond the body. Even in *Haṭha Yoga*, after transcending the *āsanas* and *kriyās*, the higher meditative aspects are *tantra*. The dominance of physical orientation rather than spiritual orientation, in popular yoga, has given predominance to *āsanas* and *kriyās* in *Haṭha Yoga,* which work at a lower level than *tantra*. Calling it as the whole yoga is a misnomer.

Tantra, used for unethical or selfish purposes (*adhārmic*), has led many people to distance themselves from *tantra*. However, *tantra* with surrender to God with the understanding that we are simply instruments of the cosmic flow leads to the higher and complete understanding of yoga.

Tantra Yoga approach includes physical alignment which is the predominant focus of *Haṭha Yoga*. However, in *Tantra Yoga* physical movements may be done in sync with breathing cycles, visualizations, *mudrās*, and even mantra vibrations. Academic scholars who lack depth in spirituality externally see *Tantra Yoga* primarily associated with mantras and worship. That is a limited view.

The nādis and chakra concepts, the use of mantras, and physical alignment practices done with movement in sync with breath and visualization are distinctive in the Tantra Yoga approach relative to other approaches in yoga. The physical alignment process done with movement is called ***Prāṇakriyā***. It is interesting to note that some of the recent masters of *Haṭha Yoga* having discovered the movement aspect have created a new term called *Vinyāsa* yoga, which is encompassed in *Prāṇakriyā*.

Tantra Yoga is generic without religious connotation although applied in every religion. However, the Yoga philosophy conception of the first creation coming out of God which is just programmed energy called *Prakṛiti* or *Śhaktī* has been adopted into certain religious systems.

Everything in the observed universe coming out of the first programmed entity, *Prakṛiti* or *Śhaktī,* is sometimes religiously worshipped as the Divine Mother. In these religious traditions, it is thought that the Divine Mother would lead to the Divine Father or God. This has special relevance for the *Kuṇdalinī Yoga* system which is discussed in a separate chapter.

PERCEPTION FROM SUBTLE TO GROSS

While commonly people coming from popular *Haṭha Yoga* think of the physical and gross leading towards the subtle, one of the deeper principles of relationship among the levels of embodiment is that the subtler layers control and organize the grosser layers. This can be experienced in yoga practice in the spontaneous occurrence of a *mudrā*, which is the physical body following a change in the subtle energy channels (*nādis*). For example, when one is very relaxed in *Śhavāsana*, you may notice a subtle attraction between your thumb and forefinger which eventually brings them into *Chit-mudrā.*[79]

Yoga's Requirement of *Dharma*

Unlike faith-based systems, yoga is the approach of direct experience without assumptions. In a traditional sense, yoga philosophy is not needed for the yoga practitioner. However, the Yoga Sutras provide guidance for the practitioner, especially in the third *pāda* where extraordinary abilities may manifest, so that the practitioner is not confused. The Yoga Sutras clarify that no matter what extraordinary abilities one may experience, these abilities are meant only to perform one's duty as part of the cosmic flow, and not meant for pursuing one's desires.[80] This idea of each person's special role in creation, i.e., one's duty, is called *Sva-dharma* (One's own *Dharma*). *Dharma* literally means that which supports the cosmic flow. The clear understanding of yoga is that one is only an instrument of the cosmic flow. Thus, the life of a yogi, with whatever abilities one obtains, must only be used to fulfill one's purpose of life that is intuitively divined moment-by-moment without preconceptions.

This clarification is very essential because the ability to go beyond the body, if used for personal desires, goes into misuse of such ability. These are the negative aspects of *tantra* and Voodoo systems which have no place in yoga, and which have resulted in many people shying away from the term *tantra*.

[79] Swami Veda Bharati's book: Philosophy of Haṭha Yoga

[80] The distinction in yoga between desires and cosmic duty is that desires are borne out of sensory attractions, while the cosmic duty is intuitively perceived when there are no internal desires. Such internal desires can create biases in intuitive receptivity where one begins to mistakenly think these desires or preconceived notions are actually intuitive guidance of the cosmos.

The Special Place of Kashmir Shaivism in *Tantra*

Kashmir Shaivism is considered a complete expression of *tantra*. The idea of completion is that there is integral expression of cosmic reality beyond the body through connectivity and intent – i.e., the nature of creation and existence of the individual and everything, and the role of the individual and the final state of release (*kaivalya)*. Incidents expressed in the book by Swami Rama "Living with the Himalayan Masters" speak to such astounding abilities of projecting intent. However, from the perspective of higher realization the ancient (7th century CE) book "Vijñyana Bhairava Tantra", describes 112 practice methods of Kashmir Shaivism and the associated *Trikā* (Three-fold) philosophy of *Śhiva*, *Śhaktī* and the individual human being. The *Trika* philosophy fits into the Yoga Sutras concept of *Puruṣha*, *Prakṛiti* and the seeker.[81]

Questions and Discussion Topics

1. Is there a pitfall in comparing electromagnetic wireless communication with *tantra*? How is *tantra* equivalent or different?

2. Reflect on the practice of blessings that is common in many traditions. What makes blessings effective or not? Use the idea of two elements – the message and the medium of connectivity – in your analysis along with sources of effectiveness or lack of effectiveness. Consider who within the tradition you know are qualified to give blessings and why that may be the case.

3. Consider the practice of invocation of a highly evolved being (saint, *Devatā*, angel, etc.) either for meditation or some religious service that you have observed. Analyse what happens in the invocation process and the intent it serves.

4. Is the experience of *tantra* – going beyond the body – good or bad? Is it necessary for higher realization in yoga?

[81] Some scholars of Kashmir Shaivism find the equivalence with the Yoga Sutras as problematic because of their strict perception of monism.

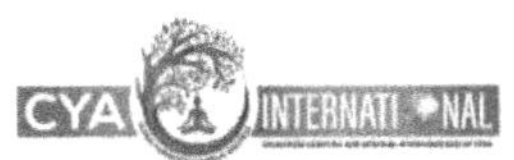

CHAPTER 23:

Kuṇdalinī Yoga System

The *Kuṇdalinī Yoga* system, as portrayed in popular writing, is a zone of many conceptions. Many of these conceptions are not validated and often discarded by discerning yogis, who also cull out the core and valuable essence of these conceptions more sensibly. To add to the confusion, there is one school of yoga that uses it as a trade name. To understand this system, we need to begin with the meaning of the word *Kuṇdalinī*. Also, any theoretical conception cannot be inconsistent with the Yoga Sutras.

In Sanskṛit, the word *kuṇda* means a hole (that can hold something). Also in North India, a horoscope is referred to as the *Kuṇdalī* of the person – the idea that it holds the factors that govern the flow of one's life. Thus, *Kuṇdalinī* should be understood as the awareness or force of one's existence that makes us who we are at each moment in time.

Accordingly, the *Kuṇdalinī Yoga* System focuses on the evolutionary expansion of awareness where the ultimate expansion is the awareness of, or merger into, God. In this system, creation starts from *Śhaktī* (primordial energy), often referred as the Divine Mother who gives birth to creation. This is the concept of *Prakṛiti* of the Yoga Sutras. Therefore, all of creation is considered as the nature of the mother or female (also referred as *Māyā* or illusion – the idea that something is transient). The inner cause of every being is considered the father or *Śhiva* element, called *Puruṣha* in the Yoga Sutras. Thus, *Kuṇdalinī* is represented as female merging with the male, i.e., God, in its highest expansive awareness.

Understanding the Awareness of *Kuṇdalinī*

Fundamental to understanding the awareness of the *Kuṇdalinī* is knowledge of the *kleśha* of the Yoga Sutras, the *varṇa-āshramas* of the Vedic system, and the *chakra* system of *tantra* discussed in the fifth chapter of this book.

The five-fold *kleśha* noted in the Yoga Sutras (2:3) are the initial programmed composition of each entity. As the Yoga Sutras (2:4-5) note that *avidyā* or lack of understanding of the nature of existence is the singular *kleśha* element that allows the other *kleśha* elements to run loose, and to act and react creating new *karma* that propagate further births.

At any given time, one's existence is anchored by three elements:

a) ***Level of Avidyā*** (or the opposite *Ātma Vidyā*) – this is the innate awareness of the soul of the nature of existence,
b) ***Bundle of Programs*** – this is the remaining *kleśha* and *karma* of yoga,
c) ***Cosmic Connectivity*** level represented in the de-stressed state from adequate sleep or meditation and being true to one's conscience.

This essentially presents itself in a person in one of four broad outlooks which are called the *varṇa-āshramas* associated with their nature called *varṇa-dharma*[82]:

- Survival-based thinking with inability to think beyond immediate sustenance – This comes from no awareness beyond the body and no thinking ability to plan forward. This outlook is called ***kśhudra*** nature in the Vedic system. The word *kśhudra* in Sanskṛit means small or insignificant. In the Vedic system people with such orientation are considered the order-takers of society that support the society with necessary work that does not involve much thinking, with society taking the social responsibility of meeting their needs of sustenance.
- Self-centered thinking beyond the immediate sustenance – This outlook is called ***vaiśhya*** nature that seeks to control resources for one's own benefit. *Vaiśhya* comes from the root word *vaśha* which means control. In the Vedic system such orientation makes one a profit-motivated businessperson, where society has the responsibility to ensure that such self-centered profit motivation does not tread on the well-being of others in the society.
- Thinking about others beyond oneself – There are two levels here depending on whether (a) one thinks in terms of a narrow group like family, friends and associates, community, nation, OR (b) thinking in a wider level of all of humanity or all of temporal living. The focus is still within the observed and material world. These two levels of thinking beyond oneself are called ***kśhatriya*** nature. The word *kśhatra* refers to domain. The lower *kśhatriya* has a narrow domain of focus, while the higher-level *kśhatriya*, often referred as *chakravarty*, thinks of the whole world as their domain. People with the *kśhatriya* outlook are the rulers, administrators and soldiers of society who protect the interest of society as a whole, whether in a narrow or broad domain. In the Vedic system, they are considered the guardians of society who work without self-interest and solely in the interest of society, especially to prevent exploitation of the *kśhudras* by the *vaiśhyas*.
- Thinking beyond the physical world – There are four levels in this type of outlook.
  - First is the ***seeker*** of what is beyond death and before birth. The search is for the meaning of temporal existence (and its relationship to spirituality).
  - Second is the ***believer*** who feels convinced about the nature of temporal and spiritual

[82] *Varṇa* means outlook and *Dharma* means one's duty that is consistent with the cosmic flow, thus supporting the cosmic flow (i.e., the divine intent).

existence based on what has been learned from readings, associations, and one's own mental analysis.
- Third is the ***renunciate***, who is convinced by one's belief that issues of the temporal world don't matter. Thus, one stays unaffected by anything with an attitude of 'letting go'.
- Fourth is the ***Realized*** person, who realizes the purpose of birth, engages in one's duties, and understanding the cycle of *karma* is unaffected by anything.
These four levels are considered ***four levels of brāhmanas***[83] (meaning those who seek or know the nature of existence).

These eight levels bundled into four categories of broad outlook are mapped into the *Chakra* system. Each *chakra* represents the type of thinking or outlook, governed by the gene-expression (*Samāna* along the *Suṣhumnā Nādi*) as noted in Chapter 5 of this book. Each *chakra* also affects organ systems in the region of the *chakra*. It is said that where – in which *chakra* – the awareness resides is where the bulk of the energy of a person is functioning. The eight chakras (See Figures 5.3 and 5.4 in Chapter 5) are associated as follows:

1. Root *Chakra*, ***Mūlādhāra*** of the *Tantra* System, located in the perineum, is associated with the *kśhudra* nature.
2. Sacral *Chakra*, ***Svādhiṣhṭhāna*** of the *Tantra* System, located in the middle of the body between the pubis and the sacral bone, is associated with the *vaiśhya* nature.
3. Navel *Chakra*, ***Maṇipūra*** of the *Tantra* System, located in the middle of the body between the navel and the spine, is associated with the lower level *kśhatriya* nature focused on a narrow domain.
4. Heart *Chakra*, ***Anāhata*** of the *Tantra* System, located in the middle of the chest between the breasts, is associated with the higher-level *kśhatriya* nature focused on the world as a whole.
5. Throat *Chakra*, ***ViŚhuddhi*** of the *Tantra* System, located in the middle of the throat area, is associated with the seeker nature, the first level of *brāhmana* inquiry.
6. Head center, ***Ājñyā*** of the *Tantra* System, located in the middle of the head, is associated with the believer nature, the second level of *brāhmana* inquiry.
7. Crown center, ***Sahasrāra*** of the *Tantra* System, located in the middle of the top of the head, is associated with the renunciate nature (third level of the *brāhmana varna*).

[83] *Brahmanas* is the Sanskṛit of the anglicized word Brahmin.

8. Spiritual heart, ***Hṛidaya*** (*Ātmā*) of the Vedic System,[84] located just behind the lower part of the sternum towards the front part of the body, is associated with the realized nature (fourth level of the *brāhmana varna*).

Thus, the progression of expansive awareness is thought to proceed through these levels. And the ascendence from one level to the next may happen in one lifetime or over many lifetimes. Thus, in this spiritual system, the *varna* is not caste as often thought, but rather the transitory nature, that can also change within a lifetime, in the progression towards realization.[85] In the field of psychology, this is often expressed as value system or outlook towards life as distinct from personality.

Non-Validated Conceptions

There are some popular conceptions, that are not validated, that have spread through writings by various individuals. These are:

- The *Kuṇdalinī* is the force that exists in three and a half coils in the base of the spine,
- There are seven *chakras* that are along the spine,
- The *Kuṇdalinī* rises through the spine piercing through each *chakra* and finally meeting the unmanifest (*Śhiva* entity) above the head,
- Once stirred, the *Kuṇdalinī* can rise rapidly and can create moving pain and other destabilizing sensations.

Yoga Sutras and the Vedic System are our best guide to evaluate such claims.

Verse 30 of Vijñyāna Bhairava Tantra associated with Kashmir Shaivism states (as translated):

> The twelve (centers) should be pierced successively through proper understanding of their (associated) twelve letters. Thus, becoming liberated from the gross, then the subtle, one by one, at the end (of its journey) the *Kuṇdalinī* becomes *Śhiva*.

---

[84] The eighth *chakra* is endemic to the Vedic system and is called the seat of complete awareness, *Sannyāsa*. In later times, influenced by *Sāṅkhya-Yoga* Philosophy (and Buddhism), the combined thought process of *Haṭha Yoga* and *Tantra Yoga* brought the seven *chakras* system that is commonly seen in the Kuṇdalinī system. Along with that came many distortions: (a) concept of *Sannyāsa* as renunciation, (b) no sense of one's duty (*Sva-Dharma*) towards the cosmic flow, (c) concept of *Brahmacharya* as celibacy, and (d) the Yoga Sutras labelled as *Mokśha Śhāstra*, instead of *Dharma Śhāstra* leading to *Mokśha*.

[85] In Kashmir Shaivism and in the Vedic system it is thought the first level of sustenance, with limited ability to think, has no chance to attain the highest realization within one lifetime. In Kashmir Shaivism the word used is "*Anupāya*" or no solution, and in the Vedic system such people are not invested with the sacred thread which is considered the initiation to meditative practices. However, all the others are eligible for the sacred thread, even though there is a general wrong perception that it is for the *Brāhmanas*.

Clearly these twelve centers have no correspondence with the seven or eight *chakras*. Even accounting for the concept of the three *granthis* or Knots (*Brahma Granthi*, *Viṣhnu Granthi* and Rudra *Granthi*) noted in Tantra traditions, it does not add up to twelve.

Further the Yoga Sutras provide clear guidance on purification of the *nādis* by keeping the attitude of a dispassionate observer even as we engage in worldly duties, and the process of inquiry in meditative connectivity (*Samyama*) as the way to Realization. The progression may happen in stages, but not necessarily in the context of one lifetime.

This is amply expressed in *Śhiva* Sutras of Kashmir Shaivism that states that there are four categories of individuals whose paths are different. This explains why Ramana Maharishi reached enlightenment simply by asking himself "Who am I?" which for the general population leads nowhere. The four categories of Kashmir Shaivism are expressed as follows:

- Those with *nādis* fully cleared – They ask the question mentally and they instantly have the answer from the Supreme source of everything. This is called ***Shāmbhopāya*** (Solution of *Shambhu*) of Kashmir Shaivism – the direct connection to *Śhiva* from fully cleansed *nādis*.
- Those with some *karma*, whose *nādis* require some cleansing – Here the recommendation is to do mantra meditation that cleanses the *nādis* and takes one to the Supreme Awareness. This is called ***Shāktopāya*** (Solution of *Śhaktī*). Here *Śhaktī* or the divine mother that creates everything by the play of energy, with mantra vibration, clears the gateway to experience the unmanifest God (*Śhiva*).[86]
- Those with some *kleśha* and *karma* and need more *nādi* cleansing – This approach requires one to go through the wringer of life to fulfill the programs of our creation. This is called ***Āṇavopāya*** (Solution for *Aṇu* referring to matter or smallest particle connoting material attachment) in Kashmir Shaivism and can be associated with the concept of *Karma Yoga* or *Kriyā Yoga*.
- Those with significant *kleśha* and *karma* that cannot be purified in one lifetime – Here there is no Realization in this lifetime. In Kashmir Shaivism, this is called ***Anupāya*** (No Solution).

Based on this understanding of Yoga Sutras and Kashmir Shaivism, popular concepts of *Kuṇdalinī* are not tenable. When a person experiences destabilizing pain or sensation from any mantra or spiritual practice, we call it the manifestation of disturbance caused by vibration force in uncleared *nādis*. Such excessive experiences can lead to incapacity or even premature death,

[86] Based on understanding from the Yoga Sutras, mantras create temporary cleansing of the *nādis* that makes one receptive to *Ātma Vidyā* or cosmic knowledge. As this knowledge of the nature of the higher existence grows, one become non-reactive except where duty is called for, and thus creating no new *karmas* expends all the existing programs to fully purify the *nādis* and reach the state that those with *Shāmbhopāya* could achieve.

and such forceful practices are not recommended. This is the reason some higher practices of yoga are not for general instruction, but rather imparted with selective guidance.

It is important to note that much of spiritual literature comes from those who start experiencing beyond the body, and not necessarily from the state when the highest is reached. So even the work of Realized Masters like Shankaracharya, written before full Realization, are not exempt from this pitfall. In stanza 9 of Shankaracharya's *Saundarya Laharī*, he states the concept of the *Kuṇḍalinī* rising through seven *Chakras* and reaching the Ultimate. He also states in the second verse of *Vivekachūḍāmaṇi* that women are unqualified for learning the higher knowledge although, at a later time, in his respect for the female he named one of his '*Daśhanāmi*' Swami order after Mandana Mishra's wife. We know from history that until his experience with the *Chāṇḍāla* (cremation keeper) in *Maṇikarnikā Ghat* in Varanasi, he was not fully Realized, even though he had had heightened spiritual experiences. These unvalidated *Kuṇḍalinī* conceptions should be understood in this light.

Conclusive Understanding of the Value of the *Kuṇḍalinī* System

The real value of the *Kuṇḍalinī* System is to point toward our progressing awareness (or value system) through living. From low level of thinking to self-centered thinking to society-centered thinking to existence-centered thinking are the stages of expanding awareness. Where our thinking resides is where most of our energy will flow. So indeed, focus of energy and thinking are two sides of the same coin. It is important to remember thinking drives the focus of energy, and if one attempts to force the energy towards a higher level of thinking it will necessarily pressure the *nādis* and create tremendous stress and unwanted side-effects. From time immemorial ancient Masters of Yoga have realized the interrelationship between the physical body and the psychic forces.

For clarity between different points of view, it is important to note that this interrelationship between the physical body and the psychic forces, along with conceptions and misconceptions of *Kuṇḍalinī* are well represented in the *Haṭha Yoga* texts of the last millennium. While the concept of *Śhiva* and *Śhaktī* are brought into these texts, they are significantly influenced by the non-theistic view of the *Sāṅkhya-Yoga* philosophy of those times which is distinct and different from the theistic Yoga philosophy. Yoga philosophy goes back few more millennia and is in sync with the Vedic tradition.

Thus, the Vedic and Yogic concept of purpose of living for the cosmic flow (*Sva-dharma*) has been diluted in popular representation of *Kuṇḍalinī* Yoga and the *Haṭha Yoga* system. The Vedic and Yogic purpose of yoga is realization of the nature of existence which includes one's duties (*Dharma Śhāstra*) without attachment (to results) and the natural outcome is liberation (*Mokśha*). The influence of the non-theistic *Sāṅkhya-Yoga* philosophy on the *Haṭha Yoga* system has deviated the focus to liberation (*Mokśha Śhāstra*) alone rendering the purpose of worldly activities as irrelevant and useless, with no meaning for the cosmic flow. Hence there is no surprise that the *Haṭha Yoga* texts do not follow the *Ashṭānga* system of Patanjali dropping the concept of *Yama* and *Niyama* and the role of *Īśhvara Praṇidhāna*. *Gorakśha* is upfront in his *Gorakśha Ṣhataka* in calling his instructions for *Mokśha* as giving up all experiences of the world with *Haṭha Yoga* (Sutras 1-3). This directly contradicts Krishna's Vedic view in Chapter 18 of the *Bhagavad Gita* where he clearly distinguishes between one who gives up worldly actions (*tyāgī*) versus one who engages in worldly actions with understanding and without attachment to results (*sannyāsī*). Thus, for the learning of yoga, *Haṭha Yoga* practices and the *Tantra Yoga* approach must be selectively applied and understood within the yoga system of Patanjali.

Questions and Discussion Topics

1. Reflect on yourself and others whom you know very well over many decades. Can you relate the evolutionary process of *Kuṇdalinī* going from self-centered nature to higher natures? If so, please note the points in the lifetime when the changes happened. Also, note significant events in life – usually troubling events – that result in advancement in the nature (or value system).

2. Do you think this concept of *Kuṇdalinī* is useful in any way for your practice of yoga?

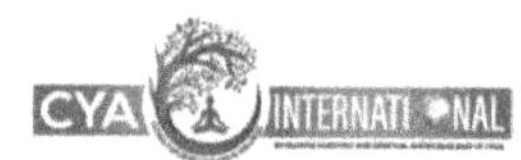

CHAPTER 24:

Tantra As Integral to Yoga

Yoga is all about connecting into the Cosmic flow (*Prakṛiti*) and then into the Cosmic Intelligence (*Īśhvara/Puruṣha*). Mechanism of connection outside the body is *tantra.* Therefore, *tantra* is core and integral to yoga, when yoga is understood as attaining *Samādhi* or Cosmic connectivity, and therefrom directly experience and realize the nature of existence.

Obviously when yoga is understood as a set of postural or breathing exercises, then of course it may be perceived as unrelated to *tantra.* When yoga is understood in the higher experience of meditation and cosmic connectivity, postural and breathing practices are only seen as yoga exercises that serve as stepping-stones to help meditation.

Tantra as integral to yoga can be best appreciated in the following contexts.

Samyama of Yoga Sutras is *Tantra*

The *Samyama* process described in the third *pāda* of the Yoga Sutras that enables one to intuitively sense and attain higher abilities is *tantra. Samyama* is the integration of *Dhāraṇā, Dhyāna* and *Samādhi*, the last three of eight-fold (*Ashṭānga*) yoga.

As described in the Yoga Sutras:

- *Dhāraṇā* is the point of focus that leads to *Dhyāna.*
- In *Dhyāna,* there is complete quietness and stability of the mind, as a result of the purified *chitta* and *nādis* that is required to begin the connectivity with the cosmic flow.
- In *Samādhi*, when the consistent wave of connectivity with the cosmic flow collapses the triad of observer (the practitioner), process of observation and the subtle object observed (point of focus) into a singularity, it opens access to the cosmic flow and cosmic intelligence where intuitive perception occurs. (Ekāgrata Parinama – YS 3:12).

The key ingredient in the process is the vibrational wave to connect (beyond the body) with the cosmic flow (*Prakṛiti*) and the cosmic intelligence (*Puruṣha*) – through the purified *nādis* and the message carried from the intent of *Dhāranā* (*saṅkalpa*) – which results in the intuitive perception which comes in response. This is *tantra.*

Yoga Concept of Three Bodies and Role of *Dharma* Assumes *Tantra*

Yoga's concept is that of three bodies: gross or physical (*sthūla*); subtle or vibrational (*sūkśhma*); and causal or spirit (*kārana*). The spirit that carries the program content of the being communicates to reach the physical body associated with it. The communication happens through some form of subtle vibration. Upon entering the live body and getting access to its energy its activation as pulsating vibrations is measured in traditional medicine systems as the subtle body. These vibrations on a moment-by-moment basis make the physical body act within the physical and physiological domains. In the higher yogic state, one is expected to be connected cosmically to intuitively understand one's purpose of life and fulfill that purpose without reactivity – what is called *Dharma Megha Samādhi* in the Yoga Sutras (4:29). That connectivity to fulfill one's purpose happens with vibrational waves, which is *tantra*.

From a traditional medicine perspective deviation from one's *Dharma* can cause ill-health. Conflict between the physical body and vibrational (subtle) body is resolved by *ā*sana and breathing practices, whereas deep-rooted conflicts that require elimination of conflicts between the causal and vibrational body require mantras and meditative practices which go into the *tantra* domain. The power of positive thinking, typically called the placebo effect in medicine, is also *tantra*.

Tantra is Apparent in Certain Yoga Practices

Use of mantras and *saṅkalpa* (affirmations) are *tantra* in normal yoga practices. Also, in traditional martial arts, which are essentially rooted in yoga, where one anticipates or senses without the normal five senses is considered *tantra*.

Questions and Discussion Topics

1. Have you experienced instances in your life where you did not have strong intentions, but rather mental queries, but after deep sleep or deep meditation the answers to your queries seemed answered and at a later point in time you validated them to be true? How do you explain this in yogic terms?

2. Some yogis give blessings and initiations that are palpable and make a difference for people instantly. Have you known any such yogi who suffers from continuing ill-health? If so, how do you explain such ill-health for this presumably elevated soul?

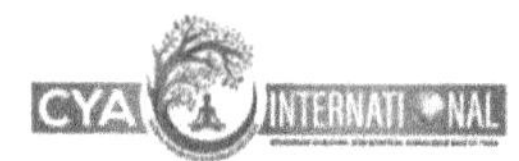

CHAPTER 25:

Prāṇakriyā

Yoga practices that work directly with the subtle energy, *Prāṇā*, are often referred to as *Prāṇāyāma*, although these are often limited to practices involving breathing through the nostrils. There are many others, done in *Śhavāsana*, or during other postures and these are also referred as practices of *Prāṇā-kriyā* (process of or practice with *Prāṇā*) or *Prāṇā-vidyā* (science of *Prāṇā*). This degree of sophisticated view comes from the *tantra* tradition.

This can also be associated with Sutras 2:1-2 of the Yoga Sutras, that explains *Kriyā Yoga*. *Kriyā Yoga* or Yoga of Action is explained as the practice that is intended to pursue towards *Samādhi* with the realization that the physical body with its programs (*kleśha*) is impure. The key elements of this *Kriyā Yoga* practice can be explained as follows:

- *Īśhvara Praṇidhāna* or Surrender to God implies no attachment (or reactions) to results of actions as explained in the Bhagavad Gīta by Krishna. This is because one has mentally surrendered every action to God.
- *Svādhyāya* is one's personal effort to inquire, contemplate, and understand what the physical body encounters and how one should deal with each situation. [This process enables one to be true to one's conscience, and eventually when the *nādis* are clear with high level of purity it leads to *Samyama*.]
- *Tapa* is the heat produced in action that purifies (from burning of *karma-kleśha*) when done with *Īśhvara Praṇidhāna* and *Svādhyāya*. i.e., the *nādis* are cleansed to allow for greater communication beyond the body.

Thus, every activity in life can be thought of as *Kriyā Yoga* when done with *Īśhvara Praṇidhāna* and *Svādhyāya*. Effectively that requires all actions be done with awareness within as fulfilling one's purpose in life (*Sva-dharma*). And nothing can be done with the physical body without the breath flowing and igniting energy through cellular respiration. This is the essence of *Prāṇā-Kriyā*. As an additional descriptor, Yogi Amrit Desai calls this "meditation in motion" – an apt description of how every activity in life should be for a yogi. Accordingly, in the *Tantra Yoga* system it is common to engage in physical practices which includes *āsanas* with movement, that are called *Prāṇakriyā*.

Questions and Discussion Topics

1. Are *Prāṇakriyā* and *Kriyā Yoga* one and the same? What are the commonalities and what are the differences?

2. Can normal beginnings from *Haṭha Yoga* lead to the *Prāṇakriyā* experience? If so, when and how does it manifest?

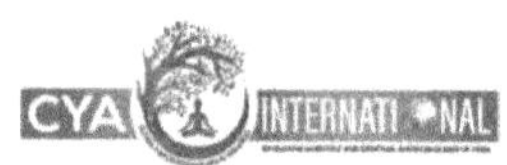

CHAPTER 26:

Chakra Vibration Practice

In the *tantra* concept each *chakra* is said to have different number of petals and all petals of all chakras together cover all the alphabets of Sanskṛit.[87] However, for vibrational purposes one vibration is used for each of the seven *chakras*. Vibrating in each *chakra* appears to be very effective in removing conflicts between the subtle and causal bodies – what we may call as balancing the *Samāna* with *Udāna* connection or keeping one in sync with one's life purpose. Since many illnesses manifest from this level, daily practice of *chakra* vibrations is considered very helpful.

There are two schools of thoughts on the right vibration for each *chakra*. In fact, the difference of opinion is in the sixth *chakra* in the middle of the head. One school uses OM in the sixth and seventh *chakra*. However, Alan Finger[88] uses *Ksham* in the sixth *Chakra* and OM in the seventh chakra. From the perspective of effectiveness in opening the energy flow, Alan Finger's version appears to be more effective and is presented here.

Vibrations for each *Chakra*

Following are the vibrations for each *chakra*. Each of the first six *chakras* ends with the vibration written as AM but is pronounced like UM like in umbrella.

1. Root *Chakra*, *Mūlādhāra* of the Tantra System, located in the perineum, is associated with the vibration LAM.
2. Sacral *Chakra*, *Svādhiṣhṭhāna* of the Tantra System, located in the middle of the body between the pubis and the sacral bone, is associated with the vibration VAM.
3. Navel *Chakra*, *Maṇipūra* of the Tantra System, located in the middle of the body between the navel and the spine, is associated with the vibration RAM.
4. Heart *Chakra*, *Anāhata* of the Tantra System, located in the middle of the chest between the breasts, is associated with the vibration YAM.

---

[87] The original text is *Ṣhaṭ-Chakra-Nirupaṇa*. It is also translated in the work of Arthur Avalon: The Serpent Power.

[88] Alan Finger is of South African origin where he learned *Chakra* Vibrations from his father, Mani Finger, and many yogis who used to visit his family. His book: ***Chakra Yoga: Balancing Energy for Physical, Spiritual, and Mental Well-being***--includes a CD with guided meditations. Alan Finger and Katrina Repka, Published December 13th 2005 by Shambhala ISBN1590302559 (ISBN13: 9781590302552)

5. Throat *Chakra*, *ViŚhuddhi* of the Tanta System, located in the middle of the throat area, is associated with the vibration HAM.
6. Head center, *Ājñyā* of the Tantra System, located in the middle of the head, is associated with the vibration KSHAM.
7. Crown center, *Sahasrāra* of the Tantra System, located in the middle of the top of the head, is associated with the vibration OM.

Repetitions in each *Chakra*

The vibrations in each *chakra* must be repeated multiple times until the *chakra* is clear. Not everyone can discern the clearing and most people may choose to vibrate 3 to 5 times in each *chakra* while those who can discern will have different number of repetitions for each *chakra*. The discernment is done by observing at each repetition, how far above the vibration resonates, even though the focus is only on the specific *chakra*. When the resonance pierces the top of the head and goes above the head, the *chakra* is recognized to be fully clear.

Use of *Mudrās* in each *Chakra*

Mudrās may be used to increase the effectiveness of the vibration in each *chakra* – i.e., allow for the vibration to ascend more rapidly. However, the *mudrā* will lock down the vibration within the body and stop at the top of the head and not pierce through. Once the *mudrā* allows the vibration to go to the top of the head, the *mudrā* is released, and the vibration is used another couple of times until the resonance piercing the head is sensed.

The *mudrās* used are based on the Ayurvedic understanding of each finger associated with each of the five elements and each of the lower five *chakras* associated with each of the same elements.

1. Root *Chakra*, *Mūlādhāra* associated with the earth element – Press the little finger with thumb.
2. Sacral *Chakra*, *Svādhiṣhṭhāna* associated with the water element – Press the ring finger with thumb.
3. Navel *Chakra*, *Maṇipūra* associated with the fire element – Press the middle finger with thumb.
4. Heart *Chakra*, *Anāhata* associated with the air element – Press the index finger with thumb.
5. Throat *Chakra*, *ViŚhuddhi* associated with the space element – Make loose fist with thumb pointing upwards.
6. Head center, *Ājñyā* – Make loose fist with thumb pointing upwards (as in throat *chakra*).
7. Crown center, *Sahasrāra* – Make loose fist with thumb pointing upwards (as in throat *chakra*).

These *mudrās* are kept in both hands, each hand comfortably placed on the knees, with the palms facing upward.

A further enhancement that some may find helpful is to keep the hands in the horizontal plane with the *chakra* where the vibration is focused. For the root *chakra*, the hands may be on the two sides close to the level of the seat. For the sacral *chakra*, it can be in line with the thighs. Thus, the hands rise higher and higher with each chakra in the two sides of the body, slightly in front of the body. Even as the hands rise, the *mudrās* as noted above can be kept, and for the last two repetitions of the vibration the fingers can be released with the palms simply open upward.

Application of *Chakra* Vibrations

Unlike some of the other practices that are sensitive to food and time of day, *chakra* vibrations can be done anytime, although being light in the stomach is always helpful for a deeper experience. In general, the best time for *chakra* vibrations is morning upon waking up and before going to sleep, so that one balances the *Samāna* with the *Udāna* connection in the beginning and end of the day.

This practice is particularly helpful for mental health conditions. [Mental health conditions are associated with deviation from one's life purpose.]

Questions and Discussion Topics

1. Sit in a comfortable spine-aligned position. Close your eyes and observe how you feel within the body and mind. Observe any tightness in any part of the body or a feeling of denseness anywhere in the body, but particularly the head. Then, start doing the *Chakra* vibration practice. If you can feel the rising resonance in each *chakra*, keep the repetitions going until it pierces through the head. If you do not feel the rising resonance, do 10 repetitions in each *chakra*, with the last two without the *mudrās*. Then observe how the tightness or denseness you felt earlier has transformed. Express the transformation in your own words. If you are part of a group, do this again separately with the whole group and document your shared experiences.

2. Consider the mechanism of yoga from chapter 5. How do you explain the transformation from this practice in terms of the *chakras*, *nādis* and the five *Prāṇās* (*Udāna, Samāna, Prāṇā, Vyāna* and *Apāna*)?

The essence of Tantra is meditative connectivity into the higher reality beyond the physical world.

But even higher is reaching the source of knowledge of all of existence, which is the ultimate liberator for the seeking soul!

PART V –THE SOURCE OF ALL KNOWLEDGE IN YOGA

27. The Ultimate Realization of Yoga
    - Becoming Self-Realized
    - Distinctions in Meditative Connectivity
    - Importance of Seeking
    - Distinguishing Between a Religious Seeker and a Yogic Seeker
    - Unity Among Philosophical Divergences
    - Place of Yogic Practices Towards the Goal of Self-Realization

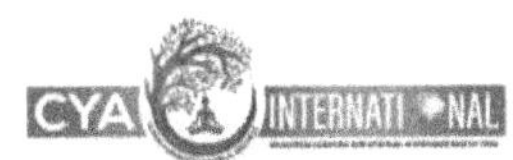

CHAPTER 27:

The Ultimate Realization of Yoga

The Yoga Sutras, in Sutra 1:25, states that God (*Īśhvara* or Supreme *Puruṣha*) is source of all knowledge. Further Sutras 1:26 to 1:29 speak about the relationship between God and sentient beings. The Sutras are presented below.

1:25. tatra niratishayam sarvajñya-(tatva)-beejam
तत्र निरतिशयम् सर्वज्ञ-(तत्व)-बीजम् ॥१-२५॥

There (referring to *Īśhvara* – God – as noted in the previous Sutra 24) is the unsurpassed source (seed) of all knowledge.

1:26. sa esha poorveshām-api guruh kālena-anavachchhedāt
स एष पूर्वेषाम्-अपि गुरुः कालेन-अनवच्छेदात् ॥१-२६॥

He (God) is also the Guru (teacher) of those (the people) of the past, uninterrupted by time. [Implication: God is the foremost and the real Guru, who is unconditioned by time.]

1:27. tasya vāchakah prāṇāvah
तस्य वाचकः प्रणवः ॥१-२७॥

***Prāṇāva* (the sound OM) is his/her/its (God's) communicator.** [*Prāṇāva* literally means the nature of the smallest particle that is divinely connected.]

1:28. tat-japaha-tad-artha-bhāvanam
तत्-जपः-तत्-अर्थ-भावनम् ॥१-२८॥

By vibrating (in meditation) on that (mantra OM) reveals its intended meaning.

1:29. tataha pratyak-chetanā-adhigamaha+api+antarāyā-abhāvaha+cha
ततः प्रत्यक्-चेतना-अधिगमः+अपि+अन्तराया-अभावः+च ॥१-२९॥

From this every *Chetanā* (sentience of living beings) comes forth and also obstacles are not present.

The implication of these Sutras, and other sutras that corroborate the implication, is that all living beings have a concurrent (dual) connection both into the cosmic flow of *Prakṛiti* and the cosmic intelligence of *Īśhvara*. The connection into *Prakṛiti* is the source of entanglement in *Karma*. Whereas the connection into *Īśhvara* (Supreme *Puruṣha*), who is the source of all knowledge, is the pathway for removal of ignorance about the nature of existence. When the ignorance of the nature of existence is removed one becomes non-reactive to the body and mind which are part of *Prakṛiti*. Thus, one has an attitude of acceptance of everything we experience in the world and wherever there is a duty to be performed as per the programs of *Prakṛiti*, we do without reactivity.

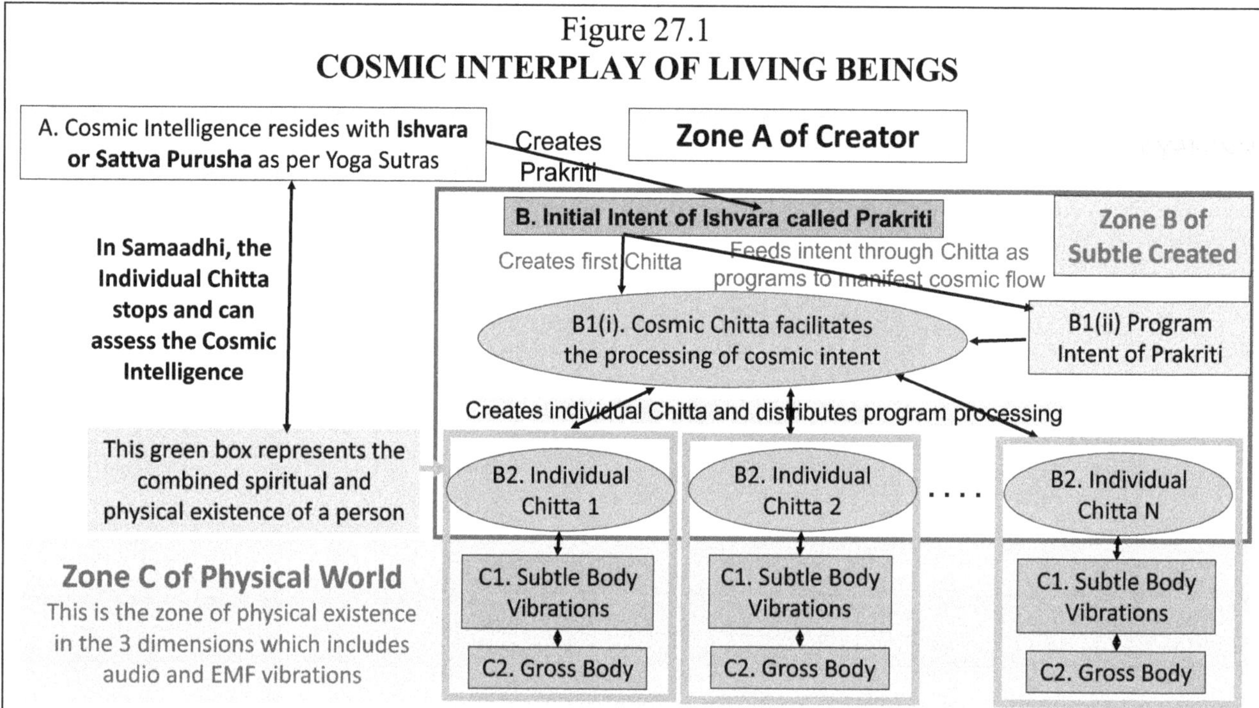

Figure 27.1
COSMIC INTERPLAY OF LIVING BEINGS

The flow chart above distinguishes three zones: Zone A of God, *Īśhvara*, Supreme *Puruṣha*, etc.; Zone B of subtle elements of *Prakṛiti*; and Zone C of the experienced Physical World which is also part of *Prakṛiti*.

These three zones cannot be confused with the Causal, Subtle and Gross bodies. In this Chart, the Gross body and Subtle body with vibrations are in Zone C of the Physical World, and the Causal Body is in Zone B labelled as B2 Individual Chitta. [Technically the Subtle body originates from Zone B and enters as electromagnetic vibrations in Zone C.]

Each Living Being is represented within the green-framed boxes with three elements:
- B2 as the Individual Chitta (along with its cosmically allocated programs is the Causal Body);
- C1 as the Subtle or Vibration Body measured in the electromagnetic spectrum;
- C2 as Gross Body.

Three green-framed boxes are representation of the billions of living beings in the created world, with the last, green-framed box having the B2 Individual Chitta labeled as N to indicate N numbers of living beings.

The green background box in the left area of the image points to each individual entity (in the green-framed box) while connected to Zone B is also concurrently connected to Zone A, which is the source of all knowledge.

This dual connectivity is only for living beings and not for non-living entities. *Chitta,* being the processor, is integral to everything created including non-living entities. However, *chetanā* which is described in the above Sutras is in the nature of living beings, and it ensures a direct connection with God (*Īśhvara*) with potential to access Supreme wisdom since God is the source of all knowledge. Figure 27.1 in the previous page provides a flow chart of the cosmic interplay of living beings.

Becoming Self-Realized

The word Self-Realization is used often as part of spiritual quest. In yoga, it has a special meaning that has the following components:

- One has continuous, unbroken connectivity at all times with Zone A (in Figure 27.1).
- One has imbibed the complete knowledge of existence to realize that each being is only an instrument of the cosmic flow. In other words, we are only actors in the play produced by God (*Īśhvara*) and directed by *Prakṛiti.*
- As a result, one plays one's part without reactivity. This implies no new *Karma* are created.

The process of Self-Realization as the Yoga Sutras of Patanjali explains happens in stages:

- First, one needs to cultivate meditative practices to allow one to remain as an observer at least through the duration of meditation. In initial stages, there can be intrusive thoughts when one is focused in meditation – what we call wandering of the mind. This is considered natural. The recommendation is to go back to the point of focus when one realizes the mind has wandered.
- Second, with regular daily practice one reaches a stage when one quickly enters the state of no intrusive thoughts upon beginning meditation. This is characterized as lack of reactivity during meditation. The Yoga Sutras of Patanjali says the regular practice over an extended period of time creates a new program within that ensures that other programs are prevented from activating when the meditation program begins. Thus, non-reactivity grows in stages and purifies the person. Sutra 1:16 says that this happens because of the Supreme *Puruṣha*, which is the connectivity with *Īśhvara.*
  [1:16. tat-param puruṣha-khyāteh+guna-vaitrishṇyam
  तत्-परम् पुरुष-ख्यातेः+गुण-वैतृष्ण्यम् ॥१-१६॥
  Because of that Supreme Puruṣha one becomes unaffected by the Gunas (nature of flow of energy).]
- Third, in stages, this non-reactive nature pervades the being all the time. Concurrently the connection with the Supreme *Puruṣha* along with the process of query within leads to imbibing the highest wisdom from the Source.
- This results in Self-Realization where all questions are answered, and one understands all created beings only as instruments of the cosmic play.

Distinctions in Meditative Connectivity

Meditation on a created object of *Prakṛiti* in Zone B or C in figure 27.1 is different from meditation on something subtle with no assumptions or meaning. Any meditation on anything created in Zone B or C can lead to quietening of the mind – like in many forms of mindfulness meditation. This leads to meditative connectivity within the subtle zone (spirits) in Zone B as stated in Sutra 1:19 of the Yoga Sutras. However, until the point of focus has no assumption or meaning, one cannot escape out of Zone B to reach Zone A. This is a careful distinction Patanjali makes in distinguishing between *Samāpatti* and *Samādhi* in the first *pāda*.

Importance of Seeking

While one can connect with Zone A (in Figure 27.1) unless one asks questions one will not receive the answers. In the Yoga Sutras, *Samyama*, in the third *pāda*, is the process of getting answers. In the first *pāda* of the Yoga Sutras, Sutra 1:17 indicates that the process to Self-Realization must begin with questioning.

> 1:17. vitarka-vichāra-ānanda-asmitā-(roopa[1])-anugamāt samprajñyātaha
>
> वितर्क-विचार-आनन्द-अस्मिता-(रूप)-अनुगमात् सम्प्रज्ञातः ॥१-१७॥
>
> ***Samprajñyā* (complete intuitive knowledge of Self-Realization) comes from questioning, reflection, deep peace within (in highest meditation – *Ānanda* of *Samādhi*) and with self-sense of one who experiences (*Asmitā*).**

In the *Vedānta* system, the concept of *Mumukśhu* (being a seeker) is considered very important. Unless one seeks one will not get the answers.

In spiritual progression, difficult circumstances in life typically become the point of initial query: why me? Why is this happening?

Distinguishing Between a Religious Seeker and Yogic Seeker

The key distinction between a religious seeker and a yogic seeker is that a religious seeker comes with the baggage of assumptions while a yogic seeker comes from the land of no assumptions. A religious seeker can only realize as far as their assumptions. But the yogic seeker can reach the highest, being true only to what one experiences without any assumptions. As experiences unfold, the yogic seeker keeps an open mind recognizing possibilities, but not concluding, of what the highest realization may be.

In initial stages, religious belief and discipline can help contain the wandering mind. But eventually they must be discarded, to become open, to experience the highest truth without assumptions. It is often said in the Buddhist tradition that if you meet the Buddha in meditation, slay the Buddha. Otherwise, the Buddha becomes the impediment from reaching the highest.

The one exception that does not serve as an impediment is visualization of the highest as the source of all knowledge and the intelligence of creation that is outside anything created. Patanjali points out in Sutra 3:50 that only by knowing the source as different (from the created) one can access all knowledge.

> 3:50. sattva-purușha-anyatā-khyāti-mātrasya sarva-bhāva-adhishṭhātritvam sarvajñyātritvam-cha
>
> सत्त्व-पुरुष-अन्यता-ख्याति-मात्रस्य सर्व-भाव-अधिष्ठातृत्वं सर्व-ज्ञातृत्वं च ॥३-५०॥
>
> **By knowing particularly that Sattva Purușha is another entity (different), one gets control over every orientation and knows everything.**

Unity Among Philosophical Divergences

Coming from the zone of mental analysis, which are governed by assumptions, great divergences in opinions arise between Monism, Qualified Monism and Dualism, in the philosophy of the nature of existence. These distinctions appear because of the window of perception. Yogic understanding shows all to be equally valid.

The concept in Monism is that everything is One. The distinctions we see in all of creation are simply illusion. The idea of illusion is that everything in existence is temporary like an actor on the stage, who goes back home to his natural state when the drama is over. This philosophical view is espoused by Advaita Vedānta and Buddhism.

Qualified Monism and Dualism is the standard in most religions of the world. God is distinct and different from the created. In Qualified Monism, there is the concept of merger with God in highest realization. In Dualism, the concept is only having nearness to God.

Place of Yogic Practices Towards the Goal of Self-Realization

Among the previous sections in the book, neither the Power of Breath NOR *Haṭha Yoga* NOR *Tantra Yoga* can lead one to Self-Realization without two key ingredients:

- Seeking to know by asking within,
- Cleaning the slate of all assumptions.

Of course, the assumption made from any yoga practice is that one has learned to become a pure observer. This also implies that one is not affected by outcomes of action – in effect, it is the idea of letting go. Where does one let go? It should be to whatever is the source of everything. This is the concept of *Īśhvara Praṇidhāna* or Surrender to God.

This is the reason the summary approach of all yoga practices for Self-Realization can be Sutra 2.1 (that was explained in the context of *Prāṇā-Kriyā* and *Kriyā Yoga* in Chapter 25).

2:1. tapah svādhyāya+eeshvara-praṇidhānāni kriyā-yogaha

तपः स्वाध्याय+ईश्वर-प्रणिधानानि क्रिया-योगः ॥२-१॥

Active Yoga (*Kriyā Yoga*) is Tapah (burning of embedded program patterns), self-study/contemplation (*Svādhyāya*) and surrender to God.

Surrender to God – letting go – is the basis of *tapas*, which is purification of the program content within us. *Svādhyāya* or inquiry within is the additional ingredient for Self-Realization. However, it is necessary to approach without strong assumptions.

This is the reason Patanjali mentions that *Ishavara Praṇidhāna* is what finally leads to *Samādhi* in the context of explaining *Niyama*, the second of the eight-fold yoga, after explaining the previous four *Niyamas* that include *tapas* and *svādhyāya*.

2:45. samādhi-siddhihi-eeshvara-praṇidhānāt

समाधि-सिद्धिः+ईश्वर-प्रणिधानात् ॥२-४५॥

Accomplishment of *Samādhi* is by surrender to God.

The concept of surrender to God that is beyond name and form and is the source of everything along with seeking to know leads to the highest level of wisdom – Self-Realization.

The concept of God may appear to make religious orientation desirable. Unfortunately, one can become a victim of assumptions that prevent access to direct connection with God.

Questions and Discussion Topics

1. Explain the distinction in creation between sentient and non-sentient beings and how it affects the ability to realize the Ultimate knowledge of existence.

2. A person wakes up one morning after seeing a dream where a god-form he prays to came and foretold him what would happen. What was the source of the dream within the dynamics of existence as explained in this chapter?

3. The dream of the person in question 2 comes out to be true a few days down the road. Would your answer about the source of the dream change?

4. Can a religious seeker attain the highest Ultimate knowledge explained in this chapter? If so, how? If not, why?

5. It is said one must seek to become Self-Realized. Why is that important? How does the system of yoga or any other philosophy explain it?

The journey towards Self-Realization begins with meditative practices. There are many ways to approach them. Unless there is transcendence into *Īśhvara*, the Supreme *Puruṣha*, one cannot access all knowledge – the Supreme Wisdom!

But every seeker must begin with the first steps of meditation.

PART VI – MEDITATIVE APPROACHES TO YOGA

28. Introduction to Meditation
    - Yoga Sutras on Meditation
    - Popular Scientific Approaches to Research on Meditation
    - Preparations to Begin a Meditation Regimen
    - Cultural Practices and Different Strokes for Different Folks

29. Meditation Approach for Deeper Relaxation
    - Focus on Activity that is Essentially Physical
    - Focus on the Activity and Breath
    - Focus on the Breath Alone
    - Focus on Breath and Visualization
    - Focus on Visualization Alone
    - Integration of Sound
    - The Special Place of Music and Sound
    - Deepening the Understanding of Niyama in Daily Living

30. Meditation Approach for Cosmic Connectivity
    - Niyama-based Approach to Cosmic Connectivity
    - Mantra-based Approach to Cosmic Connectivity
    - External Stimulation Approach to Cosmic Connectivity
    - Distinctions in Transcendence in the Spiritual Domain

31. Building a Meditative Routine in Daily Life
    - Importance of Same Place
    - Best Times for Practice
    - Meditation Practice for Beginners
    - Natural Meditative Observation at the end of a Yoga Class
    - Individual Meditative Practices for Beginners

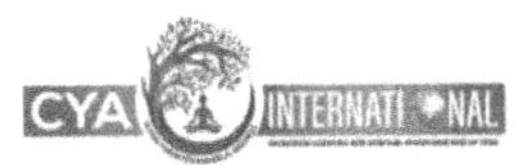

CHAPTER 28:

Introduction to Meditation

The Latin root word 'medi' means 'middle' and accordingly words like medicine, media, meditation etc., suggest the connecting role of something in the middle. So, what is the connecting role for meditation?

In meditation, one connects with one's core of existence (inner being). From a practical application, meditation can mean reflection with focus on something, quietening the mind, or it can also mean transcending awareness beyond the body, which is the focus of yoga. However, even reflection on something cannot begin without relaxation within, and some degree of self-awareness. The Yoga Sutras of Patanjali addresses all these three phases of common application of the word meditation, and the relaxation within with self-awareness. The relaxation within with self-awareness is called *Pratyāhāra*, while the three phases of meditation that follow are called *Dhāraṇā* (focus), *Dhyāna* (going beyond the mind or quietening the mind), and *Samādhi* (connecting beyond the body into the higher awareness of the cosmic flow and cosmic intelligence). These are the last four of the eight-fold, *Ashṭānga*, Yoga.

Accordingly, some schools of yoga think of meditative practices in four levels:

- Relaxation within with self-awareness
- One-pointed focus of the mind
- State of mindlessness
- Evoking Intuition in a higher state

In modern day practice of meditation among yoga practitioners, the types of meditation are classified into two categories:

- ***Mindfulness Meditation***, where the mind begins with a focus on one thing, with a goal of stopping the wandering tendency of the mind, eventually to observe the mind without reacting.

- ***Transcendental Meditation***[89], where the goal is to use focus to go beyond the inner quietness to connect with the cosmic awareness and awaken heightened intuitive potential.

Irrespective of the type of approach to meditation, functionally a quiet and focused mind leads to reduced stress, better health, greater productivity at work, a congenial interaction with colleagues, friends and family, and a general satisfaction with life. Most people pursue meditation to reduce stress resulting in better mental and physical health. However, transcendental meditation seeks higher awareness through cosmic connectivity to intuitively perceive the nature of existence, purpose and meaning of life, which in the body is temporal by nature. This objective is often stated as 'Self-Realization' or 'God-Realization.'

The field of psychology and medical sciences have conducted several research studies to objectively establish the experiences and benefits of regular practice of different types of meditation. The word meditation produced 9,121 research publications indexed in the National Library of Medicine on December 20, 2022, of which around 25% to 30% are publications based on experimental trials with subjects.

To approach any type of meditative practice the body and mind need preparation. It requires a firm resolution to allocate a time and space for meditation, and ensuring the body is balanced without discomfort, and the mind is not disturbed.

It is important to understand that the approach to meditative practices is embedded in every culture in many walks of life, where a ritualistic engrossment is called for. It could be in a religious setting, social setting (e.g. a Japanese tea ceremony) or done individually (artistic work, swimming, golf, etc.). Thus, we should view meditative potential in a broader traditional setting within the principles of yoga.

Yoga Sutras on Meditation

Having defined the four aspects of meditation – relaxation within with self-awareness, focus, stilling of the mind, development of intuition through cosmic connection – the Yoga Sutras of Patanjali (especially first and third *pādas*) can be described as the full manual of meditation: its process, the underlying factors, and the experiences. With the goal of developing heightened

---

[89] Transcendental meditation term used here should not be confused with just one method of such meditation used by the tradition of Maharishi Mahesh Yogi, but rather it falls into a category sometimes referred as 'closed-focused' meditation, while the mindfulness meditation is referred as 'open-focused.' In 'closed-focused' meditation, there is a subtle object of focus like a mantra with no meaning. In Buddhist practice this is referred to as *Shamatha*. In 'open-focused' meditation, the object is awareness of awareness, or in Buddhist tradition, *Vipāssana* (Pāli) or *Vipashyana* (Sanskṛit). This is called meta-cognition in modern neuroscience research. While *Shamatha* meditation opens intuitive potential with transcendence, the connectivity readily reveals the subtle *Prakṛiti* rather than *Īshvara*, since Buddhism is non-theistic. This is common in the initial stages of transcendence in all forms of transcendental meditation.

intuitive ability with cosmic connectivity (which is the real yoga), initial relaxation with self-awareness, focus and stilling of the mind are only considered earlier stages.

In the first *pāda* of the Yoga Sutras, which is an introductory overview of the text, the following points are notable:

- Being unaffected by the activations of our internal programs (*chitta vritti*) is the higher realization of yoga. [YS 1:2]
- This is attained by regular (and long term) practice. [YS 1:12]
- Achievement is proportional to effort. [YS 1:21]
- It can also be experienced by complete surrender to God. [YS 1:23] Sutras 1:24-29 describe God in terms that are beyond name and form. See Chapter 27.
- For common people afflicted by imbalances in physical and/or mental health [YS 1:30-31], one-pointed focus should be practiced to overcome these imbalances. [YS 1:32]
- Moderation in reaction may be the first step. [YS 1:33]
- Sutras 1:34-40 describe various ways of focusing.
- Complete engrossment into the point of focus is the first level of meditative experience. [YS 1:41]
- Awakening of intuition through cosmic connectivity [YS 1:48] is the result of one-pointed focus on something subtle that leads to engrossment and mindlessness. [YS 1:45-46]
- Such experiences can be transient, stimulated by the point of focus. [YS 1:47]
- Such transient experiences happen because the regular practice of the point of focus (cognitive behavioral stimulant) results in the building of an internal program (through neuroplasticity) that makes one unaffected by the other programs in the system (*chitta*) during meditation. [YS 1:50]
- When that too is overcome, the transient experience becomes permanent independent of any stimulation. [YS 1:51]

The second *pāda* of the Yoga Sutras discusses the root cause of our active mind-body-spirit system that makes meditation and intuitive realization difficult. Attitudinal and lifestyle optimization are considered the building blocks for progression. These include physical and breathing practices that lead to vibrational awareness within.

The third *pāda* goes into the deeper experiences of meditation. The meditative experience of the point of focus leading to mindlessness, and the subsequent arising of intuitive wisdom, is almost the entire discussion of this part of the Yoga Sutras. Sutras 1 to 6 restate and clarify the nature of the three zones of meditation (focus to mindlessness to intuitive wisdom). Sutras 9 to 12 describe in greater detail the movement from mindlessness to intuitive wisdom. Three steps are noted here:

- Cessation of thoughts; [YS 3:9]
- Establishing cosmic connectivity; [YS 3:11]

- Development of intuitive wisdom (relative to the point of focus which could be a question or a thought). [YS 3:12]

Thus, from a Yoga Sutras perspective, the following would be considered as conclusive guidance on meditation:

- One needs to discipline one's ethical lifestyle with balancing practices that include physical and breathing (energetic, e.g., *nādi śhuddhi*)) regimen.
- Daily, regular practice (at about the same time and place) on the same point of focus that has become a habit and leads to mindlessness over a period of time.
- Cultivation of moment-to-moment mindful awareness in all activities of life. This connotes purification of our programmed entity (*chitta*).
- This process leads to higher awareness that brings intuitive wisdom.

The Yoga Sutras of Patanjali is also clear that if one does not fully realize that one is only an instrument of the cosmic flow, it can lead one away from the higher realization. [YS 3:52] In particular, those with desires and strong ego may often think they have intuitive wisdom but may actually be reflecting their own biases devoid of higher wisdom.

Popular Scientific Approaches to Research on Meditation

The research publication platform indexed in the National Library of Medicine in the United States divides meditation into mindfulness meditation and transcendental meditation. The main reason for this division appears to be two great influences in this field coming to the United States: Buddhist mindfulness meditation techniques, and Maharishi Mahesh Yogi's Transcendental Meditation.

While most people think of breath related focus and Vipassana meditation techniques in mindfulness approaches, this approach is much wider. Even in the Buddhist tradition, such practices as creating mandalas and other activities done with full focus fall within this category. The field of psychology recognizes concentrative forms of meditation in writing, painting, cooking, and such expressive activities.

Typical benefits of meditation suggested by clinical research are mental health benefits[90] that suggest a positive orientation towards life, as well as cardiovascular benefits. The statement from the American Heart Association reads as: "Neurophysiological and neuroanatomical studies demonstrate that meditation can have long-standing effects on the brain, which provide

[90] Marchand WR. Mindfulness meditation practices as adjunctive treatments for psychiatric disorders. Psychiatr Clin North Am. 2013 Mar;36(1):141-52. doi: 10.1016/j.psc.2013.01.002. PMID: 23538083.

some biological plausibility for beneficial consequences on the physiological basal state and on cardiovascular risk."[91] Another summary view is that meditation serves to stimulate the body's self-regulation mechanism.[92]

It is interesting to note that in some studies long term transcendental meditators have higher levels of at least one catecholamine, specifically dopamine relative to epinephrine and norepinephrine, and in one instance higher level of fatty acids, and during meditation slightly higher level of cortisol compared to non-meditators, even though the whole psychophysiological system of meditators is in deeper relaxation.[93] This has invited scientific curiosity as to what may be happening within.[94]

The following represents another summary of physiological responses in transcendental meditation: "Based upon a wide spectrum of physiological data on TM *(transcendental meditation)*, we hypothesize that meditation is an integrated response with peripheral circulatory and metabolic changes subserving increased central nervous activity. Consistent with the subjective description of meditation as a very relaxed but, at the same time, a very alert state, it is likely that such findings during meditation as increased cardiac output, probable increased cerebral blood flow, and findings reminiscent of the "extraordinary" character of classical reports: apparent cessation of CO2 generation by muscle, fivefold plasma AVP[95] elevation, and EEG synchrony play critical roles in this putative response."[96]

---

[91] Levine GN, Lange RA, Bairey-Merz CN, Davidson RJ, Jamerson K, Mehta PK, Michos ED, Norris K, Ray IB, Saban KL, Shah T, Stein R, Smith SC Jr; American Heart Association Council on Clinical Cardiology; Council on Cardiovascular and Stroke Nursing; and Council on Hypertension. Meditation and Cardiovascular Risk Reduction: A Scientific Statement From the American Heart Association. J Am Heart Assoc. 2017 Sep 28;6(10):e002218. doi: 10.1161/JAHA.117.002218. PMID: 28963100; PMCID: PMC5721815.

[92] Sampaio CV, Lima MG, Ladeia AM. Meditation, Health and Scientific Investigations: Review of the Literature. J Relig Health. 2017 Apr;56(2):411-427. doi: 10.1007/s10943-016-0211-1. PMID: 26915053.

[93] Cooper R, Joffe BI, Lamprey JM, Botha A, Shires R, Baker SG, Seftel HC. Hormonal and biochemical responses to transcendental meditation. Postgrad Med J. 1985 Apr;61(714):301-4. doi: 10.1136/pgmj.61.714.301. PMID: 3895206; PMCID: PMC2418240.

Infante JR, Torres-Avisbal M, Pinel P, Vallejo JA, Peran F, Gonzalez F, Contreras P, Pacheco C, Roldan A, Latre JM. Catecholamine levels in practitioners of the transcendental meditation technique. Physiol Behav. 2001 Jan;72(1-2):141-6. doi: 10.1016/s0031-9384(00)00386-3. PMID: 11239991.

[94] Since dopamine is referred as the 'chemical messenger' of the brain and nervous system associated with pleasure, support for blood pressure and blood flow to the brain, and since cortisol helps to make the cell membranes more porous for rapid cellular respiration to produce energy more rapidly, one can relate this to the yogic concept of conserving and increasing energy for permitting transcendence.

[95] Arginine vasopressin (AVP) is a peptide hormone synthesized in the hypothalamus and secreted from nerve terminals within the posterior pituitary gland. Secretion is primarily under osmoregulatory control and levels rise in plasma in response to a body water deficit and are suppressed in response to water overload. By increasing water absorption (from the kidney) AVP can increase peripheral vascular resistance and raise arterial blood pressure.

[96] Jevning R, Wallace RK, Beidebach M. The physiology of meditation: a review. A wakeful hypometabolic integrated response. Neurosci Biobehav Rev. 1992 Fall;16(3):415-24. doi: 10.1016/s0149-7634(05)80210-6. PMID: 1528528.

Preparations to Begin a Meditation Regimen

Meditation is about reducing the chatter of the mind, going towards mindlessness, and activating one's internal transmitter to connect into the cosmic intelligence. To quieten the chatter of the mind one needs to be free of overwhelming worries, which requires a disciplined and honest lifestyle. Activating the transmitter requires a lot of energy and internal focus. Accordingly, the preparation requires the first few of the eight-fold (*Ashṭānga*) yoga (*Yama, Niyama, Āsana, Prāṇāyāma*) that provide systematic guidance.

- **Living life true to one's conscience without regrets (*Yama*)** – Mind is the biggest consumer of our energy and is also the cause of mental stress in our system. If there are conflicts within us, one can never get adequate peace within to begin meditation. This calls for honest, jealousy-free living as a thinking human being who will not wantonly hurt anyone else.
  [Life is such where many people live with guilt and regrets because of self-interested living that may have hurt others. Daily lifestyle practices, rituals that require focus, usually help people to get out of it by realizing the nature of temporal existence and learning to forgive oneself. Such practices could include yoga *āsanas*, breathing practices, sports, engaging in music as a listener or performer, cooking or any artistic practice that becomes a ritual. Religious methods of forgiving oneself could also be part of it.]

- **Regularity in habitual living (*Niyama*)** makes living almost a ritual. Going to sleep about the same time every day, waking up about the same time, and having ritual practices of daily living makes one in sync with the circadian rhythm, and helps to calm and balance one's energy flow. Religion could have a role for some people as part of this. A sense of contentment and faith in God helps to keep the daily ritual and be in good balance. As part of ritualistic living, having an assigned place and time for each activity including meditation and self-inquiry is very helpful.

- **Physical toning and alignment (*āsana*)** can come from various activities. However, in yoga it should come in a way to stimulate alignment and energy, rather than tiring oneself by working out.

- **Breathing practices (*Prāṇāyāma*)**, as we have noted earlier, are perhaps the easiest way to bring balance to the mind and optimize one's energy.

Depending on the person's nature and state of imbalance, an expert may recommend different types of preparatory steps for different people. For example, walking meditation with focus on the breath, with two strides for inhalation and four strides for exhalation, can have a strong calming effect for those with disturbed minds. Ritualistic jogging or lap swimming can have the same effect. Systematic *Prāṇāyāma* practices can come thereafter.

However, the initiative must come from self-motivation. For most adults, this usually happens when they have faced difficult circumstances in life and are seeking to understand why such things happen to them. Those who come because of strong persuasion by well-wishers usually find it difficult to keep regularity in practice. Therefore, those in yoga should avoid strong persuasion towards those whom they wish well – a mere encouragement is enough. As part of life, yoga will find those who are ready according to the cosmic plan.

Cultural Practices and Different Strokes for Different Folks

Every culture has its own traditions that are helpful for stress reduction. It could be religious practices, or it could be something as simple as a social dance or group singing, or something like the quiet Japanese tea ceremony. In modern times, exercising has become a global culture. Recognizing the yogic aspects of any cultural practice and helping the learner to use that as the stepping-stone to further one's meditative interest would perhaps be easiest and most suitable.

Several examples are provided in the next chapter on Meditation Approach(es) for Deeper Relaxation, and also in the chapters in the next part of the book on Bhakti Yoga and Role of Religious Practices in Yoga, and on Yoga in Non-Religious Practices.

Questions and Discussion Topics

1. What are the steps to advance towards higher meditative experiences according to the Yoga Sutras?

2. What are the differences between Mindfulness Meditation practices and Transcendental Meditation practices? Is there any relationship with the concept of *Samāpatti* and *Samādhi*?

3. How do *Āsanas* and *Prāṇāyāma* techniques of *Haṭha Yoga* take one towards meditation? Analyse within the context of four levels of meditative quietness or awareness mentioned in this chapter.

4. How can one's lifestyle be helpful towards meditation?

5. Are scientific studies on meditation practices measured through physiology and psychology helpful in any way for a yoga instructor or yoga aspirant?

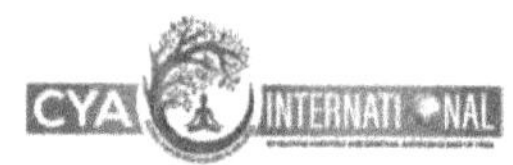

CHAPTER 29:

Meditation Approach for Deeper Relaxation

Focus on anything with effortless and complete engrossment leads to deeper relaxation. This is the meditative approach for deeper relaxation.

Engrossment on something external, called *Samāpatti* in the Yoga Sutras [1:41], only leads to deep relaxation, whereas engrossment on something subtle leads to *Samādhi* or cosmic connectivity [YS 1:44-46], which is the subject of the next chapter. The concept of 'subtle' is explained in the next chapter that distinguishes the *Samāpatti* type of meditation from the *Samādhi* type of meditation.

In common parlance, the *Samāpatti* type of meditation can be called mindfulness meditation. For most people for whom the mind tends to quickly wander, this type of practice is a good stepping-stone to purify the *nādis* (channels of communication) to allow for the higher *Samādhi* type of meditation. In fact, that is exactly the role of *Āsana, Prāṇāyāma* and *Pratyāhāra* in the eight-fold (*Ashṭānga*) yoga. So let us explore different approaches to this form of mindfulness or *Samāpatti* type of meditation. The common aspect in all these approaches is the focus of the mind.

- ***Focus on Activity that is essentially Physical*** that aligns the body and quietens the mind
- ***Focus on Activity (physical) and Breath*** that aligns the body and vitality flow, and quietens the mind
- ***Focus on Breath Alone*** that aligns vitality flow and quietens the mind
- ***Focus on Breath and Visualization*** that aligns vitality flow and the mind
- ***Focus on Visualization Alone*** that aligns the mind
- ***Integration of Sound*** (Music, Lyrics, Verbal Instructions) with focus on any of the above that enhances the impact

Focus on Activity that is Essentially Physical

This type of meditative practice involves activity done for no motivated reason other than enjoying the moment. They can range from *āsana* practice, artistic activities, religious activities to sports activities that also include what people commonly regard as exercising. Even though there may be an initial sense of motivated activity like for better health or religious fervor, the enjoyment of the activity dilutes the motivation and allows one to become absorbed into the activity – what we call 'being in the moment.' While the greatest meditative absorption comes from daily regular practice, these activities can have a meditative effect even though they may be intermittent.

Artistic activities range over a broad spectrum that can be generic or cultural.

Generic activities include painting, knitting, stitching, cooking, sculpting, diary writing, and such other activities. When a person's daily occupational activity – whether it is something more physical like tilling the land, or something less physical like gathering data and writing a report – becomes absorbing, that too can fit into this category.[97]

Cultural elements, that often border on religious customs as well, include a much wider category of activities that can include daily ritual activities and activities that are part of festivals.

- Daily ritual activities are present in most culture whether religiously associated or not. Islamic Salat practice is an example of daily religious activity that combines physical movements along with mental affirmations that absorbs the attention of the faithful.
  In South India, there is a daily practice of washing the immediate area outside the threshold of the home at dawn or sunrise time, and to draw with rice powder, a symmetrical design with a dot in the middle, on the ground. It is not a singular design, but rather the individual artist has liberty to create any design and of any size. This artistic work is called *Kolum*. While this is said to symbolize the auspicious beginning of a new day, after a while it is a daily activity done for no reason other than with complete absorption. This same type of practice is done on sites where religious or auspicious activities are to be performed. This is also called as *Alpana* and *Rangoli* (when done with colors) in North India, and fits within the same category as Buddhist *Mandalas*.
- Festival activities in most cultures, that may also be religiously associated, may involve ritual walking, bathing, cooking, etc. done individually or as a group. Examples are there in every tradition. Religious activities that involve physical action have this same meditative effect for the believer who gets absorbed in it. Pilgrimage is one such type of activity.

Sports activities range over a broad spectrum.

- Individual Sports - Jogging, running, biking, swimming, and such form of repetitive movements that are generic in nature done for at least 20 minutes non-stop can have this effect of absorption, even though people may engage in these activities motivated by health reasons. Unconventional sports like hiking, mountain climbing, white-water rafting or gliding can serve the same purpose once absorption takes place after the initial jolt.

---

[97] This can happen only when one does the activity <u>without pressure</u> of demands from others or from one's own expectations.

- Partner and Team Sports – While they may begin competitively, when full absorption occurs in physical movement and mental interaction with the sport and the team players, it can lead to the same effect.

Meditation effect is possible from absorption in any activity. This can happen in every activity we do during the day as we evoke our yogic nature. As Sutra 1:40 from the Yoga Sutras states engrossment can happen with focus on anything minute or anything big.

1:40. paramāNu-parama.mahattvāntah+asya vasheekāraha

परमाणु-परम.महत्त्वान्तः+अस्य वशीकारः ॥१-४०॥

One can be drawn in by the smallest (atomic particle) to the largest magnitude.

FALLACY OF STEP COUNTERS

The infancy of medical physiology is most present in the fad of step counters and the idea of burning calories. While it is true that intake of calories exceeding those burnt result in putting on extra weight, the role of mindfulness in impacting weight control is completely lost.

From a yogic standpoint, steps don't count, but rather the mindful absorption in walking leading to deep relaxation and inner awareness is the essence. The deep relaxation within, results in the dual aspect of sensory realization of the right food and joyful satiety, and the optimization of the metabolic rate. With optimized metabolic rate and mindfully guided eating, there can never be excess calories.

Focus on the Activity and Breath

One of the most effective mindfulness practices is walking meditation noted in the previous chapter. This involves focusing on the breath and taking twice as many strides in exhalation as in inhalation (e.g., two strides with inhalation and four strides with exhalation). The combined focus on the physical movement and the breath integration, with the eyes glued to the path of walking prevents mind-wandering.

The Tantra approach of *Prāṇakriyā* in *āsana* practice seeks to fulfill the same objective. Tai-chi in its practice does the same. There can also be other practices that fit within this category.

Focus on the Breath Alone

Mindfulness practice on the breath alone (without physical movement) requires a good posture that keeps the spine straight. The various breathing practices noted in the second part of the book "The Power of Breath in Yoga" are amenable to this practice. Also, the Buddhist technique of *Ānā-Pānā* breath fits within this category.

Focus on Breath and Visualization

Vipassana meditation of the Buddhist tradition is a good example of breath and visualization. Another similar meditative practice is to visualize inhaling vitality and exhaling out unwanted residue and cleansing our inner being.

YOGA NIDRĀ – A DEEP RELAXATION PRACTICE

Yoga Nidrā, presented to the US Military as I-Rest, has been very effective for Post Traumatic Stress Disorder (PTSD), and in many ways has characteristics of Cognitive Behavioral Therapy (CBT). However, the ability to evoke CBT in the case of PTSD comes from the deep relaxation that allows one to be an observer without reacting to traumatic memories.

While there are different variations in the practice, in both steps and duration (varying from 30 minutes to two hours), the common element is focused relaxation of the muscles of the body, building of self-awareness and learning to be a pure observer. The relaxation of the muscles can initially involve some mild physical motion along with breath, and thereafter it is only being an observer. In the AHYMSIN tradition, there is focus on specific points in the body where one mindfully relaxes.

Focus on Visualization Alone

Guided meditation techniques that are solely based on visualization, or any meditation technique that focuses on a pleasant imagery (like a mountain, waterfalls, etc.) falls within this category. In meditative practices of *Haṭha Yoga* visual observation with steady focus with intention of absorption is called *Laya Yoga.*

Integration of Sound

It is common to see people jogging with earphones playing their favorite music. In group or festival activities it is common to have thematic background music. Dance forms, whether it be ballet or Bharata-Nātyam or the whirling dervishes (Mevlevis) of Turkey, have music as an integral component. Verbal instructions are generally part of guided meditation practices. Such sounds combined with other engrossing activities serve to deepen the absorption into the activity.

DEEP RELAXATION FROM POWER OF DANCE FOR A PSYCHIATRIST

Psychiatrists have the highest suicide rates among physicians[98]. In our experience, we have found that a high percentage of psychiatrists become weird or off-centered in social interaction after decades of psychiatric practice. We were surprised to find a completely balanced psychiatrist during one of our Continuing Medical Education courses. Upon sharing with her what we observed with other psychiatrists, and observing her as different, we inquired about what made her keep her balance.

She affirmed that the daily unwanted vibrations she gets from her psychiatric practice would make her unbalanced. However, what saved her daily was her one hour of *Bharata Nātyam* practice immediately upon return from her patient practice. She would turn on the music and just dance for one hour and she would be fully relieved of all the unwanted vibrations, and then carry on her daily life as a householder, mother, and normal person. She noted that without her daily *Bharata Nātyam* practice she would be a psychiatric mess.

This is a real-life experience of Rajan Narayanan from over a decade of teaching physicians that include a significant number of psychiatrists in Life in Yoga's Continuing Medical Education program.

The Special Place of Music and Sound

Music or chanting with lyrics, where the listener or singer focuses on the lyrics leads to mindfulness meditation. However, when the focus is only on the sound, then it becomes subtle, especially if you can feel the sound within even when the external playing stops. Thus, music or sound vibrations have a special place where it can be mindful and deeply relaxing, or can also lead to transcendence, evoking intuitive capability.

---

[98] General population has a suicide rate of about 10 per 100,000, while for physicians it is around 30 per 100,000 and for psychiatrists it is about 60 per 100,000. https://www.corporatewellnessmagazine.com/article/addressing-the-alarming-trends-in-suicides-among-healthcare-professionals https://en.wikipedia.org/wiki/Suicide_among_doctors#:~:text=In%20the%20United%20States%20of,double%20that%20of%20general%20population.

MEDITATIVE ORIGIN OF *RĀGAS* (MELODY)

The traditional classical music of India is organized around *rāgas*,[99] traditional melodic and harmonic structures that were heard in the meditation of seer-musicians in much the same way as mantras. In this way, *ragas* are intended to modulate *rasa* (mood or emotion), and in this way can serve a therapeutic as well as an aesthetic purpose.

This same type of effect has been suggested in all traditional music systems of the world.[100]

Deepening the Understanding of Niyama in Daily Living

Much of *Niyama*, the second of the eight-fold yoga, can be understood in the context of mindfulness meditation where motivation and reaction to activity is diluted. By becoming absorbed in daily ritual activities with an attitude of surrender to God, the *Niyama* process results in purification of the *nādis*. The combined aspect of seeking to know (*Svādhyāya*) and surrender to God (*Īśhvara Praṇidhāna*) results in the transcendence and evokes intuitive wisdom in *Samādhi* [YS 2:45].

Questions and Discussion Topics

1. Can any activity be made into a mindfulness practice? If not, why? If so, how?

2. Is there a difference in the meditative relaxation between mindful slow walking watching the breath and jogging or running listening to rhythmic music? If not, why? If so, how?

3. Try cooking with meditative absorption into the cooking. Then, compare the effect on yourself and the food when cooking is done without meditative absorption – when your hands are moving adding ingredients or chopping or grinding while your mind is on a phone conversation or a television program. Detail the observed results.

4. If you were guiding an aspirant, new to yoga, on the practice to adopt for meditation, how will you determine what is the best mindfulness, relaxation practice for the aspirant?

5. What are the differences between Mindfulness Meditation practices and Transcendental Meditation practices? Is there any relationship with the concept of *Samāpatti* and *Samādhi*?

---

[99] *Rāga* in the Yoga Sutras refer to attractions. In the music world it is the attraction that captivates the *Chitta* into meditative absorption.

[100] Danielou A. (1995). **Music and the Power of Sound: The Influence of Tuning and Interval on Consciousness.** Rochester Vermont: Inner Traditions

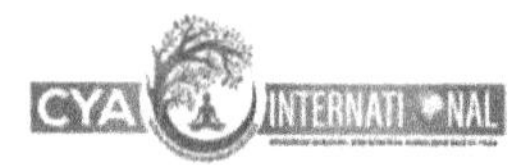

CHAPTER 30:

Meditation Approach for Cosmic Connectivity

The concept of focus on something <u>subtle</u> leading to *Samādhi* that evokes intuitive wisdom is noted in the Yoga Sutras[1:44-46]. In the third *pāda* (*Vibhuti Pāda*), the concept of *Samyama* as the coming together of *Dhāraṇā*, *Dhyāna* and *Samādhi* [YS 3:4] is explained, whereby intuitive answers to the questions focused in *Dhāraṇā* are revealed [YS 3:5-6]. All of this happens by Cosmic Connectivity as explained in the Yoga Sutra [1:48]. So, what exactly is this focus on something <u>subtle</u>?

The concept of something subtle is related to something that cannot be physical. It can be a silent mantra with no meaning or intent attached to it that vibrates in the mind, or a question related to the metaphysics of what we observe in the physical world of the past or present. Absorption into an external activity (leading to mindfulness meditation) is different from absorption into a silent mantra or metaphysical query (that leads to *Samādhi*). When the *nādis* get purified the connectivity is established, and that allows for the query to be answered intuitively.

Meditation approach to cosmic connectivity can be divided into three categories:

- *Niyama*-based Approach
- Mantra-based Approach
- External Stimulation Approach

Niyama-based Approach to Cosmic Connectivity

This is the fundamental approach recommended by the Yoga Sutras. By leading a life that upholds *Yama* and *Niyama*, one can purify the *nādis* by dissipation of the programmed elements (*kleśha* and *karma*) within. When the *nādis* are purified, the connectivity is established and the mere mental inquiry (*Dhāraṇā*) results in realization of the answer intuitively. This is the *Samyama* process noted in the Yoga Sutras.

It is important to note that unless one seeks with purified *nādis*, like in the *Dhāraṇā* aspect of *Samyama*, the answers don't come. Two examples here illustrate this point.

As stated in chapter 27, in the *Vedāntic* system, as noted by Shankarācharya, one should be a *mumukśhu* or Seeker. Without seeking, the answers may not come.

The second example is that of Ramana Maharishi. In his highly purified state of *nādis*, all he had to ask was "Who am I" and he realized it. [This is *Shāmbhopāya* of Kashmir Shaivism.] But because he had no need to go through the conventional yogic purification process, the only process for Self-Realization that he could share with other seekers was to ask within "Who am I". And for most of the world, it led them nowhere, since the *nādis* were not pure enough.

Mantra-based Approach to Cosmic Connectivity

The mantra-based approach was popularized by Maharishi Mahesh Yogi. The principle of this approach is to find a personal mantra that is the equal and opposite of one's vibration. One's vibration is the composite expression of all the programs (*kleśha* and *karma*) within when one is in a normally peaceful state. This personal mantra – harmonic vibration – neutralizes the vibrations of one's innate programs temporarily (while the mantra is in use) which allows one to establish temporary cosmic connectivity and imbibe intuitive answers. [YS 4:1]

Such an approach is a faster process than the *Niyama*-based approach. It has potential benefits and pitfalls since complete purification may not have happened. [It is not necessary to have complete purification for temporary connectivity during meditation.]

The substantial benefit from such daily practices is that one gets deep insight into one's role in living, and naturally gravitates towards less reactivity. The inner guidance from the connectivity, sometimes called the voice of the conscience, provides direction towards conducting one's role in the cosmic flow. Therefore, such meditative practices are encouraged for students from a young age.[101]

The pitfalls are two-fold in nature:

- ***Inappropriate Mantra*** - When an inappropriate mantra is used, it can create instability within the person that can reflect in physical or mental instability. If such a mistake is made, a highly spiritual master can find a compensatory mantra to cure the problem.

  Also, if a mantra is not used regularly, it may no longer work. This is because the mantra when selected is a harmonic vibration relative to the internal programs (*kleśha* and *karma*) at a single point of time that temporarily stills all other internal programs. By daily usage it creates and maintains a new program within – a meditation inducing program – that irrespective of the purification of and hence changes in the internal programs (*kleśha* and *karma*) continues to work even though it is no longer harmonic to the vibrations of the changed programs. [YS 1:50] With disuse of the mantra, the meditation inducing program of the mantra wears away over time and is no longer

---

[101] Maharishi Mahesh Yogi used to claim that this process would make one more successful in life – the idea being in sync with the cosmic flow. Accordingly, he called his organization in India Maharishi Institute for Creative Intelligence.

helpful for meditation. Once the meditation program wears away by disuse, the person's internal programs having changed will require a new harmonic vibration.

- ***Misuse of Cosmic Intelligence*** - Spiritual maturity allows one to understand one's individual *Dharma*. Without adequate spiritual maturity, when one's individual *Dharma* is not understood, it can lead to misuse of the abilities derived from cosmic connectivity. This creates a spiritual regression, and the person could become mentally dysfunctional within a lifetime, and there could be repercussions in future lifetimes as well.

  However, when a spiritually evolved master finds the mantra for a seeker, only those who are qualified will be able to obtain their mantra. This will ensure that those not spiritually qualified will be eliminated from this option. [This is the *Shāktopāya* approach of Kashmir Shaivism.] While the risk of deviation from *Dharma* is minimized for this group, it is not fully eliminated.

External Stimulation Approach to Cosmic Connectivity

There are many external stimulation approaches to enhance cosmic connectivity – some of which are temporary, and some inappropriate.

Psychedelic drugs like psilocybin and ayahuasca can provide temporary *Samādhi* state stimulating cosmic connectivity and providing intuitive answers. This is noted in Yoga Sutras 4:1. This approach has been used by some traditional healers for divining problems for those who seek to be healed. In a clinical study by Johns Hopkins University use of psilocybin by those who don't have strong belief systems and normally in good health led to life transforming positive attitudes.[102]

The downside is that some people can develop persisting hallucinations and may become dysfunctional in life. From a yogic perspective we do not recommend this approach.

Intention of Evolved Master can temporarily clear the *nādis* like a mantra and enable a person to experience connectivity beyond the body. This is called *Śhaktīpāt* and is considered an initiation. Without suitable mantra or invocation of this evolved master, in each meditation session, this cannot be sustained.

This is not a recommended approach for two reasons. A Realized Master understanding himself or herself as only an instrument of the cosmic flow will not want a seeker to develop dependence on him or her. And the seeker can also limit themselves by such dependence. Such an approach has developed because of misrepresentation of the Guru system.

---

[102] Griffiths RR, Johnson MW, Richards WA, Richards BD, McCann U, Jesse R. Psilocybin occasioned mystical-type experiences: immediate and persisting dose-related effects. Psychopharmacology (Berl). 2011 Dec;218(4):649-65. doi: 10.1007/s00213-011-2358-5. Epub 2011 Jun 15. PMID: 21674151; PMCID: PMC3308357.

Sacred places, suitable gems and stones can temporarily clear the *nādis* to allow a person to experience cosmic connectivity. Again, this would be temporary and may be used as a boost for one's personal practice in initial stages and at a later stage should be allowed to drop.

Clothing, seat and lighting a lamp can impact meditation quality. Use of silk or wool for a seat and for clothing is considered best to keep the energy of meditation focused and cohesive, and thus improve the experience of meditation. Similar use of deer skin and tiger skin[103] for the seat is considered useful. Lighting a lamp or candle and especially feeling its energy can have similar impact of improving meditation.

Environmental-Geophysical stimulants include astronomical positions (including time of day) and also such factors as vegetation, orientation, etc. Some examples are the following. Eclipses, particularly solar eclipses are considered optimal for enhanced experience in meditation. Sunrise, sunset and high noon are considered better for meditation. Orientation to east at sunrise, west at sunset and north at noon is considered helpful. Meditation under a Peepal tree or Norfolk Pine can lead to higher experience in meditation, while meditation under a Bilwa tree can be depressing towards meditation. However, use of Bilwa leaves or twigs under the seat while meditating can promote better meditation.

ROLE OF PYRAMIDAL STRUCTURES TO AID MEDITATION

The form of structure (and type of compound in the edge of the structure) influencing the flow of waves to carry intent is recognized in cosmic connectivity. Pyramidal structures are recognized to have this property. Pyramidal structures helping the body and mind to become integrated into the cosmic flow, resulting in healing and other experiences, have been noted.[104]

Almost all religious structures tend to have a pyramidal or dome-shaped structure above the sanctum.

PYRAMID OF MERKINE[105]

In Lithuania, there is pyramid called the Pyramid of Merkine, located within Dzūkija National Park, where one can feel the meditative effect of a pyramidal structure. In 1990, a young boy (whom Stephen Parker met as an adult) saw, a short distance from his house, a great light and went to investigate, thinking there might be a fire. Instead, he found an angel who instructed him to build a pyramid there for prayer and meditation. One might think that this was some kind of hallucination, except that neighbors came from some distance having seen the light several miles away, also thinking the house might be on fire. Over time, the project attracted the attention of international supporters including a group of architects who designed and supervised the building of a beautiful glass pyramid within which one can feel a meditative field.

---

103 Yogic approach is not to hunt animals for their skin, but rather to use the skin of dead animals, if at all. However, as one advances in yoga, these are irrelevant.

104 Books by Sam Osmanagich on Pyramids document some of these observations: Meditation at the Planet's Sacred Sites; A New Archaeology: Megaliths and the Energy of the Planet; The Mayan Cosmic Mission.

105 https://www.atlasobscura.com/places/pyramid-of-merkine

Invoking or imbibing another suitable entity of the past or present can provide enhancement in cosmic connectivity. Invocation of an evolved spirit as explained in the Yoga Sutras 2:44 and 1:37 can elevate one's meditative experience. Also, a life partner whose vibration is harmonic can have the same effect. This approach is considered acceptable in the initial stages. [Incidentally, all the above-mentioned external stimulants can be considered *chittas* or programmed entities noted in Sutra 1:37 that can temporarily aid enhancement in meditation, although desirability of some of them are in question.]

Grace of God as noted in Sutra 1:23 can lead to rapid and quick progress and experience of the highest. However, the conception of God must be beyond name and form, with only such attributes as the unmanifest beyond the cycle of birth and death and the source of everything and all knowledge. This is considered a desirable external stimulus. While God can be an external stimulus, it is also inherently assumed in the other approaches to higher cosmic connectivity.

While many of these can impact the quality of meditation and some of which may not be desirable, finally one should aspire to be rid of all external crutches, other than the grace of God for higher experience in meditation.

However, even a single experience of transcendence can have a life changing effect, even if it is a temporary stimulation. One's assumption about life may change permanently and take the person into the higher meditative quest by deeper purification from being a pure observer all the time. This is expressed in Sutras 23 to 26 of the fourth *pāda* of the Yoga Sutras.

4:23. drashtri-drishya-uparaktam chittam sarvaartham

द्रष्टृ-दृश्य-उपरक्तम् चित्तम् सर्वार्थम् ॥४-२३॥

(In the motionless state) The *chitta* understands everything (makes full sense) as the seer observes the coloring (or superimposition) of what is seen. [The still *chitta* allows the *Puruṣha* to be known as its presence colors the still *chitta*]

4:24. tat-asankhyeya-vaasanaabhih-chitram-api parartham sanhatya-kaaritvaat

तत्-असंख्येय-वासनाभिः-चित्रम्-अपि परार्थम् संहत्य-कारित्वात् ॥४-२४॥

Even though it (the *chitta*) has a picture of innumerable impressions, it is made to act in conjunction (with and) for a higher purpose.

4:25. Viśheṣha-darshina aatma-bhaava-bhaavanaa-nivrittihi

विशेष-दर्शिन आत्म-भाव-भावना-निवृत्तिः ॥४-२५॥

From the special sight, one is free of the idea of the self (as the doer, controller, etc.).

4:26. tadaa-viveka-nimnam kaivalya-praagbhaaram chittam

तदा विवेक-निम्नं कैवल्य-प्राग्भारम् चित्तम् ॥४-२६॥

From that low level discernment, the *chitta* gravitates towards *Kaivalyam* (freedom in isolation).

PERSONAL MANTRA SELECTION IN THE VEDIC SYSTEM

In the Vedic system mantras are intuitively sensed by an advanced yogi for seekers. However, the intuitive discovery is based on finding the equal and opposite vibration (harmonic vibration) of the composite vibration of all the programs that are running within the seeker. When intuitive abilities are not advanced enough certain rule-based approach may provide some guidance.

There are four anchor mantras for four life orientations. In young age, one has curiosity to know about everything. The overdrive of curiosity results in vibrations for which the harmonic vibration is *AYM*. In later age, one seeks to advance in career and do better in material life. The harmonic vibration then is *ŚHREEM*. In advanced age, one has fewer material interests, and one seeks to know what is beyond life. For this orientation, the harmonic vibration is *HREEM*. Finally, when one has the attitude of acceptance without reactivity living in the physical world, it is considered the indication of a completely purified *chitta*. Then, the vibration that increases meditative connectivity is *OM* that leads to Self-Realization. [These mantras are in sync with the *Varna Ashrama* view of the four roles of living in the Vedic system, and are also associated respectively with *Sarasvatī*, the goddess/spirit of learning, *Lakśhmī*, the goddess/spirit of material prosperity, and *Durgā* or *Śhaktī*, the goddess/spirit of the energy of creation, and *Īśhvara* which is the Ultimate God.]

[Typically, most adults have a mix of the four orientations, and none of the four mantras may be suited perfectly. To account for different combinations, it is said that Maharishi Mahesh Yogi devised 14 mantras.]

A secondary element of mantra selection is the level of activity in the three major and higher *nādis*. When the *Mukhya Prāṇa Nādi* (along the spine) carrying vitality is in overdrive the harmonic mantra is AYM. When there is physical imbalance (in the *Suṣhumnā*), the harmonic vibration is IM. When there is inadequate cosmic connectivity (in the *Ātma Nādi*), the vibration is OM. For these three mantras depending on the *chakras* that have imbalance using the *chakra* vibrations as prefix usually provides a suitable personal mantra.

Distinctions in Transcendence in the Spiritual Domain

Transcending in meditative connectivity essentially takes awareness beyond the physical world. As clarified in Chapter 27, when meditation focuses on any spirit, name, or form, that limits access to God, the Supreme Source, *Īśhvara*, that is beyond spirit.

The early experience of transcendence makes one more aware of the cosmic flow (*Prakṛiti*) that is outside, and also includes, the three-dimensional world we experience – the zone of spirits and the physical world (Zones B and C in Figure 27.1 in chapter 27). However, the destination of Self-Realization is beyond that into the cosmic intelligence (*Īśhvara,* Zone A in Figure 27.1). That can only be approached after complete purification and with no assumptions. This is the reason that the Yoga Sutras approach is best focusing on purification, rather than relying on external stimulants to gain temporary connection into the cosmic flow. The value of the temporary connection is to stimulate one towards the purification approach of the Yoga Sutras.

Questions and Discussion Topics

1. A person who attends your daily yoga class comes to you in a disturbed state of mind one day after being laid off from his job. He is not financially insecure but is worried about his future career and advancement in life. What type of meditation practice would you recommend and why?

2. Analyse the differences and benefits (or otherwise) between the following types of meditation techniques based on the yoga mechanism of Chapter 27 and Chapter 5. Consider spiritual connectivity and healing potential of these techniques. [If you are not familiar with the techniques you may find videos on Youtube.]
   - *Vipassana* Meditation of the Buddhist tradition
   - *Shamatha* Meditation of the Buddhist tradition
   - Brahma Kumari type of meditation
   - Harmonic, Mantra Meditation.

3. What type of meditation practice would you consider best for your regular class group? Explain rationale.

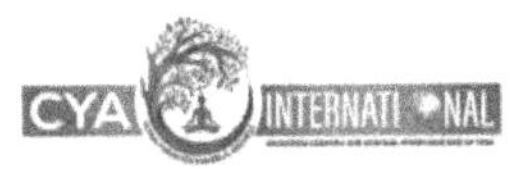

CHAPTER 31:

Building a Meditative Routine in Daily Life

Since the connection of *Niyama* (of 8-fold Yoga) with meditation has already been established, consistent with the preparations for regular meditation noted in Chapter 28, one should plan daily meditation practice – preferably two or three times a day, about the same time and preferably in the same place.

As is obvious now for an instructor, daily and regular meditation is the requirement for progressive higher experience and understanding of yoga. After each meditation session, the calmness within allows one to be less reactive and more of a mindful observer. As one keeps regularity in practice (e.g., two to three times a day), over an extended period, mindful observation becomes the general nature. Thus, one can observe mindfulness in all activities throughout the day.

For mantra-based meditation about 20 minutes two to three times a day is recommended. For other types of practices longer durations may be more appropriate and could be once or twice a day. A total daily commitment of about an hour or two for meditation (in single or among multiple sessions) is considered highly desirable for progress in yoga.

Importance of Same Place

As we meditate in a specific place daily, the meditative vibrations adhere to the place and help you to get into a meditative state faster and accelerates progress.

JAPA PLATFORM IN KERALA

In many temples in Kerala in India, it is common to have a raised stone platform with a pyramidal roof in front of the sanctum. This is called the Mantra Meditation Platform (*Japa Thinḍa*) where anyone can sit and meditate. In these old temples with innumerable devotees having meditated there, over many hundred years, the vibrations are so strong that any meditator sitting there can instantly feel a meditative lift. This is the nature of places where regular meditation is done for a long period, and hence the preference to meditate in the same place everyday.

Best Times for Practice

While there are different views related to best times – some of which suggest night-time when everything is quiet – the Vedic prescription suggests dawn, high noon, and dusk as the best times. Among the three, high noon is considered most important, then dusk and last of all dawn. The rationale is as follows.

The circadian rhythm has a natural flow where mind and energy flow are less busy immediately upon waking up. While the mind gets busier and faster through the day, the energy flow also increases trying to keep up with the mind, but usually slightly lagging behind the mind. For higher connectivity in meditation, higher the energy and quieter the mind is most effective. In the Vedic system, the noon time before lunch break is considered a time when energy is high enough while the mind takes a break for lunch from daily activity. In the evening hours at dusk, the energy level lagging behind the mind is moderately high, but less than noontime with some fatigue setting in. When the mind lets go of the daily activities, the moderately high level of energy helps meditation. However, during the early morning hours upon waking up energy level is low, while the mind is also calmer.

For practical application in modern life when lunch is often had even while working, practitioners may find it best to meditate first thing in the morning and before dinner in the evening.

SANDHYĀ VANDANA PRACTICE AND *GĀYATRĪ* MANTRA

Sandhyā Vandana Practice is part of the Vedic system that is ritual mindfulness meditation done with invocation and done three times a day with different counts of *Gāyatrī* Mantra. Its system provides an interesting insight into the use of affirmations and invocations to empower the meditation. It also provides insight into the counts of the *Gāyatrī* mantra with respect to the circadian rhythm.

The affirmations relate to *Brahmā* as the *Ṛiṣhi* or controller of the system, *Gāyatrī* as the *Chanda* or meter of the *mantra* vibration, and God or *Paramātmā* as the *Devatā* or the higher link. Then invocation of the *chitta* or spirit of *Gayatri*, *Sāvitrī,* and *Sarasvatī* is done to empower the meditation.

The *Gāyatrī* mantra in its meaning seeks enlightenment from which one is enabled to fulfill one's role in life by proper use of the enlightenment. This is the point of focus – the affirmation. In the Vedic system, the morning meditation consists of 108 *Gāyatrī* repetitions, 32 at high noon and 54 in the evening as minimal counts. The counts give perspective on the number of repetitions needed to reach the optimal level of meditation in each of the times consistent with the circadian rhythm.

Meditation Practice for Beginners

Destressing and quietening the mind for deep relaxation is the objective of mindfulness meditation practices. Such mindfulness practices are a good place to start for most beginners.[106]

Following are a few examples of easy practices for beginners. They can be divided into two categories:

- Natural Meditative Observation at the end of a regular yoga class
- Individual Practice outside a yoga class

Natural Meditative Observation happens because of destressing from other yoga practices like *Āsana*, *Prānāyāmā* and sound vibrations. The concept of destressing noted earlier in the text (Chapter 5) is that of demands on the system being less than the available energy. This can be attained by increasing vitality by aligning the *nādi* communication and better breathing, and by reducing demands on the system by quietening the mind. This happens naturally towards the end of a yoga class.

Individual Practice outside a yoga class, lacking the group effect and leadership of an instructor, requires more discipline. For beginners, to keep discipline, it may be better to focus on singular practices done for 20 to 30 minutes rather than a sequential, combinatorial practice of *Āsanas*, *Prāṇāyāma* and sound vibrations leading to meditation.

Natural Meditative Observation at the end of a Yoga Class

Two common and easy practices are the following:

Deep Relaxation Lying Down in supine pose in *Śhavāsana* is commonly done in most yoga classes following a regimen of *āsanas*. The stretches of the *asanas* done with mindfulness (where the mind is focused on the sensations of the *āsanas*) relaxes the muscles and quietens the mind. Then, in the supine relaxed lying down pose:

- One can begin observing the breath, each inhalation flowing upward towards the head and each exhalation flowing in a cascade towards the feet. Such visualization naturally stops after a few minutes.
- Then just being a pure observer of the body, as if it is distinctly different from the person, and being in that state for a few or several minutes, constitutes a good meditative ending for a yoga class.

---

[106] Even as we say this, drawing on the parallel of Kashmir Shaivism's *Śhāmbhopāya* and *Śhāktopāya*, such an approach may be too elementary and disregards individual state of being of people who may be better qualified. However, most of the world may not be in the state to begin higher practices.

Bhastrikā Practice of several rounds of 20 breaths each done at the end of a yoga class creating increased vitality naturally leads to a complete silence within, even *Kevala Kumbhaka* state (described in Chapter 15) for many people. In this state being a pure observer and staying there for several minutes is a good meditative ending for a regular yoga class.

Individual Meditative Practices for Beginners

Two easy meditative practices for beginners are walking meditation and absorption in *Ujjayī Prāṇāyāma*.

Walking Meditation is best done in an environment that is not busy with peripheral activities like traffic on a road that can be distracting or other activities that require careful observation for safe walking. A park or quiet sidewalk or even a long corridor in one's home can be a good place. With eyes simply glued downward to ensure that each step is landing on a safe place, exhaling twice as long as inhaling (e.g., inhaling in two counts and exhaling in four counts) is a good beginning. Speed of walking is not relevant – this practice has nothing to do with burning calories. The concept of counting is simply to indicate that exhalation should be longer than inhalation. Also, there will be a natural pause between inhalation and exhalation of a duration between half a second to one second. Learning to walk with natural flow of the breath, but with observation of the breath, where exhalation is longer than inhalation is the key. This practice is optimally done for more than 20 minutes, up to an hour. [Treadmills are not the best for walking meditation since they seek to determine the speed and any natural variation within may conflict with the treadmill speed and prevent the mind from staying internally focused.]

***Ujjayī Prāṇāyāma* Absorption** works well as an individual practice for some people. However, this can only be effective if the *Ujjayī Prāṇāyāma* is done with very light effort with focus on the pharyngeal area. For beginners, the primary focus should always be on the pharyngeal area for safe practice and not on the flow of the breath. With maturity in the practice, there may be a secondary focus on the flow of the breath, but the primary focus must always be on the pharyngeal area.

Questions and Discussion Topics

1. Describe your regular meditation practice. Given what you do now, do you think you can increase your progress in yoga by adopting some elements of what you have learned here? If so, what will you do differently?

2. What kind of meditative component do you include now in your classes? Are you likely to a adopt anything from this book? If so, what?

If you thought meditation is simply sitting under a Bodhi tree for Self-Realization, wake up the yogi in you, and see the meditative aspect in every facet of life!

It is about how you do, rather than what you do.

PART VII – INTEGRATIVE UNDERSTANDING OF YOGA IN DAILY LIFE

32. Role of Group Effect and Collective Consciousness in Yoga
    - Group Effect and Collective Consciousness
    - Creating Collective Consciousness Remotely

33. Bhakti Yoga and the Role of Religious Practices in Yoga
    - Consecration in South Indian Temples
    - Orthodox Christian Meditation Through Icon Gazing
    - Hesychastic Meditation in Orthodox Christianity
    - Daily Salāt in Islam
    - Mevlevi Sema Ceremony – "Sufi Moving Meditation of Whirling dervishes"
    - Group Worship at Sabbath in Jewish Tradition
    - Mantra in Kabbālāh, the Mystical practice of Judaism
    - Daily Prayer in Zoroastrianism
    - Śhrī Vidyā System
    - African Voodoo (Vodou) System
    - Spiritual Cleansing in the Shinto System
    - Rituals for the Departed in Different Traditions
    - Dealing with Religious Adherents in Yoga

34. Yoga in Non-Religious Practices
    - Team or Group Activities
    - Being a Spectator
    - Distinguishing Non-Yogic Motivated Group Effect from Yogic
    - Spectrum of Activities Promoting Nādi Śhuddhi
    - Role of *Dharma*
    - Role of Repetitive Activity
    - Tai-Chi as Mindful Practice
    - Traditional Martial Arts

35. Integrative Health from Yoga (of body, mind, and spirit)
    - Yoga and Common Health Issues
    - Yoga and Autoimmune Conditions
    - Health is Only a By-Product of Yoga

36. Role of Yoga in Global Environmental and Socio-economic Balance
    (Discussion of the spiritual eco-system understood by yoga and how human greed has created an imbalance. Cases discussed: Health Care; Financial Systems; Food Supply; Role of Media; Wireless Technology; Energy Production and Utilization; Shift from Cost-Plus Pricing to Value-Based Pricing.)

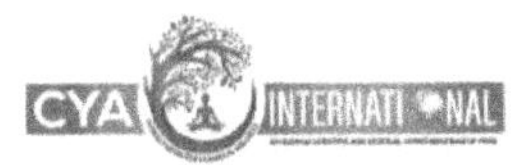

CHAPTER 32:

Role of Group Effect and Collective Consciousness in Yoga

In the first chapter of the book, in the context of effect beyond the individual, we stated the suggestion by Maharishi Mahesh Yogi about the reduction in crime rates in an area where 1% of the population are practicing transcendental meditation. In the meditation part of this book, we have noted the power of invocation of an elevated spirit that increases the power of meditation, i.e., increasing meditative connectivity. We have also noted that the presence of a person with elevated connectivity can impact others who are nearby. In a group meditation session, that can elevate the connectivity of the whole group.

Also, within the social setting, effects of social gatherings whether for a music concert or for a party, the herd mentality of the group effect (which unlike meditation may not be peaceful or elevating) is noted. The same kind of effect happens in workplaces as well when employees fit within a work culture and work as an effective team.

This is also the role of group worship in religious settings, as also in group meditation.

The group effect through collective consciousness works both in mundane elements of the world and for spiritual elevation. Understanding the process, and appropriate application, can be beneficial for the instructor and the group that is being led by the instructor.

Group Effect and Collective Consciousness

When one's focus becomes integrated with a common focus of the group, it leads to a group effect that is called collective consciousness, that is considered more than the sum of its parts. In a workplace or team sports, it helps the team participants to function as one unit and be more productive. As explained in the *Tantra Yoga* segment of the book, the ability to propagate has two components: the waves that connect and the message they carry.[107] This is the process of collective consciousness through group effect. However, application in meditation for spiritual elevation is a different matter from worldly achievements.

In a meditation session, the following are helpful elements to increase the transcendental effect of meditation:

---

[107] The term 'charisma', used for leaders who can influence gatherings, is this ability to propagate.

- Preparatory deep relaxation and clearing the *nādis* (at least temporarily and to some degree) through appropriate *āsana*, *Prāṇāyāma*, and *chakra* vibration practices.
- Singular group intent that is *Dhārmic* (consistent with the cosmic flow).
- Active connection into the group consciousness.

While a singular group intent passively allows for connection into the group consciousness, active connection makes the effect even stronger. The following exercise is one example of this approach.

Since individual meditative connectivity happens through the top of the head, focusing on the awareness above the head and visualizing a group awareness and mentally connecting into it ensures an active connection. Steps described below are illustrative of this process.

- Begin by sitting in a circle facing the center.
- Mentally 'let go' (of all ideas and concepts to clear the mind) and feel the awareness ascend above the head.
- Visualize the presence a few inches above the head as a ball of light – sometimes called Soul Star in spiritual settings or *Sudarśhana* in Indian spirituality.
- Visualize a larger ball of light in the middle of the group (in the middle of the room) at a slightly elevated level.
- Mentally have all the group meditators connect the ball of light above their head into the bigger group ball of light.
- Instantly all members of the group would feel a sense of elevated connectivity.
- An additional step may be to mentally connect the ball of light above each person into every other person in the room. This may have added effect in elevating the group intent provided it does not feel like too much mental work. An alternative is to hold hands with the immediate neighbors in the seated position.
- Since the intent is to 'let go' and let the cosmos guide, the intent would be *Dhārmic*.

THE SPECIAL ROLE OF HAND

In some group meditations and evocations of group consciousness, hand holding of the group, in a seated or standing position, in a circle is observed. Hands are considered special in conveying energy, and also hold a special place in Tantra.

Reiki and other types of energy healers use the hand as a sensory organ of energy, and also as a communicator of intent for healing. It is common in religious rituals to make gestures and convey actions with the hand to convey intent. Hand is also used for conveying blessings.

DIG-BANDHANA – SEALING THE DIRECTIONS

When leading a class or a group meditation session, you can help to create this collective consciousness by performing what is called in *Tantra Yoga* as "*dig-bandhana*," ["sealing (*bandhana*) the directions (*dik*)"] as a way of focusing the group consciousness. You can do this by sitting with your class at the beginning and mentally drawing three circles of light around the group. You can also include the upward and downward directions to contain all of the space in the three dimensions. There are more advanced versions of this practice that allow you to touch the consciousness of any number of people. Once you have performed the *dig-bandhana*, then invite the guru-force of *Īśhvara* to take its seat in your mind. You may find yourself teaching things you didn't know that you knew!

Creating Collective Consciousness Remotely

It is entirely possible to create collective consciousness when the participants are in remote physical locations when the focus is common and synchronous. In this day and age when remote group meetings have been enabled through internet technology, it is even easier. However, for it to be enabled, every participant must be engaged with full mental focus at the same time. While this can be true for any activity including business meetings, in a meditative setting with a spiritual focus, the presence of one member with higher cosmic connectivity can elevate the consciousness of everyone. Further, the *Dig-Bandhana* concept noted in the blue box above, also applies in such settings of remote participants.

Let us take the example of yoga practices by video conference. Often, participants from their locational settings may be interrupted by people and more often by phones, and they end up having brief conversations even as the group session is continuing. In order for creating an effectively collective consciousness in such group sessions, such interruptions must be avoided. It is essential for participants to emulate the setting in a physical location, even though they may be present remotely.

Questions and Discussion Topics

1. Explain the mechanism of group effect leading to higher experience in meditation when the group sits together but does not actively affirm to integrate in meditation.

2. Explain the mechanism of group effect leading to higher experience in meditation when the group actively affirms to integrate in meditation.

3. Can the group effect from active affirmation to integrate in meditation along with intention of performance help a team in team sports? If so, take any team sport and explain the process and mechanism to deliver positive results.

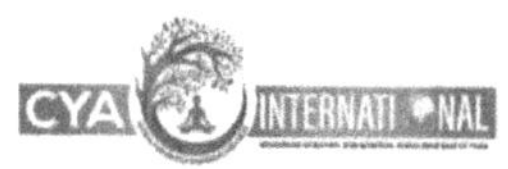

CHAPTER 33 –

Bhakti Yoga and the Role of Religious Practices in Yoga

Impact of yoga practices, in every aspect of living within an individual context and within a group context, has been discussed. That provides significant insight into the yogic application in religions.

There are several aspects in the zone of religions.

First is the role of *Bhakti Yoga*. As noted in the first chapter, there are three ways in which the mind becomes less reactive to what it observes, and in that purified state one can commune (in yoga) with the cosmic flow (*Prakṛiti*) and cosmic intelligence (*Puruṣha*). One of the three (ways) is *Bhakti Yoga*, the mental state of surrendering everything to God and thus becoming less reactive to what hits us externally. [The other two approaches are the physical cleansing of *Haṭha Yoga* and the vibrational cleansing of *Tantra Yoga*.] The true state of *Bhakti Yoga* is regarded as faith in God or the Supreme force (beyond name and form) irrespective of religion, and not necessarily associated with religious practices. However, religious practices that build a personal discipline may be considered stepping-stones towards the true experience of *Bhakti Yoga*.

The added element in religious setting, within the culture of its origin, is the role of priests as communicators into the cosmic intent, and the role of sacred places, objects, sounds and other environmental variables that affect the vibrations/waves of communication.

It is best to take examples of individual and collective practices from different religions to clarify this understanding.

Consecration in South Indian Temples

Consecration[108] of any South Indian Temple is a classic example of integration of *tantra* aspects of yoga including group effects, vibrations, and the power of intent.

However, it is important to recognize the role of the installation in a Hindu temple, that is generally referred to as an 'idol' in English, or an object of worship. This is a very limited view when one understands the Sanskṛit word *Vigraha* that is used referring to these so called 'idols'.

[108] Consecration in a Hindu temple is called *Prāṇa-Prathisṭa* or establishment of the *Prāṇa* or vibrations of the Deity.

Vigraha is *Viśheṣha Graha*, meaning a Special Holder (of cosmic connection). By going close to it or invoking it, one experiences a higher level of cosmic connectivity. This corresponds to the Yoga Sutra 1:37 that says one can experience the yogic connection by connecting into a programmed entity (*chitta*) that is bereft of desires. The *Vigraha* is a programmed entity with no desires but with the cosmic connection that a devotee can connect into.

The temple consecration is mainly about the consecration of the *Vigraha* and everything around that. The objective is to increase the connectivity of this *Vigraha* as a programmed entity so that it can be a place that enhances spiritual connectivity, even if only for a short period, for the devotees.

The components that work can be broken into the following elements:

- The temple structure and the immediate housing of the *Vigraha* has an approximately pyramidal structure on the top to enable cosmic connectivity as noted in Chapter 30 (Meditation part of the book).
- The *Vigraha* which is normally carved out of a stone block starts its journey where the sculptor invokes the divinity for guidance to get the right carving. The programming of the *Vigraha* begins from there.
- Then it is transported to the temple site and placed in a pool of water to cleanse off any unwanted vibrations coming on to it during transportation.
- It is dried and laid out on soft bedding, and devotees are encouraged to offer rice with both their hands. The hands convey the vibration of the intent of the faithful devotee through the rice into the *Vigraha*. This further strengthens the program of the *Vigraha* through the devotees grouped as a whole.
- Then the priests begin their role and through a 40-day period of daily ritual worship that includes intent, chanting (mantra vibrations) and offering into a holy fire pit (*Yajñya*, *Homa* or *Havan*) which has a string around it that is connected to the *Vigraha*. For the sensitive, if the string is touched by mistake during the consecration there would be a static shock, very similar to the sensation of the holy scroll in a synagogue or holy objects in any other place of worship. This ritual of the 40 days further strengthens the *Vigraha*.
- In the final day of the installation, it is essential for the devotees to come in large numbers and offer their mental devotion to the Lord and the installation. The power of intent increases the connectivity of the *Vigraha*. With sanctified water poured over the *Vigraha* by the chief priest with chanting (vibrations), the consecration is completed.
- Then, the chief priest walks out of the sanctum and goes straight out, about 30 feet, carrying a mirror held slightly above the face level where he can see the installed *Vigraha* behind him. He makes a mental affirmation (*saṅkalpa*) that if the consecration is complete, then let the mirror crack. Immediately a crack appears on the mirror indicating the full empowerment of the *Vigraha* as intended, and the mirror is discarded after that.

Thus, it is easy to see how the group effect, role of priest, power of intent and vibrations, all work towards creating a holy *Vigraha* that works to elevate the cosmic awareness of devotees. The whole process is yoga concepts in action.

APPLICATIONS OF TRANSFERING INTENT AND ITS IMPACT

The consecration of a South Indian temple described here is essentially *tantra* in motion, singularly by the chief priest and collectively by the devotees along with use of appropriate vibrational aids, that increase the connective power of the *Vigraha*. Because the intention is to increase its connective power, there are no other intents attached to it. Any form of worship or mental offering without any desire empowers the point of focus. This is the reason for daily worship rituals, that are mandatory in such temples, to compensate for anything that may dissipate the strength of the connectivity. When people offer such mental worship to other human beings, they end up empowering increased connectivity to such people whom they call "Gurus" or "leaders". Thus, even a person with low cosmic connectivity with others worshipping him or her can increase his/her spiritual connectivity and growth.[109] This is also the approach of collective prayers to heal someone, except the role of intent is different.

Now, just as an entity or object may be imbued with higher cosmic connectivity with intent, it can also lose the connectivity with inappropriate vibrations. When people go to temples for relief of their worldly problems and seek fulfillment of their worldly desires, they can dissipate the strength of the connectivity of the *Vigraha*. The daily rituals of the temple, and annual observances, help to limit the damage. However, to compensate in a stronger way, in South Indian temples, a reconsecration is done every 12 years.

The same type of phenomenon happens to spiritually connected individuals when they bless others who seek worldly desires. However, for a highly purified soul, the blessing is always to connect with God and fulfill the purpose of one's life; and never to use his/her connectivity to fulfill the worldly desire of the seeker. When spiritually connected people use their power of projection motivated by emotional attachment, the reactive program (*karma*) makes them less pure, and they lose spiritual connectivity.

Such transfer of intent and how it affects a person is best described by two historical events.

The 16th century Mughal king of India, Babur, was told his son Humayun would not survive an illness with which he was seriously ill. Babur prayed and is said to have taken on Humayun's illness, and while Humayun rapidly recovered, Babur declined rapidly and died in a few days.[110]

Another such story of the 16th and 17th century is that of Melpathur Nārāyana Bhattathiri of Kerala in India, associated with his famous composition, Nārāyaneeyam, and the Guruvāyur temple. His teacher, Achuta Piśhāraḍy, was suffering from rheumatoid arthritis and was completely bed-ridden. He chose to take the malady by intent from his teacher as gratitude for his learning, and while his teacher recovered in a few days, he was afflicted by the disabling condition during the same period. Then, it is said, he stayed in a disabled state for 100 days praying in the temple of Guruvāyur, and slowly recovered as he composed 10 versus every day in the name of the Lord which resulted in the 1,000-verse Nārāyaneeyam.

---

[109] In political philosophy, the concept of divine right theory of monarchs can be considered the role of worshipful recognition of the monarch by the subjects which endows the monarch with the higher connectivity. In modern day elected systems, the elected leader when accepted by the population may exhibit the same effect.

[110] https://farbound.net/was-it-a-fathers-love-that-killed-mughal-emperor-babur-babur-humayun-transfer-illness-medieval-beliefs/

Orthodox Christian Meditation Through Icon Gazing

Within the cultures of the Eastern Orthodox Church, Oriental Orthodoxy, Roman Catholicism, and certain Eastern Catholic churches, icon gazing is a religious meditative practice. Icons, which are carefully constructed diagrams of Divine figures and realized beings, are used as a visualized prayer in Orthodox Christianity in much the same way as the use of *yantras* as a visual form of mantric practice in the *Tantra Yoga* tradition. The construction and painting of icons is also a practice of mindful prayer. This can be understood in the context of Yoga Sutra 1:37, where focusing on a being, bereft of attachments, can deliver higher experience in meditation.

ROMAN CATHOLIC MASS AS A TANTRIC RITUAL

Swami Veda Bharati has described the Roman Catholic mass as a tantric ritual, containing all the subtle elements reflected in the *chakras*: earth in the fragrance of flowers and incense, water in the communion offering, fire in candles on the altar, air in the incense and space in the flowers on the altar.

This is also typical in Hindu worship of *Vigrahas* where representation, of all the five elements, is used, where the space element is denoted by the sound of bells.

Hesychastic Meditation in Orthodox Christianity

In Hesychasm, in Eastern Christianity, practitioners seek divine quietness (Greek hēsychia) through the contemplation of God in uninterrupted prayer. Such prayer, involving the entire human being—soul, mind, and body—is often called "pure," or "intellectual," prayer or the Jesus Prayer. The practice of the meditative prayer involves following the flow of breath between the navel and the nostrils while repeating the prayer, "Lord Jesus Christ have mercy upon me, a sinner." The goal is eventually to pray without ceasing, waking or sleeping, as described in the classic book *The Way of a Pilgrim.*

Daily Salat in Islam

Daily Salat, done five times a day by the faithful, is a constant reminder that one's being in the body is for the sake of God. It can be thought as leading towards *Īśhvara Praṇidhāna*, the *Bhakti Yoga* element of the Yoga Sutras. The Salat combines the element of *dhikr* (glorification of God) as the point of focus, along with mental affirmation of forgiveness and direction in one's life with God's blessings. The standing, bending, seating position (on *Vajrāsana)*, and prostration can remind one of the various *āsanas* designed to stimulate the *nādis* physically, and opening the palms and looking into them and rubbing the face can be understood as the integration of the cosmic intent into our physical being.

A typical Salat sequence, with different number of repetitions during each of the five daily sessions, is the following.[111]

- Begin with the affirmation 'God is great' to clear the mind to focus on God.
- The posture of Standing along with recitation of the prayer.
- The posture of Bowing down and acknowledging Allah has heard the prayer.
- The posture of Prostrating as surrender to God (Allah).

After the required repetitions (of the above), the final element involves the last long sitting position with recitations in the praise of God before ending the prayer session.

A YOGA VIEW OF SALAT PRACTICE

ASPECTS OF SALAT PRACTICE	ACTION ELEMENT	YOGIC VIEW
MEDITATION ASPECTS	Surrender to Creator with recitation. Promotes inner peace, encourages calmness by focusing on the recited prayers.	*Īśhvara Praṇidhāna* of Yoga allowing for clearing the mind and be stress free. Focus on nature of God.
PHYSICAL ASPECTS	Standing posture providing spinal alignment; forward bending (*ruku*) for pelvic flexibility; prostration with head touching the ground (*sajdah*); sitting between heels supported by thighs and knees (in *Vajrāsana*).	Optimizing flow of vitality to ensure better body-mind integration in prayer.
PSYCHOSOMATIC ASPECTS	Forward bending position and prostration actively promotes humility and surrender to God.	Integration of body, mind, and spirit in surrender to God

[111] https://www.al-islam.org/articles/laws-and-practices-how-perform-daily-prayers provides details of Islamic Salat. Respectful of the Islamic tradition of not sharing the details of practices, the yogic aspects are generically observed in our writing.

Mevlevi Sema Ceremony – "Sufi Moving Meditation of Whirling Dervishes"

Associated with a Sufi sect practice in the Islamic tradition is the moving meditation practice of the Sema (whirling) Ceremony. Founded by the great Muslim poet Jalaluddin Rumi in the 13th century in Konya (Turkey), this is a mystical expression of Islam in the well-known order of Sufis called Mevlevis. Their practice of remembering the Divine name, *dhikr* or *zikr*, is performed with a body prayer consisting of a turning dance while meditating on an initiated mantra which is one of the "99 Beautiful Names of Allah" from the text of the same name. Hence their characterization as "whirling dervishes." The word dervish, meaning mendicant, is derived through Persian and Turkish words, from the ancient Indo-Iranian word *Drigu* found in Zend-Avesta.

The ceremony consists of the noble eulogy to the Prophet Mohammed, flute solo, prelude, the Circling of *Veled* and four segments (*selam*), which form an integral whole and contain different Sufi meanings.[112] Thus the practice includes power of intention (thought/invocation), sound (music) and movement. Since proper repetitive movement must be synchronized with breath and proper alignment of the body, it appears to be a complete practice of yoga. Further, the effect of the transcendence of those practicing is also perceived by the audience. Thus, there is also the group effect and the spectator integration as well in this practice.

Group Worship at Sabbath in Jewish Tradition

Light and intention in music and prayer at sunset on Friday are the key elements of a Jewish Sabbath observance. The lighting of lamp indicating the fire of life, which is the energy that sustains life, signifies the energy that can allow for activating our cosmic communication. Along with the power of intention in prayer and group energy such communication is enabled.

YOGIC SPIRITUAL SIGNIFICANCE OF THE TORAH SCROLL

While in religious Judaism, much attention is paid to the material and person involved in the handwritten scroll, the yogic spiritual significance can be described as follows:

The careful preparation of the material and person to construct the Torah Scroll is comparable to the careful preparation of the stone to create the *Vigraha* for consecration in a temple or the careful construction of icons used for gazing in the tradition of the Eastern Orthodox Church. The qualified *sofar* (scribe) who does it with devout focus, in effect, transfers the power of intent as in *tantra*. Any discerning yogi who goes near the scroll in a synagogue can sense similar vibrations to the *Vigraha* in a consecrated temple.

---

[112] https://aregem.ktb.gov.tr/TR-139582/mevlevi-sema-ceremony.html

Mantra in Kabbālāh, the Mystical practice of Judaism

The concept of the creative vibrational power of divinity is fundamental in Judeo-Christian tradition. Within the mystical practices of orthodox Judaism, the attribution of specific creative energies to phonemes of the Hebrew alphabet is almost the same as in the Indian *Mantra Śhāstra*, especially the way that the Kashmir Shaiva Tantra system utilizes the sequence of the Sanskṛit alphabet as an algorithm for the process of manifesting the universe in energy and matter. The main Kabbālistic texts are the Sefeer Yetzira and the Zohar.

Daily Prayer in Zoroastrianism

In Zoroastrianism, direction of light, sound vibration and intent are part of the meditative ritual practices that can be equated to the yogic process. The following excerpts are illustrative.

The Zoroastrian Heritage[113] site notes:

"Reciting a *manthra* can become a form of meditation and meditation is now widely recognized, even in medical circles, as a method of maintaining a state of mind that permits the human body to marshal its healing faculties. . . . . . Praying and meditating at a retreat helps remove distractions and provides more time for the process to be effective. It provides the practitioner the opportunity to slow down the process by focusing on every word and the person's breathing during the intonation of the ancient words."

The site also notes: "While it is advantageous to know the meaning or intent of the *manthra* being recited, even when the ancient words are poorly understood, reciting a *manthra* has a calming, soothing effect that allows the mind to refocus itself." The potential of *manthra* vibrations to open "the portals to the spiritual realms enabling access to spiritual healing" is also noted.

COMMONLY RECITED PRAYER IN ZOROASTRIANISM ILLUSTRATING POWER OF INTENT ALONG WITH VIBRATIONS

ASHEM VOHU in Avestan [MP3 Audio]

Avestan	English Translation
ashem vohû vahishtem astî; ushtâ astî ; ushtâ ahmâi hyat ashâi vahishtâi ashem	Righteousness (Asha or Ashoi) is the highest of all good; it is happiness; Happiness is to him, who is righteous for the sake of the highest righteousness

113 http://www.heritageinstitute.com/zoroastrianism/worship/healingprayer.htm

Implied Statement: Righteousness is the best good and it is happiness. Happiness is to him/her who is righteous for the sake of the best righteousness. [Righteousness is the concept of *Dharma* of Yoga that supports the cosmic flow.]

YATHĀ AHU VAIRYO (AHUNWAR) PRAYER (most sacred manthra of Zoroastrianism) Avestan [MP3 Audio]

Avestan	English Translation
Yatha ahu vairyo Atha ratush ashat chit hacha. Vangheush dazda manangho Shyaothananam angheush Mazdai Khshathremcha Ahurai a Yim drigubyo dadat vastarem	Just as a temporal ruler is all powerful among people, so too is a spiritual teacher due to his righteousness. The gifts of Vohu-mano (good mind) are for those who work for Mazda, the Lord of life; the strength of Ahura is given unto him who to his poor brethren giveth help.

[This is the concept of living life for the purpose of God and the cosmic flow.]

Śhrī Vidyā System

One of the systems of tantric religious practice that includes yoga concepts is called *Śhrī Vidyā.* It is associated with religious worship of the Divine Mother who gives birth to all of creation.

Śhrī refers to everything that is created. The common meaning in Sanskṛit is "beauty, splendor, majesty." In a philosophical sense, it can also mean "poison or toxin" rooted in the sense that the emergence of creation from the unchanging and unmanifest into the manifest is because of an apparent reduction in consciousness (as a programmed entity). The Yoga Sutra equivalent of *Śhrī* is *Prakṛiti* or the first cosmic program (cosmic consciousness referred as the One *Chitta* in the Yoga Sutras 4:5). This first cosmic program as explained in Sutra 4:5 of the Yoga Sutras becomes many to fulfill the purpose of creation. Thus, in the tantric worship practices, *Śhrī* (also written as *Śhree*) is viewed as the divine mother that gives birth to the creation we know and is worshipped as *Tri-pura-sundarī*, "the beauty of the three worlds (earth, sky and the heavens, the subtle worlds beyond), or, as Swāmī Veda Bhārati used to say, "Miss Three Universes."

Vidyā denotes knowledge and wisdom, especially related to the nature of existence.

TRI-PURA-SUNDARĪ AND *ŚHRĪ VIDYĀ*
From a yogic standpoint, *Śhrī* or *Prakṛiti*, as the administrator of creation, is the administrator of the three worlds referred as the causal, subtle, and gross bodies discussed in Chapter 5 (also referred in Chapter 27). In this worship practice it is viewed that the Divine Mother is the gateway to experience *Vidyā* and realize *Īśhvara*.

This system sees a particular *yantra*, called the *Śhrī Chakra*[114], as a map of the vibrational energy fields of the human body-mind-spirit complex. The *yantra* is understood to be simply the densest form of the One *Chitta* and the entire universe – thus establishing the equivalence of the microcosm and the macrocosm. One of the *tantra* texts (*Prapañchasāra*[115]) says, "whatever is out there (in the wider universe) is also in here (within the individual); What I do not find here I will not find there either." Thus, in one sense, the meditative science of *Śhrī Vidyā* involves learning the depth of that equation and how to work with it.

MERU

There is a three-dimensional, pyramidal form of the *Śhrī Yantra* or *Śhrī Chakra* which is called it's *Meru* form. It is commonly used in making the ritual offering in formal *Śhrī Yantra* worship.

Śhrī Vidyā practices are usually described in terms of three paths: *kaula*, *miśra* and *samaya.* As *Swāmī Rāma* described the *kaula* path as one involving practices of external ritual worship, the *samaya* path as one where the rituals are all conducted within the mind in meditation, and the *miśra* path as a combination of the two. There are many details and subtleties to the system which are well beyond the scope of this book. However, the fundamental approach is to create conducive vibrations with matter, mind, and activity to elevate the practitioner into higher awareness to move towards realizing the nature of existence, the divine mother and the cosmic oneness.

The meditative practices involve detailed visualizations of various aspects of the *Śhrī Chakra.* In some schools there are also aspects of tāntric ritual worship that involve the coming together of two *chittas* that are viewed as harmonic vibrations that help to elevate both into higher consciousness. This is the idea of a spiritually elevating marriage. However, such rituals are ordinarily forbidden since it requires a very high level of mindful, emotional, and physical control to avoid lapsing into the mere pursuit of pleasure.

In *Śhrī Vidyā* one learns the difference between the *ānanda*, the eternal supreme transcendent joy and beauty that comes from doing ones *Dharma* (one's duties) that leads to higher awareness and the distractions of the mind that seek momentary pleasure. *Śhrī Vidyā* practice requires a high level of spiritual maturity and is difficult to comprehend for most students.

African Voodoo (Vodou) System

African Voodoo system is a yogic approach of communion with higher spirits (in Zone B of *Prakṛiti* in Figure 27.1 in chapter 27) to fulfill purpose of life (*Dharma*) and release spirit of ancestors (*mokśha*). [See section later in this chapter on Rituals for the Departed in Different

---

[114] S. K. Ramachandra Rao. (2005). *Sri Cakra With Illustrations* and (2008). *Sri Cakra: It's Yantra, Mantra and Tantra*. Sri Satguru Publications.

[115] A *tantra* text whose authorship is attributed to Shankarācharya that deals with both worship methods and meditation while discussing the nature of creation and experiences beyond the body. http://www.hindupedia.com/en/Prapa%C3%B1cas%C4%81ra

Traditions.] Dance, music, trance, the return to the ancestral past and above all the initiation to the sacred and occult are some of the common points between Voodoo and the rest of the other African cults.

The Agbadza (Agbadja) is a dance ritual of Togolese origin and has similarities with dances from Burkina Faso provinces of Boulgou and Ziro. The dancer who falls during the dance goes into a trance allowing the dancer to commune with the divine spirit of the ancestors. There are cases where specific spirits of departed souls can be summoned by the tam tam (gong). The spirit called is obliged to enter the dancer in trance in order to free itself by communicating through the dancer.

Some African societies wear a mask during the ritual dance. The mask connotes a spirit. During the dance, the wearer necessarily falls out of dance to enter a trance. The wearer of the mask assumes the identity of the spirit of the mask itself and communes with the divine nature.

UNDERSTANDING VOODOO SPIRITUALITY

Voodoo is a *tantra* system that from a yogic perspective focuses on the subtle *Prakṛiti* (in Zone B in Figure 27.1 in chapter 27) as a gateway to the one God (Zone A in Figure 27.1). In the spiritual world of the subtle *Prakṛiti* in Voodoo many types of entities are recognized. Two of them are comparable to other religious traditions like departed souls, and deities like angels of the Christian tradition and *Devatās* of the Hindu system. Departed souls need release. The deities are enablers of the cosmic system to fulfill the purpose of creation for those who are born in the temporal world. Each of these deities represents a specific type of energetic communication to enable specific functions of the temporal world and trace back to the one God. Rituals are designed to release departed souls and to connect with deities to enable *Dhārmic* life processes.

Voodoo is not a doll with a hole in it into which thorns have been put, as is commonly portrayed in the West. Voodoo is not a religion but has generated a culture and religion. Voodoo, like *tantra*, is a system of access to spirits that lead to God from the African traditions.

Spiritual Cleansing in the Shinto System

The self-purification process of priests in the Shinto system with bathing and meditative practices, and the purification offered to others or objects through the *Haraigushi* process follows the Tantra system discussed earlier.[116]

---

[116] https://www.britannica.com/topic/harai-gushi
https://www2.kenyon.edu/Depts/Religion/Fac/Adler/Reln275/Shinto-purification-rituals.htm

Rituals for the Departed in Different Traditions

From the perspective of the Yoga Sutras (4:33-34), the final resting state is that of being connected to God (like in heaven) or completely dissolved into the cosmic energy. However, in the interim, between the first birth and final state there can be many rebirths. If this cycle is in the hands of the individual soul (*Jīva*[117]), do rituals related to the departed have any more meaning than for the satisfaction of the grieving family?

In the Vedic tradition, there is one other state that is recognized where a *Brāhmana*[118] soul will not have rebirth but may not have reached the final state. In the Vedic tradition it is said that these souls reside in the *Pitṛa Loka* (translated as world of ancestors) and in Roman Catholicism it is called purgatory. For these souls, offerings need to be made to allow them to pass on to the final resting state. In both these traditions, priests take some responsibility to do the necessary prayers for these souls, while the children of the departed are also required to make certain offering.

How is this explained in the yogic system with the *tantra* understanding?

In chapter 23 (in the *Tantra Yoga* part of this book), the nature of a person's awareness defining the presence of the *Kuṇḍalinī* is noted. There, four basic levels of nature (total of eight including sub-levels) are explained. The *Brāhmana* soul is a soul whose predominant awareness is about existence beyond the physical world. Any person in any religion who lives life with an understanding that the essence of life is at a spiritual level beyond the physical world is a *Brāhmana* soul.[119] Living in the physical world, while predominantly spiritual, there can be worldly attachments to family members or regrets related to thoughts, words, or deeds during the lifetime. Unless these are dissolved, the soul cannot reach its final place of rest. Offerings made in this regard are meant to dissolve these attachments.

In the Vedic system, like many of the theistic systems, we live this life for the sake of God to support God's intent of the cosmic flow. Souls hanging in the *Pitṛa Loka* or purgatory are part of the cosmic flow and they need to be taken care whether the family members do it or not. All *Brāhmana* souls, while living, are expected to offer on a daily basis to all departed souls whether of their family or any family of any religion to allow those departed souls to pass on to their final resting. This is part of a daily ritual called the *Brahma-Yajñya*. For non-*Brāhmana* souls, there would be rebirth and the only facilitation required is peaceful passage to their rebirth. [For all souls whether there is rebirth or not, especially for those who die in unnatural circumstances,

---

[117] *Jīva* is a Sanskṛit term that is used to indicate a created being that is normally considered as 'live' and may go through many births before the final state. The closest English translation is 'soul', but the *Jīva* is still considered a subtle (vibration) material being.

[118] *Brāhmana* as referred in Chapter 24 and not based on birth.

[119] In reality, the awareness at the last moment in life is what matters. A person having lived life without any spiritual awareness is not normally expected to suddenly develop awareness beyond the physical world in the last breath. However, it is conceivable and possible – determined by the path of the soul.

death rituals are considered important to relieve them of extraordinary stresses (program patterns) that can prevent a peaceful transition to the next state, even if it is rebirth.]

Rituals for the departed in all traditions can be understood within this context, and this reinforces the idea that yoga is all about cosmic interconnectedness of everything.

Dealing with Religious Adherents in Yoga

Yoga is the path of direct spiritual experience. It is also recognized in Yoga that when the soul is ready, circumstances in life push them towards inquiry into Yoga. Religion and faith in God being the mental cleansing aspect of yoga, the person of faith has already begun the journey. We know from yoga that fixed assumptions limit the progress of direct experience. However, they also inculcate discipline. We need to approach religion and religious adherents with sensitivity in yoga.

At the instructor level, one should not comment on any aspect of religion and religious beliefs. Such beliefs should be considered as belonging in the individual domain of the person. When individual religious adherents have questions, it should be referred to a highly experienced yogi.

In the highest awareness of yoga, one understands that religious beliefs and practices were developed within cultural settings for well-meant reasons. Only a yogi of the highest level can answer the whys and why nots of beliefs and practices that some people may find objectionable. The highest-level yogi can answer all such questions with the highest respect for all religions. In general, such discussions should be in the individual domain when a yoga practitioner finds some religious practice for themselves or for their families restrictive. In general, such questions should not be discussed in the public domain to avoid hurting the feelings of the rigid faithful, except when called to advise on public policy for legislation. Then too, it must be expressed with sensitivity and respect.

One example in almost all religious traditions is the concept of fasting at special times. The yogi understands its relevance. Cosmic connectivity is hampered when part of the energy for the cosmic connectivity is diverted to digest food. Also, in that connected state the connectivity provides its own energy balance, and one does not feel hungry. When one cannot keep the attitude of surrendering to God continuously when fasting is observed, even when engaged in daily activities, the engagement in worldly activities can create hunger. Then, the acid in the stomach can be the cause of ulcers if such observances are regular. Therefore, the right advice for a religious adherent is that during such times of fasting one should have continuous mental awareness of letting go of everything to God. If such observances are going to last for a few days, during that time never begin a new project or new activity in your life where worldly considerations are inevitable for the mind. If the person is unable to keep that state and hunger sets in, it would be unhealthy to maintain the fast for both physical and spiritual purposes. The first suggestion should never be to discard the practice since faith should not be disturbed. Only if the person is unable to keep the practice in an effective spiritual way, in the interest of the physical, mental, and spiritual health of the person an alternative should be offered.

Questions and Discussion Topics

1. Review all the religious examples provided in this chapter. What is the common element in all the examples that promote spirituality? What are the uncommon elements in some examples and how do they help spirituality?

2. Consider the death rituals followed in your tradition. Carefully map out every step at the funeral and thereafter in the next few days or months or annually. Explain the rationale in the yogic paradigm.

3. Consider a situation where one of your yoga students is highly disturbed that one of his children is a lesbian or gay. Within her/his religious belief, s/he thinks it is sinful. How do you deal with this situation?

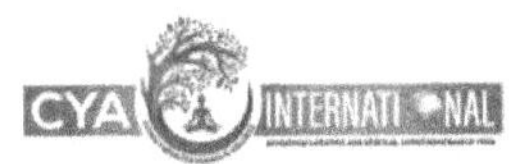

CHAPTER 34:

Yoga in Non-Religious Practices

Yoga in non-religious practices (outside conventional practices of *Haṭha Yoga*, *Tantra Yoga* and *Bhakti Yoga*) are like the meditative practices for deep relaxation discussed in Chapter 29 (Meditation Approach for Deeper Relaxation). This chapter can be thought as another, and yet a similar way, to see the yoga effect in non-religious practices. They can be categorized in different dimensions. Activities may be:

- **Actively physical** like walking, running, swimming, etc. **or Mildly Physical** like cooking, knitting, reading, being a spectator, etc.
- **Individual in nature** like swimming, knitting, etc. **or be Group or Team based** like in team sports, book clubs, study groups, etc.
- **Based on Participation or as a Spectator**
- **Evoke Connectivity, but not necessarily cosmic intuition**
- **Consciously *Dhārmic* or Just being in the Flow.**

The common element of all these practices is complete absorption in the activity. It is often described as 'being in the flow' or 'being in the zone'. This happens when the person is not motivated by any other reason to do the activity other than being in the activity. It begins by having full focus in it, tuning out external diversions, and a level of absorption described as *Samāpatti* in the Yoga Sutras (1:41-43). Thus, the activity becomes that of a pure observer, which then transcends into intuitively guided activity. Such intuitive guidance is not necessarily the higher spiritual connectedness, since that is reserved for the point of focus that is subtle (spiritual inquiry) and beyond the worldly activity – i.e., the distinction between *Samāpatti* and *Samādhi* in the Yoga Sutras. Nevertheless, such *Samāpatti* experiences, engrossment without reactivity, helps to purify the *nādis*, preparing one for the higher-level yoga inquiry at a later point in time.[120]

The nature of team participation, being a spectator, and nature of intuition and *Dharma* need further discussion.

---

[120] Initial motivation in the activity before getting 'into the zone' is what makes it worldly focused.

Team or Group Activities

Team or group activities evoke a potential that comes from group connectedness with the collective motivation of the group. This enables team players (including musicians in an orchestra) to have better anticipation and greater success in the object of the team activity. In group studies, as in book clubs or in working teams as in a job or in integrated families, it evokes deeper understanding and better accomplishment than would be possible individually. Thus, the team effect is often stated as 'more than the sum of its parts.' This group evoked potential is distinct and different from individual participation in an activity. [This book is an example. It is the collective work of a group of yogis, inspired by cosmic connectivity.]

Being a Spectator

The experience of absorption being a spectator is common in sports as well as viewing arts. Here the absorption leads to connectivity into the vibrations of what is viewed – sensing the players and the game's motion, or the expression of the artist in a painting or sculpture, or vibrations of emotions and moods of dance and music.

THE CONNECTIVITY OF DANCE – AN EXAMPLE

In the 1990's, the famous dancer Mallika Sarabhai was performing at the Smithsonian in Washington DC. The theme was ***Śhaktī***, the different aspects of ***Devi***, the feminine spirit. As she moved from one form to another, she came upon the form of *Vara Lakśhmī*, the spirit that gives *Vara* or boons. She made her left hand into a cup, and with her right hand she scooped out of her left hand and tossed the contents of her right hand into the audience. While it was only a gesture and nothing physical was tossed, many members of the audience could feel something falling on them.

When dancers connect into divine themes and become absorbed in them, they evoke that potential, which the spectators who are connected (absorbed) into the dance can also experience.

Distinguishing Non-Yogic Motivated Group Effect from Yogic

It is important to note here that connectedness in a group or as a spectator need not be positive all the time. Wild concerts, political gatherings, boisterous parties, and such group events can also lead to unwanted herd effects that are driven by motivation. Such events can have reactions related to outcomes (from *karma* being formed). They have nothing to do with yoga.

When one is a pure observer without reaction in any external activity, it leads to mindful absorption – *Samāpatti*. When the absorption is into a spiritual inquiry, it eventually leads to *Samādhi*. Irrespective of the nature of the activity or point of focus that leads to absorption, when there is no reaction, it leads to cleansing of the internal programs (*karma* and *kleśha*), and that purification enhances communication in the *nādis*.

Spectrum of Activities Promoting *Nādi* Purification

Every activity in life done as an observer without reactivity leads to purification of the (communication in the) *nādis*. In common life, without higher awareness of the nature of existence, people generally perform activities with motivation and expectation of desired results. Therefore, for higher spiritual realization, it is necessary to cultivate activities that are without strong motivation where one can be a pure observer, at least for a short time, on a daily basis. Such daily practice, yoga-type practice, begins to pervade into the other activities of life, eventually allowing one to be light on motivation on all aspects of living – as we say being in the moment in every activity.

As a stepping-stone, daily individual exercise activities like walking, running, swimming, etc. can be very helpful. In common culture these activities are promoted as motivated activities (e.g., for burning fat through exercises) and too often people tend to make it non-yogic like watching TV when on the treadmill or walking in groups with conversation going. Such ritual activities when cultivated with inner awareness rather than external awareness, prepares one to be more effective whether as an individual or as a team player in worldly interaction, while providing yogic advancement. In team sports, the most effective players are those who develop that inner awareness. The same is true in work environments and in integrated families.

Role of *Dharma*

Dharma is associated with action that supports the cosmic flow. In such practices as noted in this chapter, without a sense of *Yama* (ethics of being true to one's conscience), any intuitive sensing that enables abilities cannot be guaranteed to be *Dhārmic.*

Role of Repetitive Activity

Repetitive activities foster ability to be a pure observer leading to *nādi* cleansing. This is the nature of walking meditation described in Chapter 31, an example of an individual activity that has this yogic effect. The same type of effect can happen by mindful focus leading to absorption in a variety of activities like walking, running, biking, step-climbing, swimming, dynamic *Sūrya Namaskar*[121].

In repetitive individual activities like walking, running, etc. the intuitive awareness is less visible to the external observer. However, in team sports it becomes more visible in how a player anticipates or improvises in coordination with other team members in pursuit of the objective of the sport. For the spectator it would feel like this team player is reading the mind of the other players.

---

[121] Krzysztof Zbigniew Stec is a Polish researcher who has studied the effect of Dynamic Sūrya Namaskar.

Tai-Chi as Mindful Practice

Tai-Chi can be equated to the slow, moving, gentle yoga practices with focus on breath and inner awareness (described in Appendix 2). The key difference between Tai Chi and gentle yoga is the much slower movement of Tai-Chi and the visualization of energy flow. It fosters the ability to be an observer, without judgement, leading to *nādi* purification.

Traditional Martial Arts

Eastern Martial Arts can be thought to begin from Tai-Chi but promoting greater awareness in two specific ways. First, they promote intuitive awareness that enables quick anticipation of external threats. Second, they enable rapid muscle movement response to deal with potential threats.

Questions and Discussion Topics

1. What are the pros and cons of individual religious and non-religious activities? [As an example, you can consider daily mindful walking and any religious ritual done daily.] What elements are common and what are different? What are the impediments to further progress into higher levels of meditative awareness?

2. Consider a religious service done as a group activity in a congregation and compare it with a team sport (like soccer or basketball with many players). What elements are common and what are different? What are the impediments to further progress into higher levels of meditative awareness?

3. Consider the difference in the absorption as a spectator/viewer in a still form that is religious (like a *Vigraha* or an icon) versus a non-religious still form (like a painting or sculpture). What elements are common and what are different? What are the impediments to further progress into higher levels of meditative awareness?

4. Consider the difference in the absorption as a spectator/viewer in a non-religious still art-form (like a painting or sculpture) versus a non-religious active/live art-form (like a dance or music performance). What elements are common and what are different? What are the impediments to further progress into higher levels of meditative awareness?

5. For the same comparisons in the previous question, distinguish the effect between recorded experiencing versus live experiencing (like seeing a picture of a painting on a website versus seeing the original in a museum, like watching a dance performance on recorded video versus seeing live in-person). [Note that in live concert events a group effect may also be present that is not there in recorded viewing.]

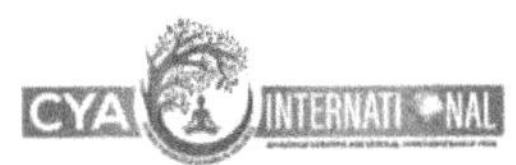

CHAPTER 35

Integrative Health from Yoga

While it is popular in recent times to talk about integration of body and mind for optimal health through the types of practices discussed in previous chapters, the real role of yoga is the integration of body, mind and spirit or more appropriately integrative performance of the three bodies of yoga: gross, subtle, and causal. Such integrative living serves to fulfill one's purpose of birth (one's *Dharma*). Thus, living life with minimal emotional reactivity as one engages with the world becomes the recipe for good health.

The limited scientific mind of western medicine focuses only on what it can see in the anatomy and physiology, and mindfully sweeping under the rug what it thinks cannot be known even if they influence health – like what is before birth or after death, what is the purpose of life, how lifestyle and treatments affect differently for different people. In the last 50 to 100 years there has been a realization that state of the mind affects biochemicals in the body, and biochemicals are used to counteract sub-optimal mental states and often creating a lifelong dependence on medications for some people. Experienced psychiatrists are asking the question why state of the mind cannot be corrected through Cognitive Behavioral Therapy (CBT) to produce the right biochemicals within the body. This, of course, requires the patient to participate in the process of healing instead of mindlessly popping a pill.

This dual limitation of the view of the medical system as only body and mind, and the expectations generated by such a view among the population, has effectively cast out the most important element: the spirit and its purpose. This has resulted in significant physiological research all over the world on different protocols of yoga practices and their effect on specific disorders.

Experienced yoga teachers know that regular practices that allow one to develop the attitude of a pure observer automatically integrates the body, mind and spirit resulting in better health and overcoming many health abnormalities. Learners here can relate to the five types of communication discussed in Chapter 5 (The Underlying Mechanism of All Yoga Approaches) and how they heal the system.

Yoga and Common Health Issues

Common health issues are healed by optimizing the flow of vitality (*Prāṇa* communication) along with the optimized communications into the musculoskeletal system (*Apāna*), fluids of the body (*Vyāna*) and the gene expression (*Samāna*). Whichever communication is the source of the imbalance for the specific condition would be the main target of practice, while also seeking complementary or collateral impact on the other three. Such an approach yields effective results for common health disorders.

Yoga and Autoimmune Conditions

Autoimmune conditions are a lot more difficult to address since the *Udāna* communication must be strong and adequate to help change the other communications to restore the overall distortion of the system. Allergic reactions that cause asthma, insulin resistance in diabetes, cancer, etc. fall in this category.

Health is Only a By-Product of Yoga

One should not lose sight of the intent of yoga, which is realization of the nature of existence and purpose of life, which in turn has a transformative effect on the individual, which has positive impact on health. It also has collateral positive impact on the immediate family, friends, coworkers, and social connections of the individual, and thus on the society as a whole. So, is it wrong for most people to pursue yoga for better physical health alone?

Over years of experience, evolved yoga masters say that the initial motivation to start yoga practices does not matter. They recognize it is the cosmic conspiracy that when the soul is ready a motivating reason will develop that may be less than the highest spiritual objective. Thus, anyone can begin yoga for whatever motivated reason, health or otherwise. Eventually yoga leads one in stages to the highest realization, provided one does not get trapped into assumptions. Irrespective of motivation (including better health), approaching yoga with an open-mind and without expectations, will yield its best results. The results come when the soul and cosmos are ready. This is often referred in religious systems as Divine Grace.

Questions and Discussion Topics

1. The integration of body-mind-spirit unfolds one's purpose of life (*Dharma*). In figure 27.1 in Chapter 27, it constitutes B2, C1 and C2 in the green framed box, which should be in sync with the cosmic flow in B1. By connecting into the cosmic intelligence and becoming self-realized, do you think the health impact on a person would be even better than without this highest connection? If so, why and how? If not, why and how?

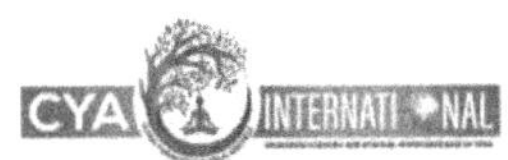

CHAPTER 36:

Role of Yoga in Global Environmental and Socio-economic Balance

The spiritual eco-system of souls – birth, rebirth, and final states – also reflects in the physical world in its environment and how humans, living organisms and non-living matter exist and transform. This is all within the cosmic connectivity of yogic existence as we understand from the Yoga Sutras – what we call as the cosmic flow (*rita*).

The cosmic flow is constantly changing. In the yogic system, as cosmic beings, we need to adapt to keep pace with environmental changes that allow us to fulfill our life purpose, and thus support the cosmic flow as planned by God's program. Sleep and meditative connectivity provide the necessary adaptation in the form of creative thinking, and in the physical dimension as strengthened immune system and adaptive capabilities. From a yogic perspective, this is what Darwin proposed as evolutionary adaptation. Of course, this is a deeper understanding than the conventional view of the immune system in the body that is known to yoga and traditional medicine systems, where the left side of the organ systems are considered the adaptive (or reprogramming capability), while the right side is considered the maintenance capability.

In the recent years, there have been rapid man-made changes in the environment:

- GMO (genetically modified) food and vegetation,
- Massive industrial pollution and its impact on the quality of air, water, soil, noise, and radioactivity levels,
- Global-warming and its impact on weather, forest fires, ocean water-levels and species dependent on these,
- Heightened electromagnetic radiation in the environment with mobile phones, broadcasts, satellite communications and even electric lines.

Such rapid changes in the last couple of generations are much ahead of the evolutionary adaptive changes of the normal human being, which occurs over many more generations. The inability to adapt fast enough creates stress in the system. Add to this the level of disinformation and information hitting on mobile devices all the time creating more churn (by reactivity) in the mind. The stresses created by these environmental disturbances manifest in the form of mental health issues and autoimmune issues.

Finally, this can all be attributed to undeterred greed (self-interest) of modern mercantilism, which has become the standard for the world. In yoga, it is called *adharma* that disturbs the cosmic flow.

In the ancient system, those spiritually connected (*brāhmanas*) advised the socially concerned (*kśhatriyas*) who ruled society to keep the balance between the self-centered greed of commercialism (of the *Vaiśhyas*) and exploitation of others and environmental resources in society. Today, all over the world, the guardians of society have sold their souls to the commercially minded. Businesses are the funders of elections, and funds buy access to the media and market research (opinion polls) that create suitable images and messaging for emotional appeal to win elections. Decisions are made in society based on how the moneyed interests are able to influence politicians and the media. Unless campaign finance reforms are done where only eligible voters can fund election campaigns and within limitations, and general 'truth-in-information' laws are put in place for election messaging or any advertising or social media messaging even for purposes outside elections, this situation will not change.

The downstream effect of such societal governance is that politicians on the one hand pander to moneyed interests to beget more campaign funds, and on the other hand to socially minded interest groups with largesse for social causes since they influence voters. Such an approach results in less taxes and more expenditure resulting in perpetual deficits in government budgets, increasing national debts, lop-sided social and economic policies, and increasing risks of volatility in financial markets.

There are too many examples to illustrate the point, but a handful are sufficient to illustrate the problem and how the process works. These are presented in the blue boxes below.

These *adhārmic* practices across the globe have today created undue stresses in societies that have caused increased individual health issues, societal issues like crime, and global societal issues as well, like global warming and rising water levels that are sinking island nations, political and religious extremism, etc. Health issues are very close to each individual and cover a spectrum of autoimmune conditions that are life threatening like cancer, and less threatening conditions like celiac, asthma and allergies related to peanut, pollen, etc.

How do we understand this situation?

Simple answer is that greed has increased self-serving activities in the name of material progress, and the eco-system has been unable to keep pace with it. The only way for the eco-system to keep pace is with spiritual transformation of society without religious divisiveness. This will help to clear the unholy relationship between government and commercial interests. Yoga is the answer.

EXAMPLE 1 – HEALTH CARE

Health Care around the world is mostly based on the Allopathic Medicine system of the Western World. While understanding of the human system is based on observed anatomy and physiology, which is reasonably definitive, therapy is a different matter since different people, given different underlying factors which are not fully understood by modern medicine, react differently to the same therapy for the same diagnosed health disorder. Therefore, therapeutic modalities are based on statistical probabilities with the understanding that the unfortunate may minimally need to move to another drug or suffer some minimal side-effects or the side-effects treated with another drug, or at worst case lose one's life since the drug or surgery had a severe negative reaction. To manage this risk, the system created today is called Standard of Care.

The Standard of Care established by the American Medical Association has the following implications:

- Approved Treatment - For each diagnosed condition, there is an established first line of treatment, and if it does not work the next available treatment, etc. based on large sample trials of treatments that can include drugs, surgeries, and devices.
- Liability Protection – As long as the physician is using the Standard of Care there can be no liability for the physician from any adverse outcome, because it is considered the best scientific knowledge available.
- Role of Testing and Limited Discretion of Physician – Validating diagnosis is critical for appropriate application of Standard of Care, so that the physician must do exhaustive tests (with minimal consideration for exertion of patient and cost of such tests) and the traditional role of a physician, where diagnosis is made based on externally observed symptoms of patients, is minimized.
- Funding and Validation System Not Driven by Genuine Health Effectiveness - Approach of Drugs and Device Makers is to exploit the statistically based validation system with funding for trials where there is potential for big profits. The double-blinded controlled studies with a control group and test group are considered the scientific gold standard for validating the impact of drugs or devices for specific disorders. The influence of the system is so strong that some have suggested that even among government funding authorities some cost effective options may not be considered relative to options that seem like technological advancement that are pushed by the industry whose interests are in big profits from patented new applications.
- No Interest in long term side-effects - Because there is no profit to be made, long term longitudinal studies of medications, devices and surgeries are typically not pursued.
- No Interest in 'Placebo-effect' – The original reason for the control groups in studies was to demonstrate that the intervention investigated was truly effective. Subsequently we have learned that the 'placebo effect' by itself can be effective psychosomatic medicine. This is the power of positive thinking which can have the healing effect. But that does not bring in revenue, and so there is no interest in promoting it for patients. From a yogic standpoint, the power of positive affirmation only works for those whose *nādis* are clear enough to generate the healing communication. Clearing of *nādis* can happen from deep relaxation.

- Use of Governmental control to promote the revenue interests of the current medical system by legal impediments to alternatives and limited funding to study alternatives under the consideration of approaches that don't fit the current scientific model.
- Wisdom of Traditional Medicine Systems and Yoga are sidelined or work on the edges with limited impact. For instance, from Ayurvedic tradition, surgery is considered the last resort to save lives, since surgery can disrupt communications of *nādis* and in a small proportion of cases the disruption may not be restored and can lead to cascading health issues. Yet in modern medicine, surgery is being pushed as it brings in revenue. Gall Bladder stones are treated by surgery to remove the gall bladder, whereas in traditional medicine systems use of horse-gram (seed of *macrotyloma uniflorum*) in small quantities over a period of time is known to dissolves gall stones.[122] Hysterectomy for women with difficult conditions of the uterus (fibroids, painful periods) is often the choice since the patients and providers have little patience to work with long term changes in lifestyle.

Thus, there is no wonder, we have increased costs of health care all over the world, with not necessarily better quality of life. It has also led to thoughtless application of risk. While the probabilistic understanding is well-recognized in modern medicine, the signed off consents before invasive processes are considered standard, and doctors generally tell patients not to worry too much about it. Such views of doctors minimizing the possibility of negative outcome is based on two underlying assumptions: (a) the patient has no better alternative available within their narrow realm of knowledge; (b) mild negative reactions can be quickly corrected and addressed, and the possibility of fatality is very remote.

In effect modern medicine operates in a way that this is the best-known therapeutic science available with underlying risks of fatalities or disabling possibilities. It completely ignores the meaning of life and death, which in its view cannot be known, and is therefore functioning to address disease conditions instead of the underlying cause of true health which in a spiritual sense is related to the purpose of life. The influence of yoga and traditional medicine systems have made the role of stress management as key to healthy living more apparent in recent times. However, revenue interests and the control of the medical and pharmaceutical interests on elected law makers makes it very difficult for accelerated changes in the healthy direction. A prime example of how drug manufacturers in the USA made the law makers approve a provision in 2003 that government-funded Medicare cannot negotiate drug prices, and even in 2022 efforts to undo it is stymied by limiting it to specific drugs. In the meantime, HMOs have taken the opportunity to offer Medicare coverage since their annual drug costs through their negotiation allows for about \$3,000 of lower costs per person on average, which allows them to provide extra benefits utilizing part of the extra margin. In effect this robs the taxpayers and the public for commercial interests, in cahoots with law makers and the government.

In effect, the health care system is a source of tremendous stress on the users and providers, fully based on greed, and pushes everyone away from cosmic harmony.

---

[122] This has been tested on mice. See Bigoniya P, Bais S, Sirohi B. The effect of Macrotyloma uniflorum seed on bile lithogenicity against diet induced cholelithiasis on mice. Anc Sci Life. 2014 Apr-Jun;33(4):242-51. doi: 10.4103/0257-7941.147433. PMID: 25593405; PMCID: PMC4293752. However, no effort has been made for human trials done to the specifics of modern scientific standards.

EXAMPLE 2 – FINANCIAL SYSTEM

The abuse of the Financial System between the government and commercial banking institutions is transparent in the following ways:

- Manipulation of Financial Markets – Politicians, interested in doling out favors to interest groups in return for campaign funds and votes, intentionally run a budget deficit, since revenue raising taxes are not popular. When the national debt becomes outrageously large, the Federal Reserve manipulates to keep the interest rates so low, much below the inflation rate, that the cost of borrowing for the government is minimal, and real return on risk-free bank deposits is negative. This forces almost everyone to invest in the stock market and its exposure to risk irrespective of sophistication in investing. This artificially creates an increased market for asset managers while increasing the level of stress on the general population exposed to the volatility of the stock market.

- Unethical Profiteering of Banks - While the use of debit cards cost less than 15 cents per transaction and is easily conducted over the financial system infrastructure of the Federal Reserve, banks loot the merchants who must pay a percentage of the transaction to the banks. The value to merchants was based on an established fact that when people can pay by card and not have to carry around a lot of cash, the ease of payment increases sales for merchants. This was at a time when financial transactions were subject to bigger risks. Now the private banking sector rides on government infrastructure and risks of fraud and default are less, but the greedy banking system continues exploitative profits from merchants and the federal government. Interestingly when the Reserve Bank of India introduced RuPay through its government owned National Payments Corporation of India and the Indian government started promoting it to reduce transaction costs for merchants, VISA representing western mercantilism was complaining since their no cost cash cow was threatened.

- Exploiting the Financially Vulnerable – The credit card system with usury-level interest rates figured out that interest on balance was the biggest source of revenue and profits. So, they promote more spending with money-back schemes paid by higher rates on merchants enabling those who are financially secure and pay their balance every month to be subsidized by those who are financially insecure and keep paying high interest on their balance every month.

- Emergence of Cybercurrency – The distrust of politicians and the banking system abusing the financial health of countries has resulted in the strange phenomenon of cybercurrency with greed of individuals trading on their value with conventional currency. Even while its integrity is questionable some people have started using it. It enables easier access to cyber criminals and money launderers who have been exploiting the system.

The greed of the manipulators of financial system increases stress in society and pushes everyone away from cosmic harmony.

EXAMPLE 3 – FOOD SUPPLY

The story of food supply is the same story as the pharmaceutical industry and its side-effects. In the name of increasing food productivity, genetically modified food grown with chemical fertilizers, may well have increased allergy sensitivities in the population. This side-effect was never assessed earlier and the economic dependence of farmers on seeds from biotech companies that manufacture them has the same color of handholding between commercial interests and the government.

Allergy sensitivity is a stress on the human system that causes inflammation.

EXAMPLE 4 – ROLE OF MEDIA

The role of advertising has been well understood over the history of the world. The phrases like "out of sight, out of mind," "keep lying over and over again consistently, and even lies will be perceived as the truth" are traditional adages that describe the role of political propaganda and the role of promoting brands and product sales. While the message is one part, the media that carries it is the important second segment. In this age of internet marketing, targeting based on demographic and psychographic profile of individuals is the icing on the cake for successful disinformation and information. The success of Trump's Big Lie about the stolen election in 2020 is a striking example. In effect, the disinformation of media distorts the minds of people, and many people get addicted to such content.

The self-centered use of media for disinformation, along with easy availability of firearms, has created polarized societies, increased crime levels, and has increased the stress level within society.

EXAMPLE 5 – WIRELESS TECHNOLOGY

In this age of wireless and mobile technologies, the level of electromagnetic radiation on health is another concern. Of course, as adaptive beings of the cosmos, we get used to everything and they cease having negative effect provided we have stress-free relaxation to adapt. In bio-meridian (*nādi*) readings Life in Yoga Institute has found that for the older generation mobile phones and fit-bit watches may increase stress in the body. However, for the younger generation who are used to it, removing it may increase stress.

EXAMPLE 6 – ENERGY PRODUCTION AND UTILIZATION

Excessive use of energy has become common place (e.g., disposable products), and use of fossil fuels and other industrial gases have resulted in global warming that is being discussed these days. Disposable products are a major contributor for excessive use of energy, since their production, distribution and disposal require substantial use of energy while adding to waste contamination. The resistance of countries based on commercial interests has been significant.

EXAMPLE 7 – SHIFT FROM COST-PLUS PRICING TO VALUE-BASED PRICING

The tradition in economic policy before the advent of the computer and internet age was that free-market economics would ensure competition to keep prices at a level where it would cover operational costs and a normal real rate of return on investment of about 6%. In industries like electrical power distribution, considered natural monopolies, where it was not economically or logistically feasible to have different lines of competitors going into buildings, the Public Utility Commission would regulate the allowed rate of return on investment and fix the price. In the field of economics, it was understood that between monopolies and free competition (based on a large number of providers of goods and services), there was the phenomena of other market distortions that would limit competition and impact pricing. The most prominent among them are oligopolies where a handful of providers control the industry. In traditional pricing philosophy, there too some limited regulation was warranted that ensured fair pricing.[123]

The advent of the computer and internet age created a paradigm that has not yet been fully digested within the tradition of economic philosophy of fair pricing. A computer application like a word processing software requires only a one-time investment, like writing a book.[124] Thereafter, when it is sold in small numbers or in millions or billions, the revenues largely go towards profits. But unlike a book,[125] when files (documents) created by an application requires others to have the same application for ease in managing tasks, it creates a pressure for all or most users to buy the same application (making competitive applications of less value). Thus, while the output of Microsoft Office is technically portable for other applications for review and editing for others to work on, it is practically inconvenient. Thus, Microsoft Office as a product creates limitations in competition and their pricing creates a situation where the return on the initial investment is no longer near the normal. [The frequent releases of new editions with minor improvements are only a technical excuse to justify big profits.] While this was only an example, this is characteristic of many providers that have emerged by leveraging the computing and internet systems.

In turn, this creates speculation among investors as to which provider will become the winner and where to fund as a venture capitalist, providing fuel to motivated greed creating a great deal of stress. The stress is in two constituencies: employees that work in such companies, especially during the stages before they become market leaders; investor community which directly or indirectly includes a sizable share of the population. In time, the same kind of stress becomes the corporate culture across the private workforce. There is no wonder that we see the health consequences of such stress factors in society. Society has not yet figured out how to balance entrepreneurial dynamism to further societal progress without making it into an exercise in mindless greed that damages society.

---

123 This is the role of the Federal Trade Commission in the United States.

124 Like a book, later editions can have additional or improved content which requires further investment. For simplicity in conveying the point, that need not be addressed here.

125 Textbook requirements in educational courses and participation in book clubs are an exception which appear to be similar to computer applications but are much less in impact.

Questions and Discussion Topics

1. Take any example of conflict or distortions in the economy anywhere in the world that you see reported in the news in the last three months. Study the underlying factors and explain how yoga will view the problem and provide the structure for correction. [As this book is being finalized the Russian war on Ukraine is a good example to study.]

As you start experiencing yoga in every aspect of living, you develop a sensitivity towards your impact on others and the world around you, and the importance of being true to one's conscience in everything we do.

As T.S. Eliot notes (Choruses from the Rock): "Where is the Life we have lost in living?
Where is the wisdom we lost for the sake of knowledge?
Where is the knowledge we lost for the sake of information?"

Dalai Lama's Lament About the Modern World

We have bigger houses, but smaller families.
We have more degrees, but less sense,
More knowledge, but less judgment,
More experts, but more problems,
More medicines, but less health.
We've been all the way to the moon and back, but we have trouble crossing the street to meet the new neighbor.
We build more computers to hold more information to produce more copies than ever, but we have less communication.
We have become long on quantity, but short on quality.
These are the times of fast food, but slow digestion; tall man, but short character;
Steep profits, but shallow relationships.
It is a time when there is much in the window, but nothing in the room.

PART VIII – FUNCTIONAL AND ETHICAL REQUIREMENTS IN LEADING A YOGA CLASS

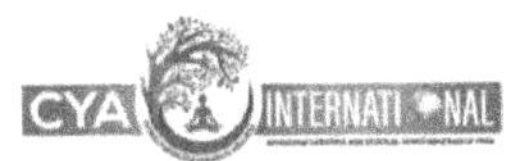

CHAPTER 37:

Functional and Ethical Requirements

While conducting a yoga class, functional and ethical elements include the environment of the facility, and the conduct and presentation of the instructor.

Facility

When preparing to lead a class, an instructor must make sure that the physical environment is conducive to learning and safe for practice. For an *āsana* class, one must make sure there is a large enough space where students can maintain a comfortable distance from each other. The space should be clean and uncluttered to avoid potential for stepping or colliding onto something that may hurt. Good lighting and air circulation, and adequate acoustics are also important. Arrangement in the room should be such so that the instructor can maintain optimal eye contact with all the students to hold their attention. (Some people like to come into class and hide in a corner or behind a pillar.) Any additional materials that may be needed, for the type of yoga class one leads, should be made available: chairs with good back support for those who need them, yoga mats, shawls, and yoga props like bolsters, straps, blocks, etc. and any audio, video and graphic aids that may be useful.

Presenting the Instructor

First impressions are important. It will condition the whole relationship with the students. Wearing light, peaceful colors that suggest clarity and calm is desirable. Clothing should be modest according to the culture of the location. For example, in many Muslim countries, women are expected to wear a covering over their hair. In some places these rules may be even more specific. In India, people generally avoid short pants and tend to keep arms, shoulders and ankles covered, especially among women. In some of these cultures, not following these rules can invite harassment or worse for women. Modest clothing is always a good idea to minimize distractions from the yogic content of the class.

A good teaching approach is to first explain the practices that will be done. This will make sure there is guidance on safe practice and the benefits and qualifiers, if any. It is a good idea to demonstrate each practice before asking the class to do the practice. Thereafter the instructor may do the practice along with the class and as needed provide verbal cues to reinforce the correct method. Once the class is in a smooth flow, the instructor should focus on observing each person in the class and make verbal or physical adjustments and suggestions as needed. It is very helpful for students to receive expressions of positive feedback when they are doing well: "Yes!" "Right!" "Good!" It is very common for people to feel a need for confirmation that they are doing well.

Punctuality, especially for the instructor, is important for several reasons. It demonstrates commitment to the students. The students' punctuality helps them develop their habit of discipline in practice. Asking everyone to come a little early gives time to settle the body and mind before beginning the class.

Interaction with Students/Attendees

Sensitivity in Comments - Many people tend to observe themselves as if from outside the body, ignoring their internal states, and to make critical comments about what they observe. This mental habit often helps one to sustain painful moods and emotional states. This same mental habit may be expressed relative to what one observes in others. However, as an instructor, one should be sensitive to how attendees in the class may feel, and words should not result in discouragement. It will be best to reduce this tendency by refraining from making critical remarks. Instead asking a struggling student, "How does that feel," and by focusing on catching people doing it right and commenting on that may serve as positive reinforcement. In fact, if the student is not doing something that violates safety, it may not be necessary to point out faults. In most of these cases, within a few weeks of regular attendance, the student by observing others or with minor cues from the instructor will find their optimum.

Touching Students - Whether and how to touch students is a question often asked by new instructors. While touching appropriately in some situations may be warranted to protect the safety of the student, when safety is not a concern it may be best to observe and provide verbal cues for the student to find how the posture fits in their body.

When touching is required, it is important, again, to know the student and to know the local culture. In some cultures, people of opposite genders never touch each other casually. It is impossible to know who among the students may have experienced physical or sexual trauma that may make them exquisitely sensitive to touch. One way to deal with this initially is simply to be clear about the way touch may be used in the class and give the students permission to say no. When approaching a student to adjust the posture, one must ask whether it is OK to offer an adjustment and one must be specific about the part of the body that will be touched. In any touch, one should avoid touching sensitive parts and remain in neutral territories. The preferred solution, when possible, is to do the adjustment verbally without touching. If a person can keep the back straight in a seated position, by avoiding postures that are difficult to do correctly, touching can be completely avoided. Further, as the *nādis* cleanse what was not possible earlier will become possible in stages with regular practice.

It is important to remember that in any class or whenever people seek help with something, there is always a power relationship involved. An instructor must fully recognize that whether one sees it that way or not. While an instructor's natural focus may gravitate towards teaching, it is more important to focus on the needs of the students.[126] Any time that balance begins to get reversed it is a sign of potential trouble and needs to be thought through carefully, hopefully with the assistance of someone with greater experience.

AN EXAMPLE OF RESOLVING A SITUATION WITHOUT TOUCHING

Ardhamatsyendra is a sideward-twist āsana practice that can be difficult for anyone. This can be progressed in stages without pressuring the student to graduate to the next stage within the paradigm of correct approach to yoga, i.e., all practices must be done without strain, and should be meditatively engrossing. Graduated stages of the practice and instructions that avoid unwanted strain and bad posture, which also avoids touching, is described below.

FIRST STAGE: Cross one leg over the other and grab the knee of the leg on the top with both the hands and bring it towards the opposite shoulder only to the extent possible with mild effort, while the head turns the other way. Instruction should be given to make sure the spine does not bend (slouch) in any part of the vertebral column. Students in almost any shape will be able to accomplish this.

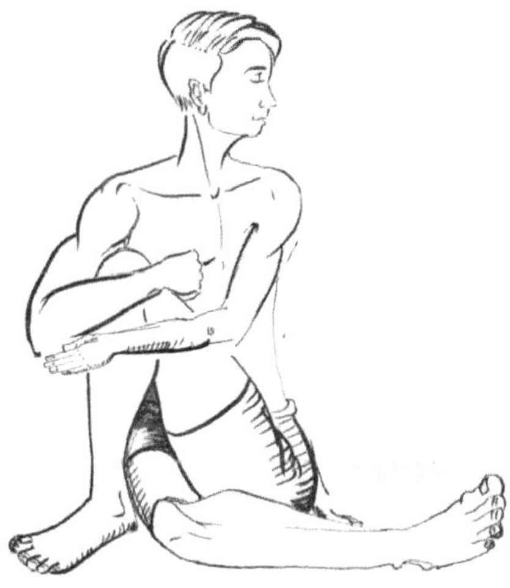

[While in *Haṭha Yoga* style the position can be held for a couple of minutes, if this also poses some difficulty, it can initially be done in *Prāṇakriyā* style. The knee being held can be pulled towards the opposite shoulder in exhalation and released in inhalation. Twenty breaths done daily for a few weeks will allow graduation to the *Haṭha Yoga* style.]

[126] Most successful businesses call this as 'customer focused' management, focused on customer satisfaction. In this case one is not selling something that comes in a box. It is a service that is delivered in close physical proximity. Great caution must be taken to ensure that one's power relationship and focus on teaching not only does not cross normal 'professional' boundaries, but also is not insensitive to the expectations of the 'customer'.

SECOND STAGE: For people who are not significantly overweight or with other obstructive disability, the knee being pulled should be coming very close towards the opposite shoulder. Under these circumstances one can be persuaded to graduate to the next step. Using the opposite hand to hold or leverage the knee, releasing the other hand and keeping it behind on the floor in the same direction as the head which has turned, completes the second stage.

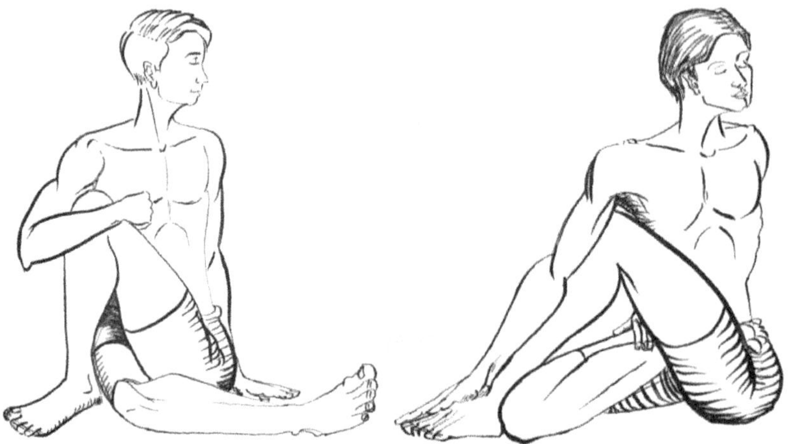

THIRD STAGE: Only when the student seems very comfortable with the knee drawn in close to the opposite shoulder, and the hand holding the knee stretching to the point of leveraging the elbow on the knee, should one attempt the third stage. In fact, the best indicator of the readiness is the nature of the breath – whether it is peaceful and relaxed in the second stage.

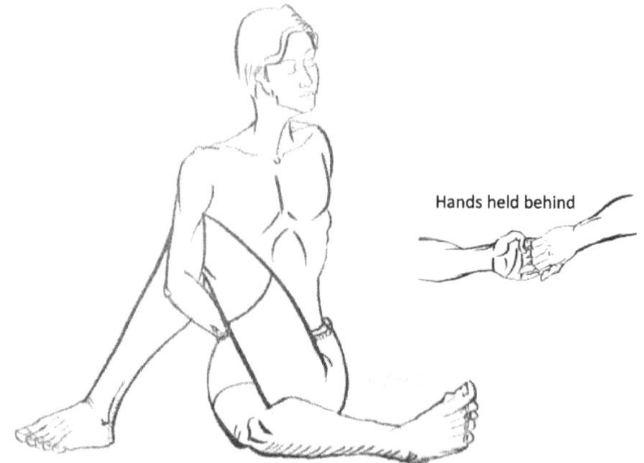

If the hand holding the knee can leverage the elbow over the knee and at the same time bring the hand under the knee, one can attempt to hook the hand with the other hand which is behind turned from the other side. If the hands are unable to connect and stay hooked, the spine is likely to bend and should be avoided. Maintaining the second stage will be sufficient.

Thus, by working in stages, watching the ease of breath, and explaining to the students that *nādi* stimulation is the key and not attaining an advanced final position, a teacher can work to avoid postures where a student is likely to struggle. Thus, touching can be completely avoided. Such a graduated approach can be adopted for any yoga practice by an experienced teacher.

Motivation and Ethics in Yoga Instruction

Monetary Motivation - Money can be a difficult area for instructors. While in modern times people think in terms of value of time and expanding business in every activity and ensuring sufficient income, such a focus can dilute one's yoga progress. Realization of one's being as a cosmic spirit, a transactional mindset can conflict with one's soulful purpose. Therefore, it is best to have another source of income for the needs of regular living. Unless society recognizes the value of yoga for human development and equates it to necessary education, and pays a salary, like teachers in any school, through governmental or other non-profit institutions, pursuing yoga as a livelihood has potential to deviate one from the higher realization of yoga.

PERSPECTIVE OF A SENIOR YOGA TEACHER ON MONEY

If you come to rely on your teaching for most of your income, you may open yourself to a bias towards endless expansion of classes or hanging on to students beyond what the students may want. One way to avoid these pitfalls is to obtain your primary income from a different job or other source. That way you are free to offer your teaching gratis when you choose to or to teach as a gift to your students and accept whatever offerings they may choose to make.

Ethics in Yoga Gleaned from Yama of the Yoga Sutras - When teaching yoga to students, ethical behavior is part of teaching the first limb of the yoga system: *Yama*. The *Yamas* are ethical attitudes and behaviors that assist students and instructors in using their relationships as part of the process of creating a clear and pleasant and stable mind that is capable of deep meditation. **Another way to put it is to be true to one's conscience** with the sensitivity beyond oneself. [Of course, this assumes that the instructor has been regular in meditative practices to have developed that sensitivity.] *Yamas* have a very important role in yoga practice through the entire system. That is part of the reason that Patanjali has placed this first in the list of the limbs of yoga.

While Patanjali describes the *Yamas* as non-violence, being truthful, not stealing, seeking to know (*Brahmacharya*[127]) and not being excessively acquisitive (greedy), all these should be understood comprehensively as being ethical and true to one's conscience.

The most important of these attitudes is non-violence. As a person grows spiritually in one's dedicated practice (*sādhanā*), one naturally grows in one's empathy, which is the ability to feel what other beings feel. This enables one to do his/her duty (*Sva-dharma*) based on the guidance of his/her conscience.

---

[127] Brahmacharya has been mistakenly assumed to mean keeping celibacy. In fact, the real meaning is "exploring creation within and beyond the physical world" or "walking in the awareness of divinity". It is generally assumed that sexual attraction can be a distraction for Brahmacharya. However, procreation is a natural process of creation and cannot be prohibited.

For instance, not being a vegetarian for someone who comes from a non-vegetarian tradition where killing animals for food has never troubled one's conscience cannot be called violence within their conscience. The moment one feels the guilt, then one must become a vegetarian to be true to one's conscience. The same is true for a soldier who kills in a war. The soldier, following one's orders from superiors, to defend one's country, having no reservations in his/her conscience does not violate non-violence when inflicting harm on the enemy. Thus, it is said that all the *Yamas* are subject to one's *Dharma* or duty to support the cosmic flow.

According to the commentary of sage Vyāsa, all *Yamas* and *Niyamas* are specialized forms of non-violence.

THE SUFI WARRIOR

This story exists in many traditions but is probably originally a Sufi story. A Sufi warrior was engaged in fierce hand-to-hand combat. He had almost defeated his foe. Just before he struck the final blow, his opponent spit in his face. The Sufi dropped his sword and walked away. Astonished, his enemy protested that it is his duty to finish the battle and strike him down. The Sufi warrior said, "When you spat in my face, I felt anger. To kill from anger is murder and I do not do murder."

Similarly, truth is as one knows it and cannot be absolute, and sometimes hiding a truth without seeking to lie to avoid pain for another person may not be considered as lying. The objective of being true to one's conscience is more important than the absolute truth. There are many instances where "the truth" has been used as a weapon to try to hurt someone else. This use of the truth is violent and cannot be comforting to the conscience. A good guideline for speech is to ask oneself whether what I have to say is beneficial (*hita*), measured and friendly (*mita*), loving (*priya*) – i.e, true to one's conscience. If one is truthful, then the mind doesn't carry the anxiety that one carries with lies.

Stealing is again relative to one's understanding of ownership, which may differ in societies and circumstances of living. As one begins to relax one's sense of ownership, one may find oneself becoming more generous with others.

The concept of seeking to know and not being excessively acquisitive are the higher dimensions of *Yama* that develop and indicate higher awareness. Seeking to know is the impetus that leads to higher awareness. Not being affected by material attachments, and not seeking to compare with what others have, reduces acquisitive tendencies which is the real indicator of higher awareness.

These really are attitudes and realizations, rather than rules. They depend on how well one cultivates one's awareness and sensitivity to relationships with others and to the particulars of one's situation. When one models these attitudes and realizations for students while teaching, it is a powerful resource for them in their own lives.

There are several areas that can be especially problematic. Lending money to students can be a problem in several ways, especially if they fail to pay it back. Receiving gifts from students in front of other students can create an impression that the student is special in some way and closer to the instructor than other students. And romantic and sexual attractions can also be difficult. It is never a good idea to have a sexual relationship with a student and in some places, this would be considered criminal behavior.

What is most important in teaching others is that the instructor is there to meet their need to learn and grow. The students' needs are the focus.

Questions and Discussion Topics

1. One of your students invites you to dinner with the idea s/he wants to engage in further discussion in yoga. Should you accept this invitation? Why or why not?
2. One of your students is planning a festival party at her/his home. Should you accept this invitation to attend this large gathering? Why or why not?
3. Your class organizes a picnic and invites you to join them. Is it appropriate to accept this invitation? Why or why not?
4. You have been asked by a wealthy person to offer an individual yoga class at her/his home and has offered generous payment. Should you accept this offer? Why or why not?

It is time to bring the diversity in the approaches and practices of yoga into the unified understanding of yoga.

Yoga is life well-lived – for everyone, everywhere, and everything.

PART IX - CONCLUSION

38. Conclusive and Summary Understanding of Yoga
    - Existence is the Nature of Yoga
    - Mechanism of Yoga
    - Goal of Yoga
    - Yoga is One, But Practice Approaches are Many
    - Yoga is the Spiritual Content of All Religions
    - Yoga Sutras as the Comprehensive Principles
    - Importance of Regular Practice
    - Recognizing Progress Without Getting Deluded
    - Yoga for Cosmic Harmony in Integrative Existence
    - Motivation and Mundane Benefits of Yoga
    - Yoga Can be Present in All Aspects of Life

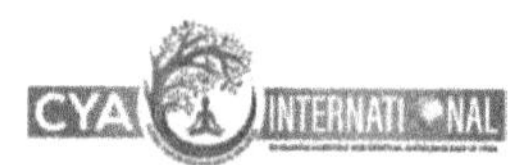

CHAPTER 38:

Conclusive and Summary Understanding of Yoga

When you understand a subject, depending on your audience and available time, you can speak on the subject in a few sentences or in volumes. Now that you have gone through the entire book, here are the different dimensions of yoga in a nutshell.

Existence is the Nature of Yoga

All of existence emanating from God is interconnected and held in a designed flow to fulfill the dynamics planned by God. Thus, all of existence is a dynamically distributed computing system, where each one of us and everything we observe (or don't), whether animate or otherwise, are nodal computing units, contributing to the cosmic flow. Live beings (like us) come with significant learning and adaptive capabilities[128].

In the scheme of creation, God stays unmanifest and outside creation. The Master creative program that comes out of God is called *Prakṛiti* and it creates the cosmic processor to run its program intent, which in turn creates small individual processors which are the different components of creation including everything living or non-living. Processors in the language of yoga are called *chittas*. While everything in creation has a *chitta*, beings that are alive have *chetanā* which is the ability to learn and adapt. While all of existence, animate or inanimate, has a connection to the cosmic *Chitta* or *Prakṛiti*, only beings with *chetanā* (live beings) have a concurrent connection with God. God being the source of all knowledge and everything, the connection of living beings to God gives them the unique ability to imbibe cosmic knowledge from God and become Self-Realized. Thus, as the Yoga Sutras of Patanjali states, God is the Ultimate Guru of everyone and at all times. The connection into the unmanifest God is called *Purușha*, and God is sometimes referred as the Supreme *Purușha*.

What we see in the three-dimensional world is the output or projection of the *chittas*. All *chittas* – individual ones and the Cosmic *Chitta* – are in the subtle domain outside the three-dimensional world and are not measurable with conventional scientific tools. The communication into the three-dimensional world starts from the domain of the *chittas,* that can be called the zone of the 'causal' body. In the three-dimensional world, it transforms into vibrations in the electromagnetic spectrum that are measurable and often referred as the zone of the 'subtle' body. These vibrations create the physical elements that we see in the world that can be called the

[128] This is called AI or artificial intelligence in the computing field.

zone of the 'gross' body. In traditional medicine systems with various sensory methods like pulse reading, and in modern times systems based on electromagnetism, these 'subtle' body vibrations entering a person's body can be measured and are used to assess the health of a person.

Mechanism of Yoga

Each live unit (like each one of us) in this system has five types of communication running within us, among which one allows for communication beyond the body. Each of these five types of communication have two aspects: communicating to maintain the system and communicating to reprogram and adapt the system to the changing environment to help better functionality to serve the cosmic intent. Three lower communications are communications to manage the earth elements of the body (musculoskeletal system) called *Apāna*, communications to manage the fluid elements of the body called *Vyāna*, and communications to manage the fire element of the body, which is the gene expression that integrates the demands of the external environment with the internal program of the body, called *Samāna*. The higher communication that can go beyond the body is the reprogramming ability of all the other communications, and thus also organ systems in the body. The intelligence of the reprogramming ability comes from the higher intelligence of the cosmos (*Prakṛiti*) and God, which naturally happens in sleep, deep rest, and in transcendental meditation. This communication is called *Udāna*. In the physical body it contributes to the immune system and repair needs of organs, and beyond the body it allows for intuitive experiences and realizations. This is where the higher realizations of yoga reside.

All these four communications are possible only if there is power (flow of energy) in the system – i.e., the body is alive. The communication that regulates power is called *Prāṇa.* Physiologically it is the central nervous system that controls the cardio-respiratory process and thus the cellular respiration that produces energy. In yoga, the higher understanding of *Prāṇa* goes beyond the cardio-respiratory process that merits deeper discussion in the teacher and therapist levels.

Goal of Yoga

Yoga is the path of direct realization of spiritual existence. The realization is that everything in creation, including each one of us, is simply an instrument of the cosmic flow. If we are true to our conscience and do whatever we confront in life with inner awareness and subdued reactivity – acceptance of what comes to us – that is the path to complete our duties towards the cosmic plan and be liberated.

Becoming liberated is the idea of going beyond rebirth which is associated with exhaustion and elimination of innate programs that are called *karma* and *kleśha* in yoga. However, the concept of Self-Realization has two ideas: (a) realizing that each one of us are only instruments of the cosmic flow to fulfill the cosmic intent of God; (b) realizing the nature of existence through intuitive perception that comes from the connectivity with God. This knowledge of the nature of existence can only come if one seeks. The concept of seeking and intuitively imbibing the answer is called *Samyama* in Yoga.

Yoga is One, But Practice Approaches are Many

Yoga as the path of direct realization is one, and that one system is called *Rāja Yoga*, which is enunciated in the Yoga Sutras authored by Patanjali. However, approaches of practices may differ. Popular yoga practices are associated with *āsanas*, with different variations associated with different popular schools. However, in the diverse domain of yoga practices, they may be approached by physical stimulation of *āsanas* and breathing practices, vibrational stimulation of sound, and mental stimulation of thought often associated with surrender to God – all designed to quieten the mental reactivity, which is the purification process of yoga that makes one become a non-reactive observer. These diverse approaches that emphasize the physical, vibrational, or mental-surrender aspects are categorically referred as *Haṭha Yoga*, *Tantra Yoga* and *Bhakti Yoga*. Each of these approaches works predominantly on some channels of communication in the mechanism, and an integrative approach is usually most effective for yogic realization.

Yoga is the Spiritual Content of All Religions

Faith and surrender to God are critical components of most religions. These components are also yogic principles. Further, the core of all religions is the spiritual pursuit of what existence is all about. Thus, the spiritual core of all religions is the yogic component, whose mechanism has been explained.

Yoga Sutras as the Comprehensive Principles

Yoga as a systematic, non-religious set of principles was enunciated in the Yoga Sutras of Patanjali in ancient India. The impetus to find the non-religious, spiritual principles possibly emanated from a search for the commonality among 33 ancient religions of India. While the spiritual principles were enunciated by Patanjali, a later or contemporary figure by name Vyāsa unified the 33 religions within the Vedic System by compiling the Vedas that included sacred hymns most likely from all the 33 religions. Thus, there is a common thread in the spiritual philosophies of Vyāsa and Patanjali. While Patanjali stays in the non-religious domain of principles, Vyāsa has the Vedic religion attached to it.

Importance of Regular Practice

Yoga is essentially experiential and not a path of academic discussion or mental analysis. It is a path that requires training to be a pure observer, which comes from daily and regular practice about the same time every day. By learning to be a pure observer, one becomes less reactive and lets the programs within slowly dissipate allowing the channels of communication to become more effective. This is called purification of the *nādis* or the channels of communication. This allows for deeper understanding of our physical, mental, and spiritual existence. However, the process of purification may be short or long depending on the individual. Anticipation is a mental barrier to being a pure observer. One must be patient with daily regular practice until the cosmos is ready to connect.

Recognizing Progress Without Getting Deluded

Progress is recognized in one's transformation – becoming more patient and less reactive. However, progress can also come in the form of intuitive and other extraordinary abilities. These are called *siddhis* of yoga described in the third *pāda* of the Yoga Sutras. One should remember that these abilities do not come to all, but only to those who have a need for them to fulfill their purpose of birth. One should not feel pride or seek emotional gratification by demonstrating such abilities, but only use them quietly where the cosmos guides to support the cosmic flow, with no personal interest of any kind.

Yoga for Cosmic Harmony in Integrative Existence

Yoga is the anchor of existence – the connector of every aspect of functioning of the Universe. Becoming realized in yoga and being in sync with the cosmic flow is the recipe for cosmic harmony and fulfillment of each individual being. While yoga can be a personal goal, in the totality of existence it has implications for how societies are ruled and managed, utilization of resources and environmental balance – all contributing to harmony beyond the individual who also contributes to it.

Motivation and Mundane Benefits of Yoga

While most people pursue yoga for mundane motivations like deep relaxation, health, ability to better focus and concentrate, be more effective/successful in physical and mental activities, there is nothing wrong with it. The reality is that in time, those who are consistent and dedicated will begin to experience the higher possibilities. Very often distress from failures in life draws people to yoga. We call this as the conspiracy of the cosmic flow when the soul is ready.

Yoga Can be Present in All Aspects of Life

Yoga is not specific to any practice or exercise. Learning to be an observer with intuitive awareness makes every aspect of living into a yoga activity. Training to become thus need not necessarily happen from conventional classes. Group or individual activities, like sports, games, jogging, swimming, cooking, cleaning, artistic activities, etc. done for no reason but for enjoyment of living in the moment become yogic training practices, which in time evokes intuitive awareness and fulfillment of the yogic objective.

Questions and Discussion Topics

1. Prepare a powerpoint presentation with charts that you can use for a 20-minute presentation to your students that provides an overview of yoga. Since all elements of yoga cannot be completed in a 20-minute presentation, this exercise will force you to separate the top-level concepts from the details. This will help you to clarify concepts of yoga in your own mind.

APPENDICES

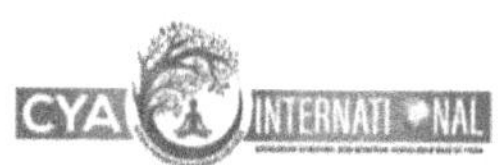

Appendix 1:

Sectional Breathing

Sectional breathing is a preparatory exercise designed to sense the three areas of the lungs to enable proper full breathing (using all parts of the lungs) as one progresses. It is designed to correct bad breathing practices that only use some parts of the lungs due to prolonged stresses in lifestyle. Typically stressed people breath only with the upper and mid lungs. For women, during pregnancy, they habitually start breathing with the upper and mid lung as the expanding foetus in the womb prevents downward expansion of the lower lungs, and the habit is sustained after childbirth. Practice of sectional breathing, by sensitizing each part of the lungs, enables one to overcome these habitual sub-optimal breathing.

As a point of note, lower lung breathing is the key area that needs revival for most people, and hence Diaphragmatic Breathing is the most important element in the three areas of breathing. Accordingly in a ten-minute practice we allocated 6 minutes for diaphragmatic breathing, 2 minutes for thoracic breathing and 2 minutes for the clavicle breathing.

Diaphragmatic Breathing - We begin with lower lung breathing with the diaphragm pushed down and the belly (abdominal area) responding to compensate.

The abdomen is of fixed capacity with the organs there held in a bag called the fascia of the abdominal area. However, the chest, unlike the abdomen, can expand in all directions as one breathes with the design of the rib cage and the peripheral muscles. As the lower lung expands with a deep breath, it pushes down the diaphragm. Since the abdominal area is of fixed capacity, it is compressed downward resulting in a bulge coming out in the abdominal area.

This practice is done as follows:

1. Starting position should be sitting up with an aligned posture[129] – back support (as seated on a chair or support of a wall) may be used.
2. Keeping one hand on the belly, begin by exhaling and drawing in the belly. The exhalation should be smooth without hurrying.

---

[129] Aligned posture refers to the natural alignment of the spine. Typically, people may say "sit up with an erect spine." The spine has a natural curve where in the lower spine the lumbar area curves in, and at the sacroiliac joint it bulges out, and then curves in again at the sacrum and coccyx.

3. Upon completion of the exhalation and a natural pause of about half a second, inhale slowly and deeply and feel the belly come out.
4. Repeat exhalation and inhalation as in steps 2 and 3 for about 6 minutes two to three times a day, and in about three weeks one will have developed enough sensitivity of the diaphragm to enable normal deep breathing of the lower lungs.

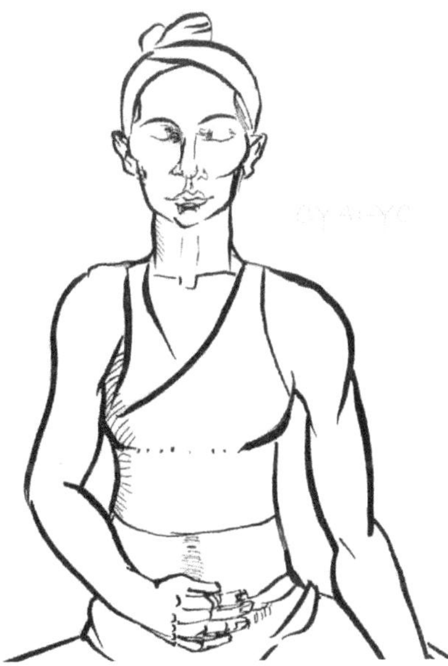

In a seated position, if it is difficult to feel the belly going in with exhalation and coming out with inhalation, as a beginning step, lying down in a supine position can make the sensitivity easier. After a week of such practice, effort must be made to sit up and continue in a seated position.

The recommendation for 6 minutes of practice is based on sufficient time, and yet not too long to draw on the patience of the practitioner. There is no adverse effect from longer and more frequent practice.

Thoracic Breathing – After the Diaphragmatic Breathing we do mid lung breathing with the chest expanding.

This practice is done as follows:

1. Starting position should be sitting up in an aligned posture and the hands stretched out in the front. Begin by exhaling completely bringing the palms together.
2. As you inhale separate the hands (without bending the elbows) and stretch them out on the two sides like wings in a full span in line with the shoulders. Observe the expansion of the ribs and the chest. [Make sure there is enough space on the two sides to avoid collision with another object or person.]
3. As you exhale, bring the hands together again as before.

4. Repeat inhalation and exhalation as in steps 2 and 3 for 2 minutes.

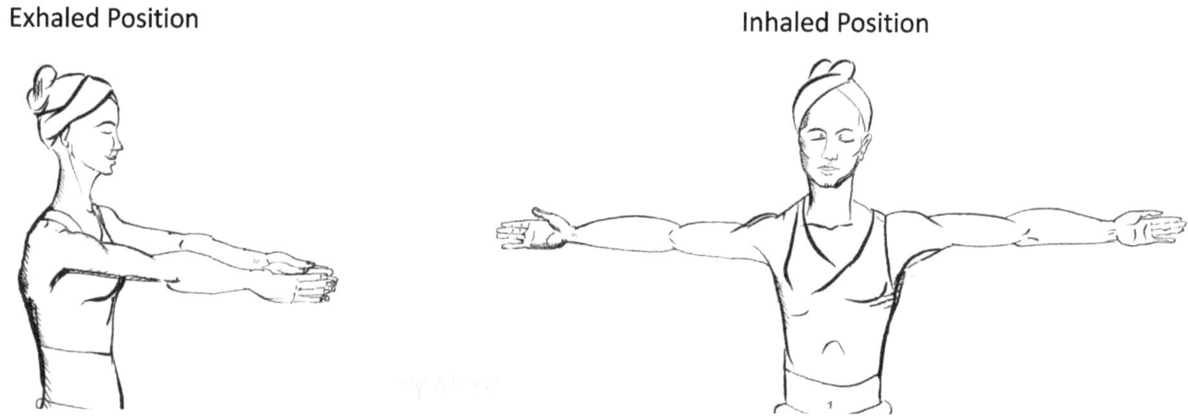

[<u>OPTIONAL ALTERNATIVE</u>: An alternative method is to place your palms over your floating ribs at the base of your rib cage (while the elbows stay on the sides of the chest) and feel the expansion of your chest as you inhale (as the elbows slightly pull backward). As you exhale, regain the starting position.]

This practice should be done immediately after the Diaphragmatic Breathing. Unlike the diaphragmatic sensitivity which many people may have difficulty in sensing, the chest expansion is easier for people to feel and therefore 2 minutes is enough.

Clavicular Breathing – Third in sequence is stretching out the collar bone (clavicle) as you inhale and relaxing it as you exhale.

This practice is done as follows:

1. Starting position should be sitting up in an aligned posture.
2. As you inhale, feel the stretch of the clavicle (collar bone). The motion will be sideways and slightly upward. The breath should be smooth and relaxed. [If you are unable to feel the stretch, you can consider lifting both your hands and stretching upward and sideways as you inhale.]
3. As you exhale slowly and smoothly, let the clavicle relax. It will also feel like the shoulders are relaxing.
4. Repeat inhalation and exhalation as in steps 2 and 3 for 2 minutes.

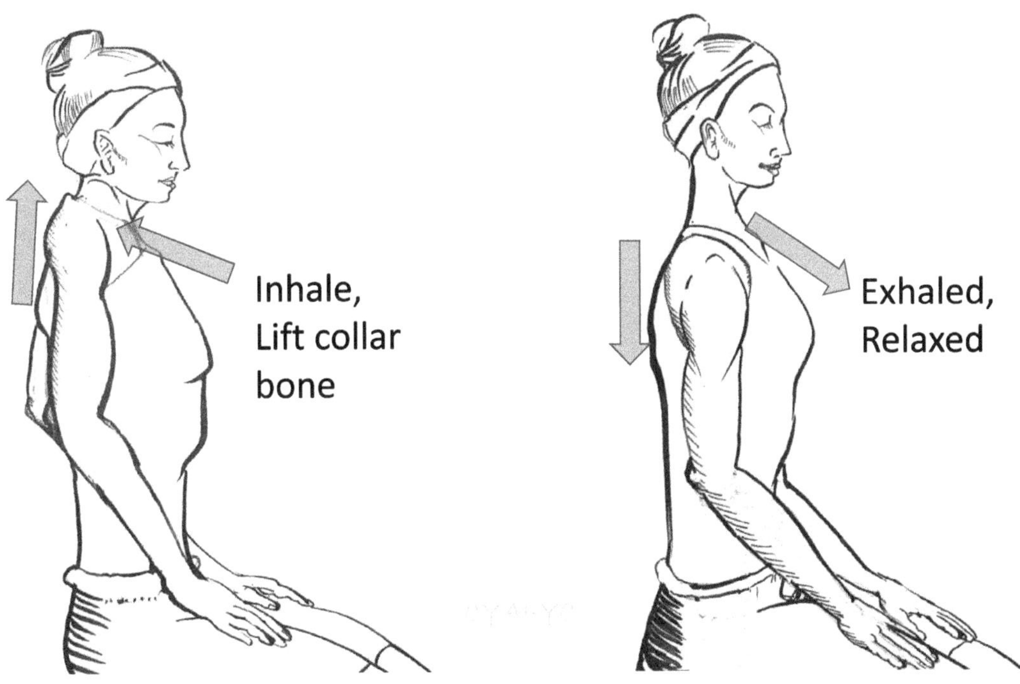

ALTERNATIVE: When done as part of the loosening exercises, inhale and stretch the shoulder upward and sideward, and while exhaling rotate the shoulder backward and bring it down.

This practice should be done immediately after the Thoracic Breathing.

As noted earlier, we focus on the Diaphragmatic Breathing more, because that is the source of weakness in most people. The other two breathing practices are not really needed for most people, other than to demonstrate the sensitivity of breathing in different parts, since most people have no difficulty with these breathing modalities.

The objective of this breathing training is to ensure that when one breathes normally and naturally, the belly should come out slightly, and the chest should expand slightly, and the collar bone should feel slightly stretched. In these sectional breathing practices, the motions are significantly exaggerated. Feeling this degree of exaggerated stretch in all the three parts will be observed only in *Bhastrikā Prāṇāyāma* where there is an active effort to inhale and exhale to the fullest.

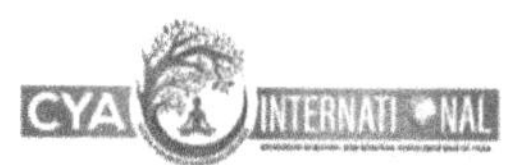

Appendix 2:

A Beginner's Regimen of Gentle Physical Practice

Any beginner's physical regimen consists of loosening the muscles of the neck, spine, hips, and joints of the limbs. This can be done from the feet to the head or from the head to the feet, and there can be many varieties of loosening exercises. When done for beginners with no physical limitations, such practices can be done on a mat. However, considering that this practice should be amenable for those with physical limitations, it should be possible to do them seated on a chair as well.

Also, keeping in mind the yoga objective of mindfulness in any physical practice with regulated breathing, and the association between the head and the mind, some prominent schools of yoga prefer to begin from the head to the toes. One such routine is presented here. It can be done fully seated on a chair. Needless to repeat, all practices must be done slowly without haste, and done in sync with breath that must be slow and long. Such practice done without strain should be safe for almost anyone who does not have a spinal injury that has not healed.

Step 1 – Mindful Relaxation

Seated in aligned posture, with back support as needed, one can quieten the mind from other distractions through chanting, music, visualization, affirmation, or breath – any point of focus. Focus on breath is the most generic, non-cultural practice.

With eyes closed, one focuses on slow deep breathing, with exhalation slightly longer than inhalation. Done for about 2 to 3 minutes will bring the awareness within.

Variations in this practice can include hand or shoulder movements. Some schools may lift the shoulder with inhalation and with exhalation rotate the shoulder backward and bring it down. Other schools may start with hands spread like wings in line with the shoulders and inhale lifting the hands above the head and bringing them together (in the *Namaskār*, prayerful position) as the head tilts backward. While exhaling hands are brought vertically downward to the mid chest as the head tilts forward. This serves as an exercise that combines some shoulder and neck movement with the breathing as well.

All practices involving motion along with breath for mindful relaxation should be longer than breathing practice alone, since building smoothness and adequate focus may take a little longer. Thus, if 2 to 3 minutes is used for a breathing practice for mindful relaxation, 4 to 5 minutes may be appropriate for a motion-based practice.

Step 2 – Neck Loosening

There are four neck loosening exercises:

- **Tilting the head sideways** bring the ear towards one shoulder with exhalation, and thereafter coming to the starting position with inhalation. Then with the next exhalation the tilt is to the other side – with the other ear going towards the shoulder. This is done with 20 breaths – effectively 10 tilts on each side.

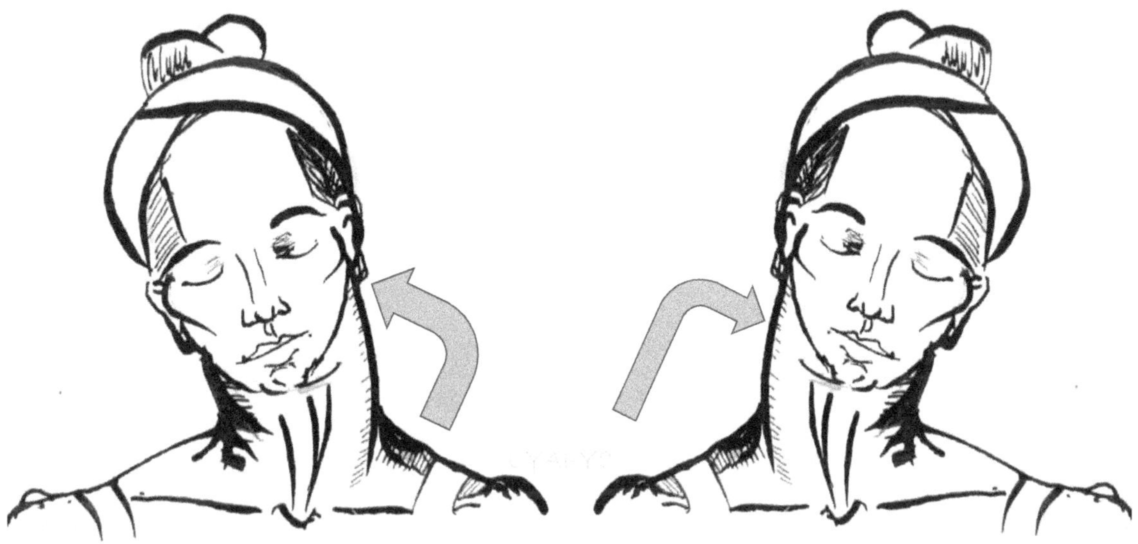

- **Turning head to the left and right** alternating with each breath – Begin with inhalation, and in sync with exhalation turn the head as if looking over one shoulder, and with inhalation coming back to the starting position. In the next exhalation the head is turned the other way. This is also done with 20 breaths – effectively 10 rotations on each side.

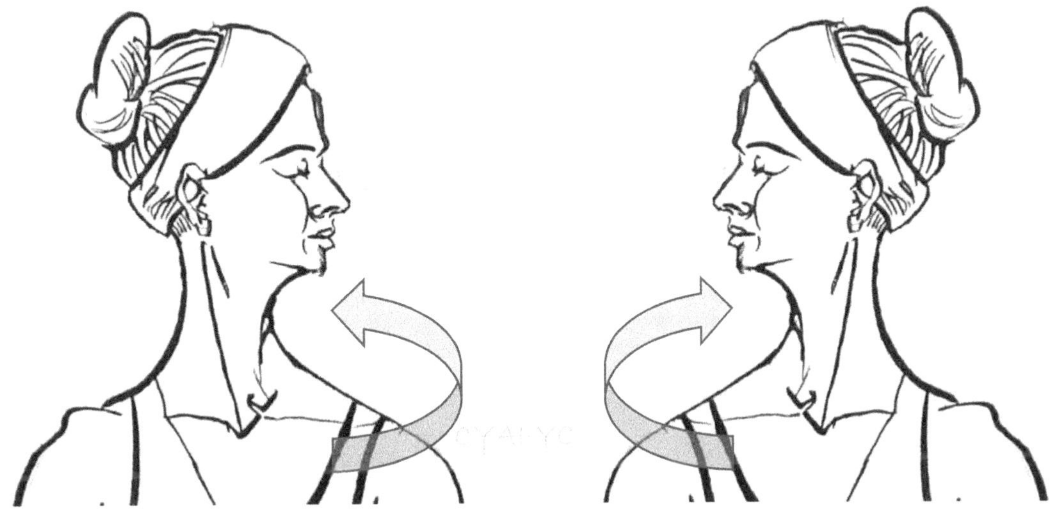

- **Tilting back and front** – Tilting the head backwards with inhalation (as if looking up towards the ceiling) and forward with exhalation (as if chin is coming towards the chest) is done for 10 to 15 breaths.

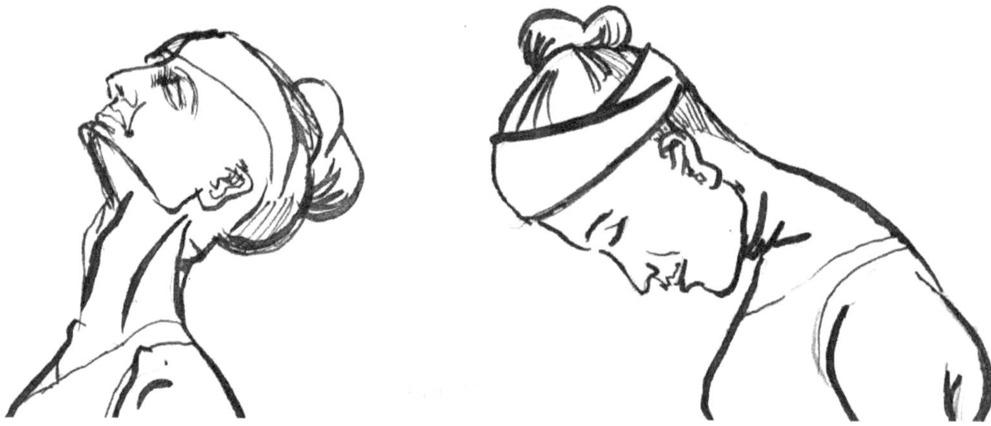

- **360-degree rotation** of the head is done, with about a third to half of the rotation done in inhalation and completing the remainder of the 360 degrees in exhalation. This is done for 10 breaths in one direction and another 10 in the other direction. It is best to begin with exhalation bringing the chin towards the chest. Then begin the inhalation going sideways around the shoulder and then backward. Then start the exhalation from the backward tilt to come back over the other shoulder down to the chest before beginning the next inhalation or at the end of the practice.

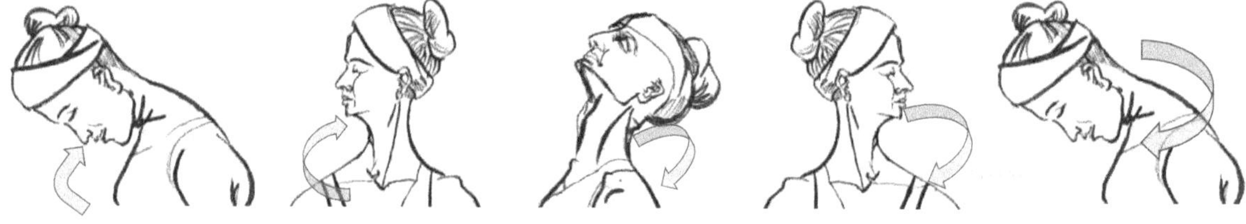

In the above illustration, after 10 breaths, the movement of the head and arrows would be reversed for the next 10 breaths.

Step 3 – Shoulder Loosening

Shoulder loosening can be done with three exercises.

- **Single shoulder lifting** – With each inhalation lift one shoulder towards the ear and with exhalation rotate backward and bring down the shoulder. This is first done for one shoulder about 10 times, and then repeated for the other shoulder 10 times.

- **Alternate shoulder lifting** – The second exercise is the same as the first, except with each breath one alternates between the shoulders. So, in 20 breaths, each shoulder rotates alternatively ten times.
- **Both shoulders lifting** – The third exercise lifts both shoulders at the same time – as opposed to one shoulder as in the earlier two exercises. This should be done for about 10 breaths.

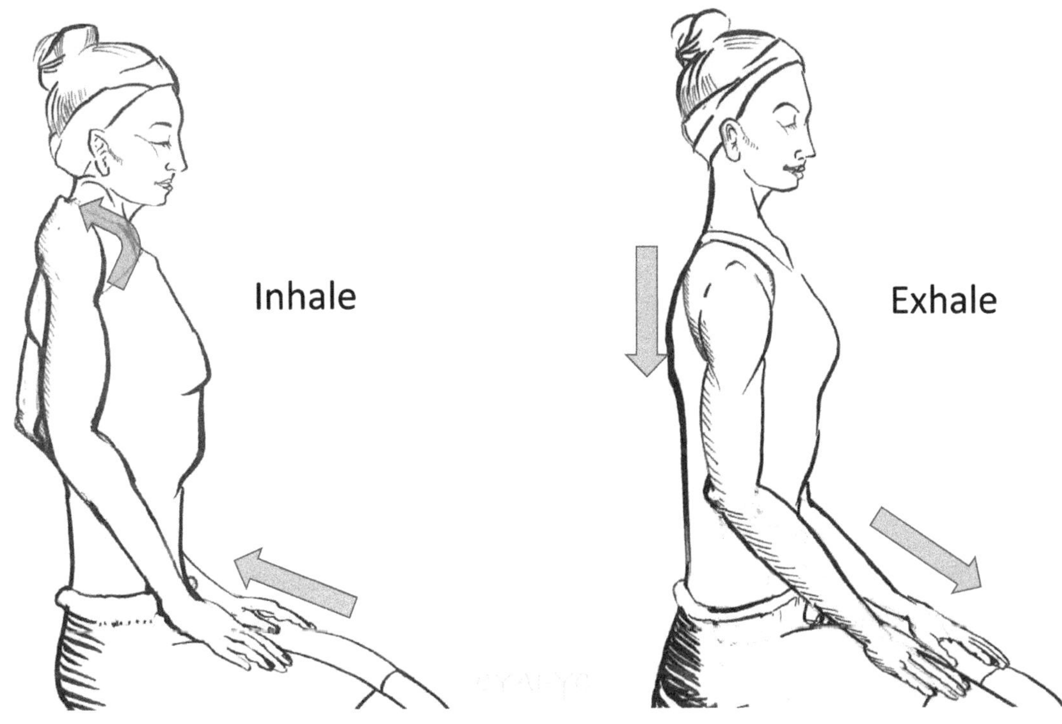

Step 4 – Hand and Wrist Loosening

There are three exercises in this sequence.

- **Wrist, Palm and Finger Stimulation** is done by first stretching out the hands in front, in line with the shoulders, with palms facing the floor. Then lift the palms upward from the wrist, perpendicular to the arms while inhaling. [Left panel picture] Also, stretch out the fingers at maximum expansion from the tip of the thumb to the tip of the little finger. Then, while exhaling, fold the thumb into the palms, close the other fingers over the thumb to form a fist, and drop the closed fist downward at the wrist, perpendicular to the forearm. [Right panel picture] This creates an up and down stretching for the wrist while also mobilizing the palm and fingers. Do this for 10 breaths.

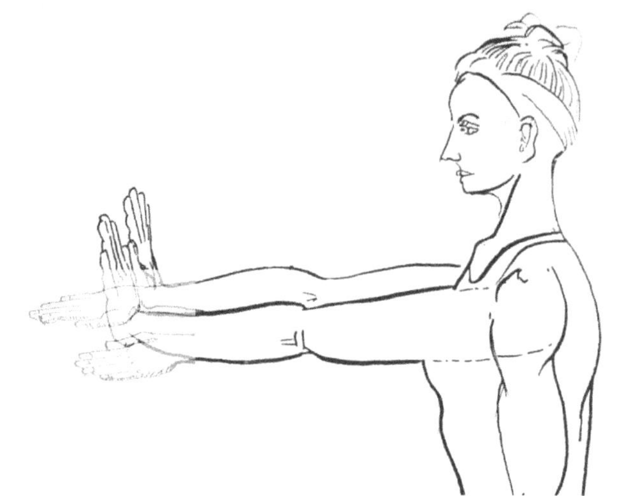
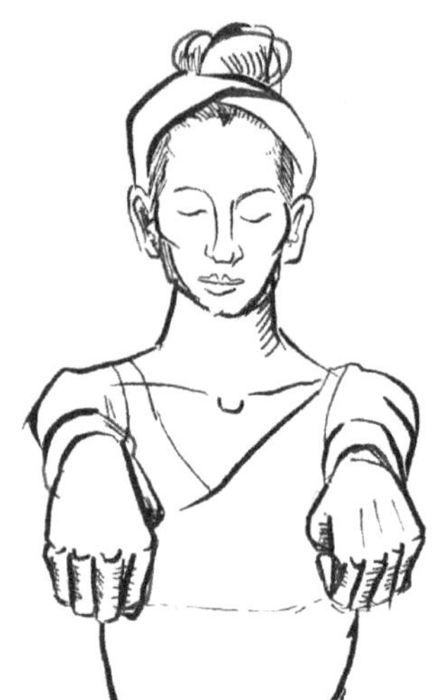

- **Fist Rotation** is done immediately after that last exhalation of the previous exercise, where the fist is downward facing. From that position, the fist is rotated in one direction, with half a rotation in inhalation and the other half in exhalation. The motion should be slow, done 10 times, with slow and long breaths. Then the direction is reversed and done for 10 breaths.
  This practice can be done with one fist at a time or with both fists together. [When done with one fist at a time, holding the wrist with the other hands enables greater stability and mobility of the wrist.]

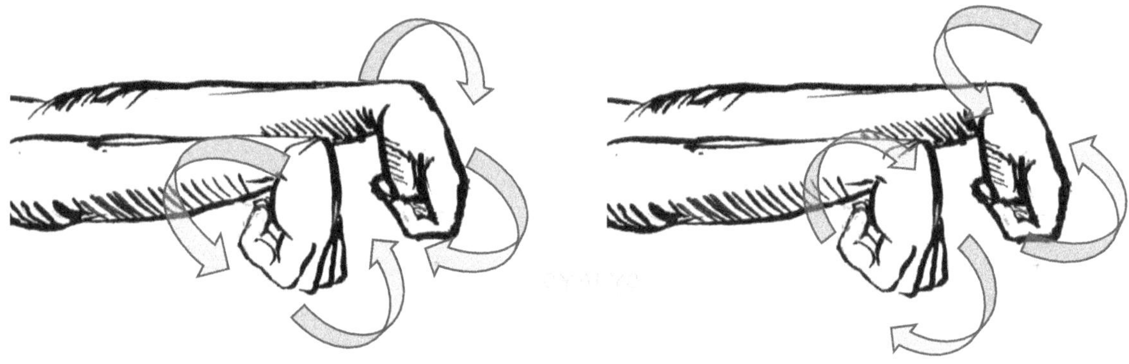

- **Wrist and Elbow Mobilization** is done beginning with elbows in line with the shoulders and the hands drawn into the upper chest (below the chin) in a loose fist. [Left panel picture below.] With each inhalation, rotate around the wrist and open out the fist, and with each exhalation complete the rotation closing the fingers into a fist again. This is done 10 times in one direction and another 10 times in the reverse direction.

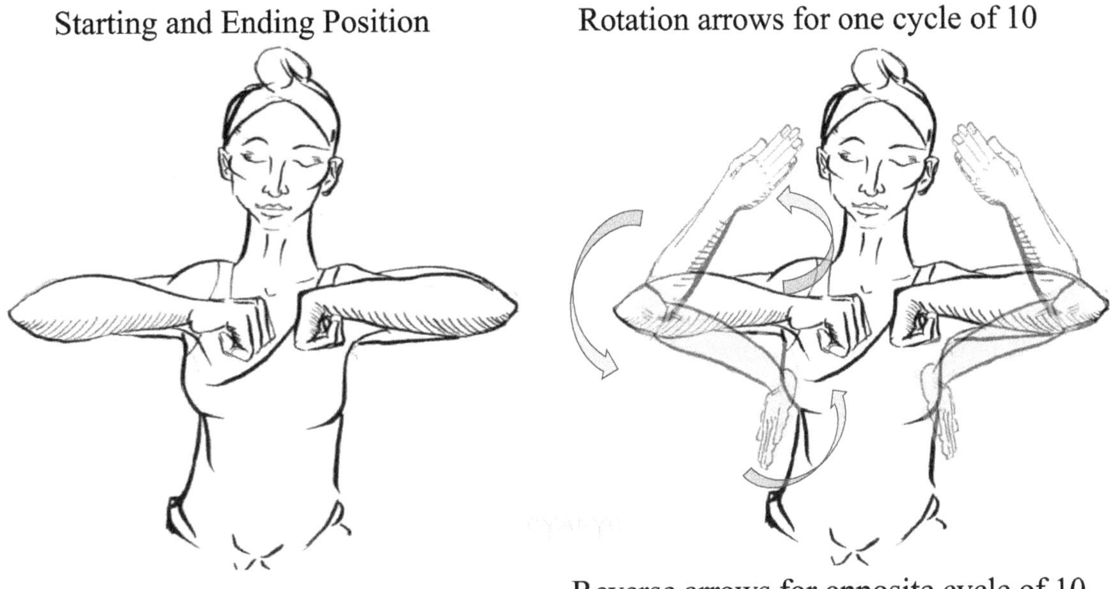

Step 5 – Spine Loosening

This is done with four exercises.

- **Upper Spine Rotation** is done beginning with interlocked palms behind the head with elbows stretched out on the two sides above the shoulders preferably at a 180-degree angle. [With aging and kyphosis, many seniors cannot attain the 180-degree stretch out of the elbows. Doing within their capacity is enough.] Then as one exhales, the upper spine, neck and head, twist to one side, and regain the starting position while inhaling. In the next exhalation, the twist is towards the other side, and coming back to the starting position while inhaling. This is done for 20 breaths, 10 times each side.

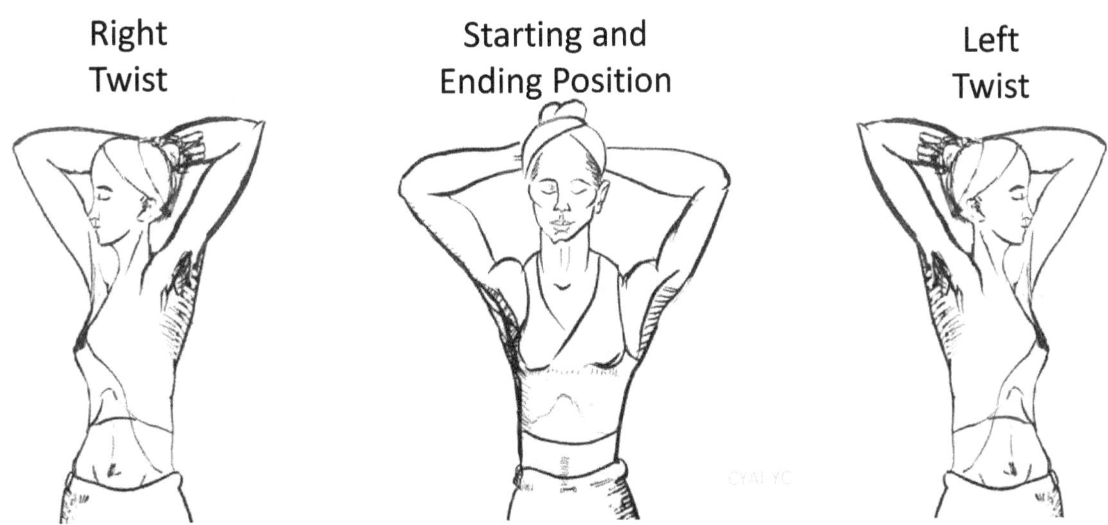

- **Sideward Stretching** is done immediately after, starting by holding the opposite elbows with the hands behind the head. With each exhalation one elbow is pulled sideways stretching the shoulder and shoulder blade along with the sideward stretch of the spine. In inhalation, one regains the vertical position before stretching the other side in the next exhalation. This is done for 10 to 20 breaths, i.e., 5 to 10 stretches on each side.

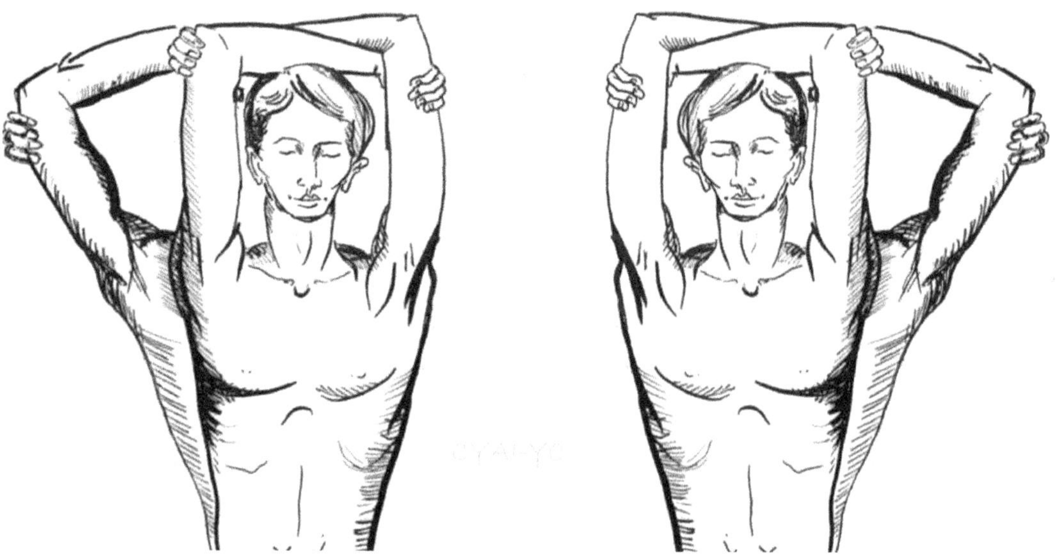

- **Lower Chest and Lumbar Rotation** is done beginning by holding the opposite elbows (or forearms) behind the back. Then with each exhalation one alternates between a twist to the left and right, while inhalation regains the starting position. This is done for about 20 breaths.

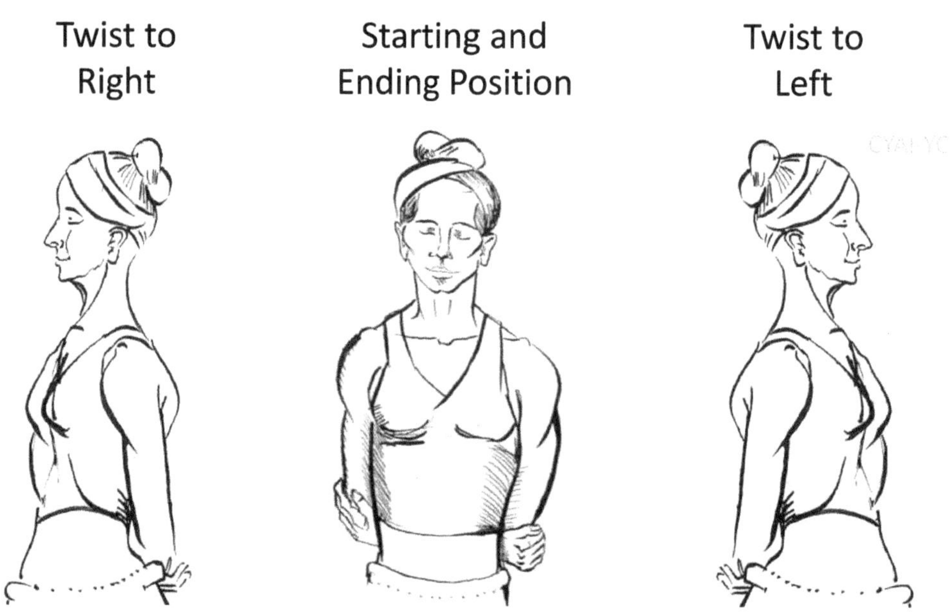

- **Backward Stretch of the Spine** is done starting by holding the hips behind the back. Then with each inhalation pushing on one hand stretch backward (slightly tilting towards that side) with the head also tilting backward. With exhalation regain the starting position. Alternating between the two sides, 20 to 30 breaths are recommended.

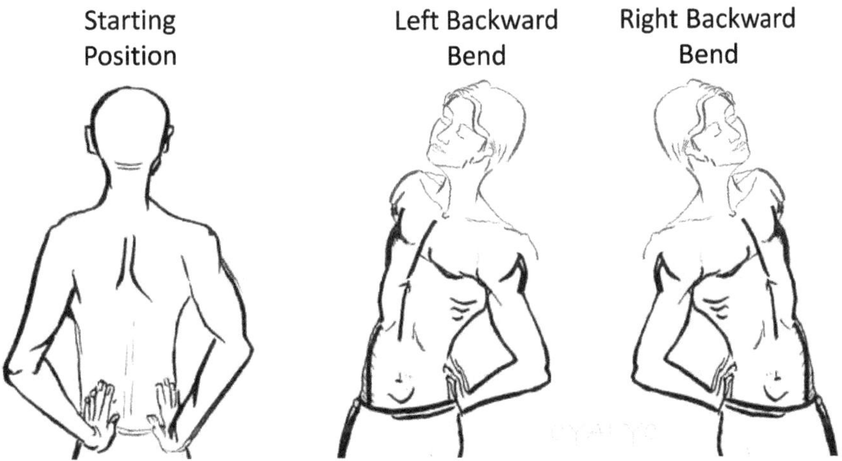

Step 5 – Hip and Lower Spine Loosening

There are three exercises here.

- **Crossing Over Knee**, where one leg is crossed over the thigh, and the knee on the top is pulled in exhalation towards the opposite shoulder while the head and upper spine twist towards the other side. This is done for one knee 10 to 20 times with exhalation, while regaining the starting position in inhalation. Thereafter the same is done for the other knee. This exercise is focused on stretching the hip, buttocks and the sacrum and coccyx region of the spine.

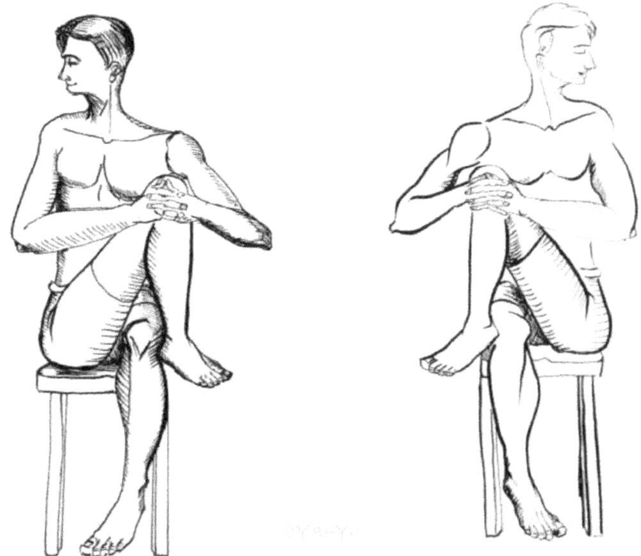

- **Pelvic Bending** is done best in a standing position with feet shoulder-width apart (or slightly wider for good balance) with the inside of the feet parallel to each other. However, for those with poor balance it can be done seated on a chair as well. Taking the hands behind, holding the opposite elbow or forearm, with inhalation one stretches back with head tilting backward, and in exhalation one bends only at the hips keeping the chin up and shoulder pulled back. This will create a stretch in the hips, and for those standing it will create a stretch from the bottom of the feet to the hips. In this position, one holds for a minute or a few minutes – about 20 to 50 slow breaths – and one can observe the slow loosening of the muscles and being able to achieve a greater bending angle after every few breaths.

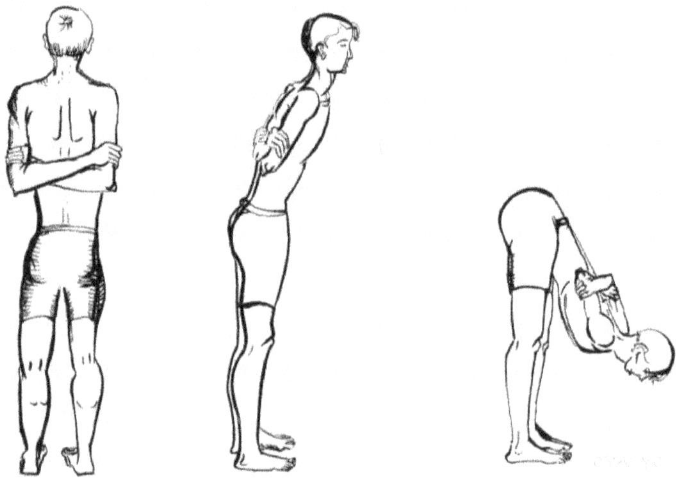

- **Hip Joint Rotation** is done by stretching out the leg without bending the knee, one leg at a time, and rotating around the whole leg (around the hip joint). Completing the 360-degree rotation in one breath, half the rotation with inhalation and half with exhalation, done 5 to 10 times in each direction and for each leg should be sufficient. For instruction purpose in a class, one can say as "stretch out your (right or left) leg without bending the knee and draw a circle in the air with your toes." [This can be done lying down or seated on a chair with legs stretched out.]

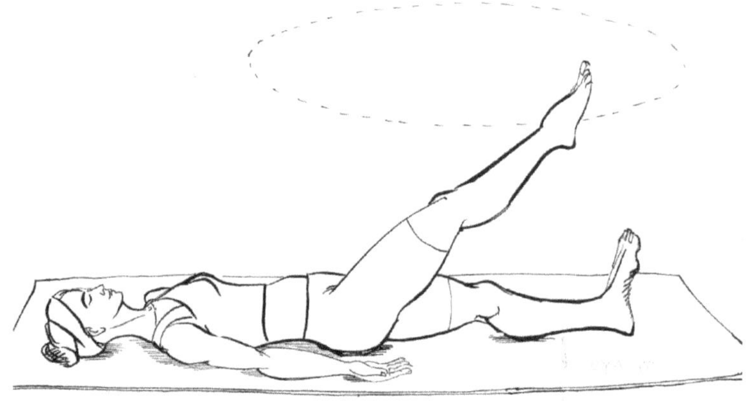

Step 6 – Knee and Feet Loosening

There are two exercises here.

- **Ankle and Knee rotation** is begun by holding under the thigh near the knee, with the knee drawn into the chest, one leg at a time. From this starting position, knee and ankle rotation can be done together or separate, one rotation with each breath. Ten rotations in each direction, and for each leg, would require 40 breaths.

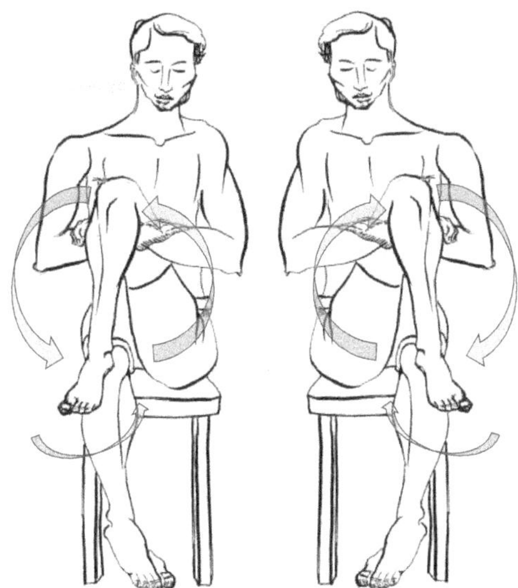

- **Feet, Toes and Ankle Stretching** can be done with both feet together at the same time. With inhalation point the feet and toes away from you and with exhalation push out the heel and curl in the toes and feet towards you. Done for 10 to 15 breaths should be adequate. Some people may like to do the stretching one foot at a time.

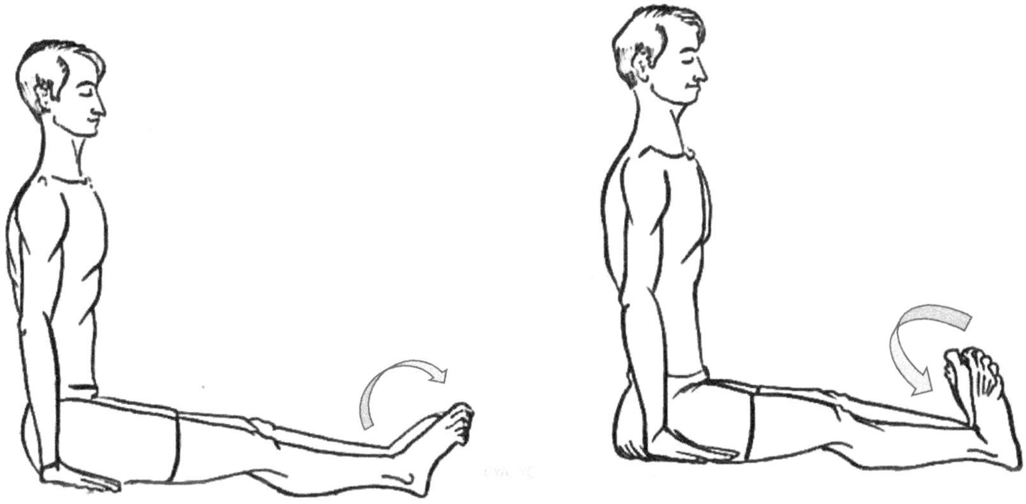

Qualification of this Gentle Regimen

The above sequence is a comprehensive approach to mindful stretching of the spine and joints. However, this can be modified as needed in the following ways:

- Skipping some exercises that may be too difficult for the participating individual/s.
- Changing the number of repetitions to the capacity of the individual/s.
- Balancing selection of practices and number of repetitions to be within time limit of practice sessions.
- Adapting as needed to chair or mat usage.

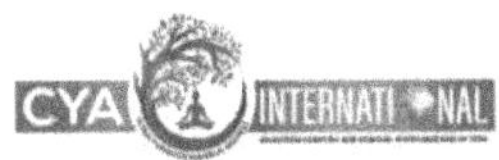

Appendix 3:

Jala Neti: Nasal Cleansing

The easiest form of *Neti*, one of the *kriyās*, is *Jala Neti* or *Neti* done with water. [The other form of *Neti* is called *Sutra Neti*.[130]] The three elements in this practice are the water, the spouted vessel, and the process.

Quality of Water

The water must have four characteristics for safe, gentle, and effective application.

- First, the water must be boiled (at least for one full minute after reaching boiling point) and cooled to be free of germs.
- Second, the temperature must be warm (tepid warm), close to body temperature. [This means temperature of hot beverages is too hot, and room temperature water is too cold.]
- Third, dissolve salt in the water, approximately one-quarter of level teaspoon for each cup of water. Any clean salt is fine.
- Fourth, you should have at least two cups of such salted water.

Boiling and cooling the water is to prevent any potential for infections[131], but the temperature and salt in the water is for creating a harmonizing effect in the nasal passages that makes it easy to do the nasal cleansing.

Spouted Vessel and Process

A spouted vessel is like a teapot. A small teapot with a narrow spout will work fine.[132]

---

[130] *Sutra Neti* is the textual description in the *Haṭha Yoga* texts. But it is too intrusive and is not recommended for the general population.

[131] Typically, there are two types of protozoa in tap water (*naegleria fowleri* and *balamuthia mandrillaris*) which can lead to infection that can be fatal. Hence boiling the water is very important. The CDC (Center for Disease Control) guidance for nasal cleansing is available at https://www.cdc.gov/parasites/naegleria/sinus-rinsing.html

[132] Search on the web for *Neti* pot will bring up sellers of such spouted vessels.

Using one cup of water in a clean (sterile) spouted vessel, insert the spout into one nostril and tilt the head the other way and lift the vessel to allow the flow of water from that nostril and drain through the other nostril.

See illustration below.

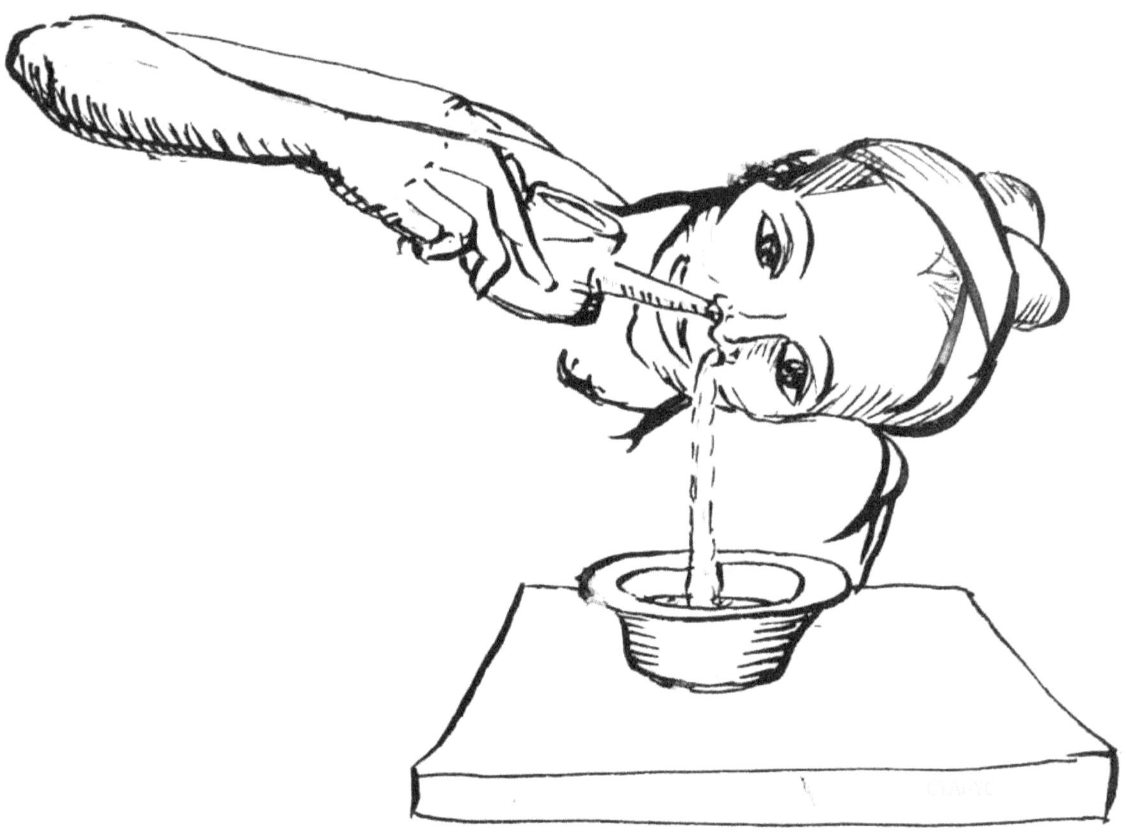

Use the second cup of water for the flow from the other nostril to drain through the first nostril.

Nuances and Concerns

When a nose is clogged, it may be difficult to do this. Otherwise, in a naturally relaxed state it should be easy to do. It is considered particularly effective in managing sinus health.

People sometimes have a concern that the water may enter the eustachian tube and whether the moisture may cause ear infection. Such instances are rare and in general with properly boiled water and doing twenty *Kapālabhāti* type of forceful exhalations immediately after the *Neti* should avoid any unwanted problems.

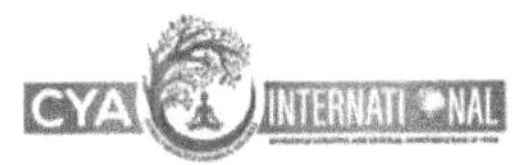

Glossary & Index

A

Adhara Mudrās अधर मुद्रा	*Mudrās* related to focus on the lower body, particularly the perineum, as classified by Swami Satyananda Saraswati of Bihar School of Yoga.	116
Ājñyā आज्ञा	It literally means to guide, order or control.	74, 131, 141
Ājñyā Chakra आज्ञा चक्र	The sixth *chakra* in the head center that is considered the controller of the lower five *chakras* and often referred as the seat of consciousness or the embodiment of the cosmic programs that an individual carries to fulfill one's purpose of life.	74
Alternate Nostril Breathing	Called *Nādi Śhodhana Prāṇāyāma* involves inhaling from one nostril and exhaling through the other and reversing as a way to balance the two hemispheres of the brain. A typical recommendation is to begin inhaling from the left nostril and exhale through the right, and then inhale from the right and exhale through the left. The breathing is done at a slow pace with exhalation longer than inhalation. It is considered effective for calming the mind.	30, 37, 50, 59, 62, 64, 74, 81, 84, 86, 112
Anāhata अनाहत	Refers to the fourth *chakra* that is in the middle of the chest in-between the breasts. It is considered the seat of emotion, humanitarian nature, and at a physical level the conduit of *nādi* communications to the chest organs.	77, 131, 140, 141
Ānanda आनन्द	The joy or bliss of cosmic awareness in Self-Realization	48, 148, 190
Ānā-Pānā आना-पाना	The precursor practice to *Vipassana Meditation* to develop sharp focus of the mind. It involves observation the sensation of breath at a single point below the nostrils.	162
Annamaya अन्नमय	Literally meaning engrossment in food awareness, this refers to physical awareness of gross matter.	47
Antar Kumbhaka अन्तर कुम्भक	Retention or suspension of breath within, without exhalation for a short period of time.	85
Anuloma-Viloma Prāṇāyāma अनुलोम-विलोम प्राणायाम	This is the commonly used name for *Nādi Śhodhana Prāṇāyāma*, which is the Alternate Nostril Breathing, described above.	55, 59

Anupāya अनुपाय	Literally meaning no recourse, is a Kashmir Shaivism term, used to describe the state of a person who must be reborn and there is no recourse available in this lifetime for Self-Realization.	132-133
Āṇavopāya आणवोपाय	Literally meaning the recourse through matter or particle, a Kashmir Shaivism term, used to describe the state of a person with much material attachment and must go through the wringer of life exhausting enough of one's internal programs (*kleśhas* and *karmas)* to attain enough purification before one can work with practices towards Self-Realization.	133
Apāna अपान	Is communication that controls the musculature in the body as presented in this book. In the reductionism of Ayurveda, it refers to communications to specific organs and functionalities in the lower part of the body.	29, 30, 32, 111, 116, 142, 199, 221
Ardhamatsyendra अर्धमत्स्येन्द्र	Is a sideward twisting *āsana*. [Illustration in blue box in chapter 37.]	104, 213
Āsana आसन	Literally meaning posture, in the Yoga Sutras, that brings stability of the body and mind to prepare for meditation. This is the third limb of the eight-fold *Aṣhṭānga Yoga.* In the *Haṭha Yoga* system it refers to various postures that stimulate the channels of communication (*nādis*) to relax the body and mind.	2, 4, 44, 45, 58, 62, 74, 86,
Aṣhṭānga अष्टाङ्ग	Means eight parts or limbs. In yoga, it refers to the eight-fold process described in the Yoga Sutras of Patanjali, that is also referred as the eight limbs of yoga.	2, 5, 105
Ātma Chakra आत्म चक्र	Is the cosmic transmitter-receiver in each person that may be referred to as the soul. It is in the region of the lower part of the sternum.	42, 52, 65, 67, 70, 73, 74
Avidyā अविद्या	Refers to the lack of understanding of the nature of one's cosmic existence and cosmic purpose of life. This is considered as the factor that promotes reactivity and desires from what the sense organs experience. It is considered a hindrance for Self-Realization.	129, 130

B

Bāhya Kumbhaka बाह्य कुम्भक	Suspension of breath after complete exhalation -- effectively not trying to inhale after complete exhalation. As a practice this is done along with holding of the three locks: (i) lifting the pelvic floor/perineum drawing in the anus (*Mūla Bandha*); (ii) drawing in the abdominal area (*Uddiyāna Bandha*); (iii) bringing the chin to the chest (*Jālandhara Bandha*).	85
Bālāsana बालासन	Often translated and referred as child pose involves a prone relaxation position for resting in between *Haṭha Yoga* postures.	105
Bandhana बन्धन	Is a protective energy shield (sheath) around a person done by affirmation for binding focus of consciousness for meditation.	181

Bandhas बन्ध	Translated as locks, it refers to constraining or drawing in of muscles to hold in or hold out breath. E.g., as used in *Bāhya Kumbhaka* above.	57, 85, 99, 114-116, 118
Bhakti Yoga भक्ति योग	The yoga approach of mentally surrendering to God. It involves engaging in all actions of living with a sense of duty for the sake of God and surrendering the results of the actions to God as well.	4, 5, 19, 159, 182, 184, 195, 222
Bharata-Nātyam भरत-नाट्यम्	A traditional form of South Indian dance that was considered a spiritual practice and used as part of temple rituals in South India until it was banned by the British in 1910. It involves *Mudrās*, *Prāṇakriyā* movements, and many aspects of the *Aṣhṭānga* Yoga process and we consider it as a complete yoga practice.	115, 163
Bhastrā भस्त्रा	Is translated as bellows (traditionally used by blacksmiths and goldsmiths to blow air to increase the heat in the fire).	70
Bhastrikā भस्त्रिका	*Bhastrikā* refers to a breathing practice of full deep breaths done like the motion of the bellows (of a blacksmith or goldsmith). It is normally done in cycles of 20 breaths to prevent fainting from respiratory alkalosis. It is one of the main *Prāṇāyāma* practices.	55, 58, 70-74, 112, 176, 229
Bhastrikā Kumbhaka भस्त्रिका कुम्भक	While literally translated as suspension of breath after breathing in and out like the bellows, the term has been used in traditional yoga texts to simply mean breathing like the bellows without suspension and is popularly called *Bhastrikā Prāṇāyāma*.	70
Bhramaraka भ्रमरक	Means a bumble bee.	77
Bhrāmarī भ्रामरी	Is the humming like a bee created in slow breathing. It is considered useful for meditative relaxation and also for sinus conditions.	56, 77-79, 112
Bhrāmarī Kumbhaka भ्रामरी कुम्भका	This is the term used in traditional *Haṭha Yoga* texts and is commonly simply referred as *Bhrāmarī,* as described above.	77
Bhriguvalli भृगुवल्ली	Is the third chapter of the *Taittriya Upaniṣhad* that describes the experience of Bhrigu.	32, 47
Bhujangāsana भुजङ्गासन	Translated as cobra posture it involves lifting up the head and chest from a prone position on the floor.	104
Brahmā ब्रह्मा	Is the program (*Deva* or angel) of creation of everything in cosmic existence. Often referred as creator, is not considered God, but rather a functionary of God.	174
Brahmacharya ब्रह्मचर्य	Refers to curiosity or impetus to learn and know more about everything in existence. *Brahma* refers to all of creation, and *charya* means movement (inquiry) within it.	20, 132, 215
Brāhmana ब्राह्मण	Those who seek to know or have awareness of all of creation, beyond the temporal world – often associated with priestly occupation.	131-132, 192, 202

Brahma-Yajñya ब्रह्मयज्ञ	Offering to all of creation including subtle elements like spirits. This is a daily practice done by yogic adherents in the Vedic traditions to fulfill the needs of spiritual beings. This is considered important for maintaining the cosmic flow.	192
Buddhi बुद्धि	The element within the cognitive space that understands, can analyze and conceptualize. This is considered the dynamic energy that allows one to become Self Realized.	125

C

catecholamine	These are biochemicals produced in nerve cells (hence called neurotransmitters) in response to levels of harmony or stress. Principal among them are epinephrine (adrenaline), norepinephrine (noradrenaline) and dopamine.	157
causal body	The program content of a person (called *kleśha-karma* in yoga) attached to the soul, present even before birth, is the causal body - - understood as the cause of birth.	26-27, 33-34, 45-47, 146
Chakras चक्र	*Chakras* are *nādi* communication hubs serving as meeting and distribution points for communication of the five types of communication understood in yoga and Ayurveda. Traditionally seven major *chakras* are recognized in common understanding of the *tantra* system.	7, 18, 25, 29-30, 41-42, 74, 89, 94, 131-133, 140-142, 171, 185
Chāndāla चांडाल	Keeper of cremation grounds - is considered normally as a person with low sensibilities impervious to the emotion of death and grossness of charred cadaver.	134
Chanda छन्दस	Meter of lyrics	174
ChandraBhedana Prāṇāyāma चन्द्रभेदन प्राणायाम	Inhalation from the left nostril and exhaling from the right nostril. Left nostril is considered *Chandra Nādi*. The word *Chandra* by itself means the moon. In *Haṭha Yoga* moon is a said to be cooling and sun (called *Sūryā*) as heating.	85
Chandra Nādi चन्द्र नाडि	Left nostril communication associated with cooling of the body systems	63
Chandra Prāṇāyāma चन्द्र प्राणायाम	Inhaling and exhaling from the left nostril	85
Chandranamaskar चन्द्र नमस्कार	A modification of the *Sūryā Namaskār* that is easier and considered gentler for the body.	103
Chetanā चेतना	The nature of a sentient, living being understood as implying: (a) ability to adapt; (b) having a dual connection with God and creation. In contrast dead matter has only connection into creation and not God.	26-27, 145-146, 220

D

Devatā देवता	Beings, in the nature of light or vibrations, that enable the senses in the temporal world. In the Vedic system this is one of three spiritual entities that impact the temporal world. The other two are *ṛiṣhis* and *Piṭras* (departed souls that are not yet liberated).	128, 174, 191
Dhanurāsana धनुरासन	Bow pose of *Haṭha Yoga*	104
Dhāraṇā धारणा	One-pointed focus to progress towards meditation. This is the sixth limb of the eight-fold *Aṣhṭānga Yoga.*	2, 115, 125, 136, 153, 166
Dharma धर्म	Duty or engagement that sustains the cosmic flow in proper order. [Also see *Sva-dharma, Varṇa-Dharma* and *Dharma Megha Samādhi.*]	9, 23, 25, 34, 59, 67, 83, 100, 125, 127, 130, 134, 137-138, 168, 189-190, 195 197, 199-200, 202, 215, 216
Dharma Megha Samādhi धर्म मेघ समाधि	The state of cosmic connectivity where one understands one's *Dharma* and can fulfill it without reactivity leading to complete purification and liberation.	137
Dharma Śhāstra धर्म शास्त्र	System of *Dharma*	9
Dhyāna ध्यान	Extension of one-pointedness in meditation practice that leads to collapse of the mind. This is the seventh limb of the eight-fold *Aṣhṭānga Yoga.*	2, 136, 153, 166
Dhyāna Mudrā ध्यान मुद्रा	Hand-finger position that helps meditation	117
Diaphragm diaphragmatic	The flat and long muscle that separates the chest case from the abdominal cavity. Controlled by the phrenic nerve its up and down movement enables proper breathing of the lower lobes of the lungs. Movement of the diaphragm	32, 44, 52-54, 72, 75, 80-81, 226-229
dig-bandhana दिग्बन्धन	*Dik* (directions) and *bandhana* (protective energetic shield), written together as *dig-bandhana* is the invocation of a protective shield around a person or a group of persons for meditative focus.	181
Dik दिक्	Directions - ten in all: eight around and above and below.	181
dopamine	a catecholamine, a neurotransmitter that keeps a person in a happy state of mind.	157
Durgā दुर्गा	Meaning one who is fierce looking or difficult to approach. This is a name used to describe the concept of the Divine Mother energy that creates and sustains all of creation.	171

E

Electro-photonic Imaging	Imaging auras by placing a finger or any organic body in an electromagnetic field. Bio-well is one example used to assess *nādis*. readings that are equivalent to three-finger pulse reading of traditional medicine systems.	26
epinephrine	a catecholamine, a neurotransmitter, also known as adrenaline, that is released in stress.	157

G

Gāyatrī गायत्री	Literally meaning that which is beyond the body, the word is associated with a helpful spirit whose invocation elevates meditation. At the same time, it also means a mantra that is associated with it called the *Gāyatrī* mantra. Also, it is considered a meter (*chanda*) of 24 syllables.	174
glossopharyngeal nerve	It is the ninth cranial nerve that works as afferent to the pharyngeal area. i.e., connecting the back of the nasal cavity and mouth to the brain.	55, 66
Gorakśha गोरक्ष	Author of the *Gorakśha Śhataka*, a text of *Haṭha Yoga*.	98, 115, 134-135
Graha ग्रह	Literally meaning that which grabs you, and in the context of astrology the influence of celestial bodies that represent the flow of one's *karma-kleśha*.	183
Granthi ग्रन्थि	Knots in the flow of *nādis*.	133
gross body	Physical or anatomical body	25-27, 29, 33, 74, 89, 146

H

Halāsana हलासन	Plough pose of *Haṭha Yoga*.	104
Haraigushi	Process of purification or blessing in the Japanese Shinto tradition	191
Hasta Mudrās हस्त मुद्रा	*Mudrās* of hands and fingers	78, 116
haṭha हठ	Force or strong resolute physical effort	
Haṭha Yoga हठ योग	The system of yoga dealing with force of the body that includes asanas, cleansing kriyas, breathing practices and meditative observation.	3-5, 18-20, 35, 37, 41-42, 45, 54, 56-59, 63, 65, 70, 75, 77-78, 80-81, 83, 85-86, 89, 92, 96, 98-105, 108-110, 112-115, 118-119, 126-127, 134-135, 139, 149, 159, 163, 182, 195, 213, 222

Havan हवन्	Term used in North India for fire-based worship with offering into the fire. Sanskrit terms are *Homa* and *Yajñya*.	183
Hita हित	Beneficial, helpful to others	216
Homa होम	Another name for *Havan* or *Yajñya*	183
Hṛidaya हृदय	Meaning the hidden core, the term is commonly used for the anatomical heart as well. In yoga, it refers to the spiritual heart, the *Ātma Chakra.*	31, 65, 132

I

Idā इडा	Left side *nādi* representing internal intent or program whose communication feed into the central channel *Suṣhumnā.*	29-30
I-Rest	US Military name for Yoga Nidra used to help with PTSD.	163
Īśhvara Praṇidhāna ईश्वर प्रणिधान	Surrender to God	5, 124, 138, 149, 165, 185-186

J

Jala Neti जल नेति	Internal nasal tract cleansing with flow of water	81, 110, 241
Jālandhara Bandha जालन्धर बन्ध	Neck/chin lock that prevents swallowing like the flow of saliva	66, 115, 118
Jñyāna ज्ञान	Knowledge or awareness	48
Jñyāna Yoga ज्ञान योग	Yoga of Knowledge that is associated with *Samyama* of Yoga and *Svādhyāya* of *Vedānta*	5

K

Kaivalya कैवल्य	Liberated state from Self-Realization	128, 170-171
Kaivalyadhāma कैवल्यधाम	Name of a well-known Yoga Institution in India	71
Kākāsana काकासन	Crow pose of *Haṭha Yoga.*	105
Kapha कफ	Literally phlegm, but also related to Ayurvedic assessment of a constitution type where the person has a relaxed attitude towards life.	81, 109
Kārana कारण	Meaning cause, it is associated with the causal body in this text.	137
Karma कर्म	Reactions that feed into one's cosmic program (causal body) that cause more life situations in this or later lives as commonly understood. However, in a comprehensive sense, it has three components: the reactions, the future situations they cause, and the	6-7, 10, 20-21, 26-27, 33, 42, 45, 47, 59, 99, 104,

Karma (continued from previous page)	duty or action that bounds one to deal with the situation. Thus, duties are also called *karma*.	108,123, 129-131, 133, 138, 145, 147, 166-167, 184, 196, 221
karma cycle	*Karma* considered as the cause of rebirth, the term *karma* cycle is used to indicate the concept of birth and rebirth in South Asian philosophies.	5, 25-26, 48
Karma Yoga कर्म योग	Often described as yoga of selfless action, it has two components: acting with inner awareness of duty with no desire in the mind, and being non-reactive to the outcome of the action.	4-5, 59, 133
Kashmir Shaivism	A philosophical and tantra system associated with Vedic traditions that is associated with the Kashmir region.	128, 132-133, 167-168
Kāya Mudrās काय मुद्रा	*Mudrās* of the body as classified by Swami Satyananda Saraswati of Bihar School of Yoga.	116
Kevala Kumbhaka केवल कुम्भक	Automatic cessation of breath in a meditative state	85, 118, 176
Kleśha क्लेश	Literally meaning blemish or fault is considered the initial program in creation of each soul – it can be thought as the initial sin associated with Christianity.	6-7, 21, 26-27, 33, 42, 45, 47, 59, 99, 104, 123, 129-130, 133, 138, 166-167, 196, 221
Kriyā Yoga क्रिया योग	Translated as yoga of action, it is another name for *Karma Yoga*. In the Yoga Sutras the same action without desire and reactivity is defined in a deeper way with its three components: purification, contemplation to understand, and surrender to God. These three components allow a person to engage in action without desire and reactivity.	5, 7, 19, 47, 59, 133, 138-139, 149-150
Kśhatra क्षत्र	Domain of people or geographic association	130
Kśhatriya क्षत्रिय	Those who care for the *kśhatra* - considered the guardians of society commonly thought as military, police and ruling class.	130-131, 202
Kśhudra क्षुद्र	Literally meaning small, referring to people who don't have logical thinking and planning abilities.	130-131
Kumbhaka कुम्भक	*Kumbha* is a pot filled with water symbolizing life and intent. Thus, *Kumbhaka* means like a *Kumbha*, referring to the body as a pot that holds life and consciousness in the *Haṭha Yoga* tradition when the breath is held without inhaling or exhaling.	56-58, 60, 65, 70, 85-86, 112, 118

kuṇda कुण्ड	Hole (like in the ground)	129
Kuṇdalī कुण्डली	That which is held in a hole, referring to the horoscope - astrological chart of a person - that holds the person's influence of *karma-kleśha*, represented by planetary positions at the time of birth, on life trajectory.	129
Kuṇdalinī कुण्डलिनी	Outlook or value system of a person based on how they perceive existence based on their *karma-kleśha.* It includes perception or outlook from unthinking to thinking beyond the physical world and is considered the evolutionary expansive process of souls in the *Kuṇdalinī Yoga* system.	127, 129, 132-135, 192
Kuṇdalinī Yoga कुण्डलिनी योग	System of yoga that focuses on evolutionary expansion in thinking - see explanation of *Kuṇdalinī.*	127, 129, 134
Kūrma Nādi कूर्म नाडि	A subtle communication channel arising from the abdominal area and coming up to the throat that is considered to bring stability and balance in the system. Physiologically, balance in the system relates to the gyros in the ear and the throat is considered as an integrative communication hub for all ENT (ear, nose, throat) issues.	74

L

Lakśhmī लक्ष्मी	The spiritual force that directs fulfillment in the material world.	171, 196
Laya Yoga लय योग	Yoga of absorption into whatever is being observed - a *Haṭha Yoga* term equivalent to *Samāpatti* in the Yoga Sutras	3, 99,163

M

Mahābandha महाबन्ध	Concurrent application of the three locks or *bandhas* – in the perineum (*Mūla Bandha*), abdomen (*Uddiyāna Bandha*) and throat (chin lock - *Jālandhara Bandha*).	115, 118
Mahāyāna Buddhism	The type of Buddhist philosophy and practices that include tantra and focuses on the experiential aspect of meditative realization. This is associated with Tibetan Buddhism. This is unlike the South Asia Buddhism called Theravada Buddhism that seeks to negate all experiences as a way for liberation.	20, 99
Mai	Is the Chinese term for meridians or bio-meridians as translated in English.	25
Makarāsana मकरासन	Crocodile or Alligator pose of *Haṭha Yoga.*	54, 105
Mana Mudrās मन मुद्रा	*Mudrās* related to the head and mind as classified by Swami Satyananda Saraswati of Bihar School of Yoga.	116
Manas मनस्	Mind	47
Maṇikarnikā Ghat मणिकर्णिका घाट	A cremation facility on the banks of the river Ganga in Varanasi, the holy city in India.	134

Maṇipūra मणिपूर	The *chakra* that is associated with the navel region that is also considered the seat of energy and initiative for action to help society. It is also associated with the digestive organs.	131, 140-141
Mantra मन्त्र	Vibration that is subtle or audible that enables transcending the mind.	4, 19, 33, 36-37, 46, 84, 123-126, 133, 137, 145, 165-168, 171, 173-174, 183, 187-188
Mantra Śhāstra मन्त्र शास्त्र	System of mantras	188
Marmas मर्म	Subtle points in the body where pressure or force that can have significant and long-lasting effect on the human system. These points are considered accessible by finger pressure and may be thought of as lying along the acupuncture meridians (most points of which are internal and need to be accessed by needles). The *Suśhruta Samhitā*, the Ayurvedic text of surgery, states 107 marma points where surgical incision is prohibited to avoid significant negative effect on the person (which could include fatality in some points).	25, 28, 96
Matsyāsana मत्स्यासन	Fish pose of *Haṭha Yoga*.	104
Mayurāsana मयूरासन	Peacock pose of *Haṭha Yoga*.	105
Meru मेरु	A pyramidal block typically crafted from mctal -- gold or brass -- that is considered the three-dimensional form of a flat plate with etching called the *Śhrī Yantra*. It is said to represent the linkage between the physically manifested world to the subtle manifestation outside the three-dimensional spectrum, as a gateway to eternity. In the system of *Śhrī Vidyā*, the Meru is worshipped as the Divine Mother. In some *Tantra Yoga* traditions, the *Suṣhumnā Nādi* is considered the Meru within everyone as the track for ascendence into higher realization.	190
Mimāmsa मिमांस	One of the six ancient philosophies associated with the Vedic traditions that unlike some of the other philosophies also include Vedic religious practices of fire-based worship. Its ritual practices are associated with the Vedantic system and Vedic religion that unfolded.	18
Mita मित	Friendliness	216
Mokśha मोक्ष	Release, commonly referred to as release from rebirth. However, in the philosophical system it is also a final dissolution or resting state (that precludes transitory states like purgatory or *Piṭra Loka*).	9-10, 134-135, 190

Mokśha Śhāstra मोक्ष शास्त्र	System of attaining *mokśha*	9, 134, 132 footnote
Mūlādhāra मूलाधार	Root *chakra* at the perineum associated with *Kuṇdalinī Yoga*	131, 140-141
Mudrā मुद्रा	Literally meaning 'seal' is used in yoga to mean sealing of a pattern of energy or communication flow. It would cover positions of body or body parts like hands and fingers that direct energetic flow and have a transformative effect on the body and mind. In modern terminology, some people refer to it as psycho-neurotransmitters.	61-62, 67-68, 78, 99, 103, 115-118, 124-127, 141-142
Mukhya Prāṇa Nādi मुख्य प्राण नाडि	Terminology probably originating from the South Indian system of sage Agastya that refers to the vitality control in the body and is more commonly referred as *Prāṇa Nādi*. It is also associated with the Central Nervous System (spine and brain) that from a physiological perspective controls the lungs and heart to enable cellular respiration that produces energy in the body.	171
Mūla Bandha मूल बन्ध	Drawing in at the perineum stimulates an upward force internally. It is considered one of the three popular locks used in many *Haṭha Yoga* practices.	115, 118
Mumukśhu मुमुक्षु	A seeker (of spiritual reality)	148, 166
Murchchhā मूर्च्छा	Literally meaning swooning, this is a *Haṭha Yoga* breathing practice that creates that sensation and is considered a cleansing and meditative practice.	85, 112

N

nāda anusandhāna नाद अनुसन्धान	Literally meaning experiencing the vibration, referring to the vibration of the cosmos in a highly meditative state.	4, 99
Nādi नाडि	Channels of subtle communication that impact the psycho-somatic-spiritual existence of a person.	4, 6-8, 18, 25, 27-35, 37-38, 41-42, 45-47, 51, 55-61, 63-64, 67-68, 70, 74, 79, 82-86, 96, 99, 102-106, 108, 112, 114, 124-127, 131, 133-134, 136, 138, 142, 156, 160, 165-

P

Pancha-Prāṇa पञ्च प्राण	Five-fold *Prāṇa* referring to *Prāṇa*, *Apāna*, *Vyāna*, *Udāna* and *Samāna*.	32, 111
Paramātmā परमात्म	The Supreme Soul or Source, referring to God.	174
Piṅgalā पिङ्गला	The right-side *nādi* bringing informational content of the external environment that feeds into the Central Channel, *Suṣhumnā*.	29-30. 60-61, 63, 67
Pitta पित्त	Ayurvedic terminology of a constitution that is fiery and dynamic.	109
Plāvinī प्लाविनी	A breathing technique associated with *Haṭha Yoga* that enables one to float in water.	85, 112
Prabhu प्रभु	Literally meaning the source of all creation, referring to God. [This should not be confused with *Brahmā* who is in a lower spiritual level as the administrator of creation.]	5, 7
Pradhāna Jayī प्रधान जयी	Literally meaning Conqueror of the Chief referring to a yogi whose awareness has transcended to a level where one has control over all of creation. Thus, *Pradhāna* refers to *Prakṛiti*.	124
Prakṛiti प्रकृति	Literally meaning a creation or composition that in its core is connected to the divine reality of God, *Prakṛiti* is the first creation of God that enables creation and manages it.	26-27, 33, 109, 122-123, 126-129, 136, 145-148, 172, 182, 189-191, 220-221
Prāṇa प्राण	Life force or vitality -- in a yogic sense it is beyond the physiological understanding of production of energy from cellular respiration.	29-30, 32, 47, 51-52, 57-58, 67, 85, 102, 117, 199, 221
Prāṇakriyā प्राणक्रिया	*Kriyā* means action. Thus, *Prāṇakriyā* is the idea of natural movement of energy that entails the actions that are in sync with one's cosmic duty (the Sanskrit term for which is *Sva-dharma*).	104, 139, 162, 213
Prāṇāyāma प्राणायाम	Regulation of *Prāṇā* or vital energy. This is the fourth limb of the eight-fold *Aṣhṭānga Yoga*.	2, 45, 52, 54-60, 64-65, 69, 71, 73-75, 77, 80-81, 84-86, 99, 102, 105, 108, 112, 114, 116, 138, 158-160, 175-176, 180, 229

Prapañchasāra प्रपञ्चसार	A tantra text whose authorship is attributed to Shankarācharya that deals with both worship methods and meditation while discussing the nature of creation and experiences beyond the body. The text has 36 chapters with 2,470 verses dealing with various topics such as creation and dissolution, development of the human embryo and birth, letters of the alphabet, *bījākṣaras* or seed-letters, *dīkṣā* or initiation and also the mantras and rituals connected with the various deities. http://www.hindupedia.com/en/Prapa%C3%B1cas%C4%81ra	190
Pratyāhāra प्रत्याहार	Inward awareness of one's vibrations that allows one to control physiological elements. This is the fifth limb of the eight-fold *Aṣhṭānga Yoga.*	2, 102, 106-107, 111, 153, 160
Priya प्रिय	loving	216
PTSD	Post traumatic stress disorder	163
Puruṣha पुरुष	The connection of each person to the unmanifest reality, God.	26, 31, 128-129, 136, 145-147, 149, 151, 170, 182, 220

R

Rāgas राग	Melodies of music. [*Rāga* is also used in Yoga Sutras to mean attraction or affinity of the mind.]	165
Rāja Yoga राज योग	System of Yoga - The Yoga Sutras of Patanjali is considered the enunciation of the system of yoga, and hence considered the document of *Rāja Yoga.*	4, 222
Rasa रस	Meaning essence of anything, and is often associated with music, dramatization, purpose of activity, and taste of something consumed.	165
Ṛiṣhi ऋषि	One who is connected into the cosmic flow or *ṛita* - the term sage is commonly used.	174
ṛita ऋत	Sanskrit term for the cosmic flow that refers to both the manifest world as well as the subtle elements that control the flow of the known cosmos.	201

S

Sahasrāra सहस्र	Literally translated as the one with thousand elements, is considered the thousand-petal lotus that arises above the head in meditation that connects beyond the body.	131, 141
Sahita सहित	Literally means that which is full of benefit, refers to *Prāṇāyāma* practices done without holding of breath. When done with holding in or out the breath it is called *Kumbhaka.*	86

Samādhi समाधि	Literally translated as complete balance of intellect refers to experience of the integrated connection of the body-mind-spirit with the cosmic intelligence that enables intuitive awareness.	25, 26, 33-34, 48, 105, 136-138, 148, 150,153, 159-160, 165-166, 168, 195-196
Samāna समान	Literally meaning the balancer, this refers to the type of communication that integrates one's internal program with the external environmental needs that makes the psychosomatic being of a person at each moment in time. This communication is thought to flow through the Central Channel, *Suṣhumnā nādi*.	29-30, 32, 67, 111, 116, 131, 140, 142, 199, 221
Samāpatti	Literally meaning 'becoming one with' something external, is the state of engrossment into some object or activity.	140, 159-160, 165, 195-196
Samskāras संस्कार	Another term for the program content of a person (called *kleśha-karma* in yoga) that makes a person's psychosomatic profile.	118
Samyama संयम	The process of intuitive realization that comes from queries in meditation. In yoga, this is said to be the integrated results of *Dhāraṇā*, *Dhyāna* and *Samādhi*, the last three of *Ashṭānga* Yoga.	5, 133, 136, 138, 148, 166, 222
Sandhyā Vandana संध्या वन्दन	Refers to a practice that includes meditative invocation and affirmation designed to transcend beyond the physical domain. This is practiced as a thrice a day ritual – early morning, high noon and at sunset – among those given the sacred thread in the Vedic system along with the use of the *Gāyatrī* mantra.	174
saṅkalpa and pure saṅkalpa संकल्प	Commonly refers to affirmation with intent, but pure *saṅkalpa* is the direction of actions in one's purpose of living that comes as cosmic intent as intuition in the highest meditative connectivity.	125, 136-137, 183
Sāṅkhya सांख्य	One of the six ancient philosophies of the Vedic tradition.	18
Sāṅkhya-Yoga सांख्य योग	A Buddhism inspired philosophy created by integrating selective segments of *Sāṅkhya* and *Yoga* philosophies of the Vedic tradition.	20, 134
Sannyāsa संन्यास	Have complete awareness or connection into the totality of existence, including the cosmic flow and cosmic intelligence of God.	132 footnote
Sannyāsī संन्यासी	One who has attained *Sannyāsa* is the original meaning. In modern day world, it is misunderstood as one who renunciates worldly living wearing a saffron robe.	135
Sarasvatī सरस्वती	The spirit that governs intelligence to understand what one attempts to learn.	171, 174
Sarvangāsana सर्वाङ्गासन	A yoga pose that impacts all parts of the body, referred as Shoulder-stand in English writings.	104

Sattva सत्त्व	The nature of smooth flow in activity without desire motivation or reaction – the nature of a pure observer. This is referred to as the nature of purity.	6 footnote
Sattva-Purușha सत्त्व-पुरुष	This is the *sattva* nature of the connection with the unmanifest source of everything. This is considered the nature of God and used as a descriptor both for God and such purified souls who are permanently linked with God. It describes the state where one goes beyond the cycle of *karmas* and rebirth.	149, 4 footnote
Saundarya Laharī सौन्दर्य लहरी	A text of 100 verses authored by Shankaracharya that speaks to his poetic and emotional experience of the Divine Mother, *Tri-pura-sundarī* or *Durgā.*	134
Sāvitrī सावित्री	The spirit of light that takes one's awareness beyond the visual light – the subtle communication into another dimension. Invocation of this spirit is used in the *Sandhyā Vandana* practice.	174
scalar waves	The resultant waves from the collapse of vibration by two sources of vibrational energy, when one is harmonic to the other.	123
Self-Realization	Realization of the nature and source of existence.	9, 33, 47, 147-151, 154, 167, 171-172, 221
Setubandhāsana सेतुबन्धासन	Translated as bridge pose, involves the backward bend raising of the trunk of the body.	104
Śhaktī शक्ति	Literally meaning energy, in a spiritual sense it refers to the primordial energy that is the source of all subtle and gross creation. In religious setting, this is also called the Divine Mother.	20, 126-129, 133-134, 171, 196
Śhaktīpāt शक्तिपात्	Transmission of energetic vibration, typically related to a highly evolved teacher intentionally transmitting the vibration to a seeker to experience higher meditation.	168
Shāktopāya शाक्तोपाय	A Kashmir Shaivism term, referring to using mantras or vibrations as the means for a person to connect into the cosmic intelligence to become realized. This is considered the appropriate means for a second category of people who have some light *karmas* remaining.	133, 168
Śhalabhāsana शलभासन	Locust posture of *Hațha Yoga.*	104
Shāmbhopāya शाम्बोपाय	A Kashmir Shaivism term, used as the means of Self-Realization for those who are in a fully purified state.	133, 167
Shanmukhī Mudrā षण्मुखी मुद्रा	Literally translated as six-faced *mudrā* or facial *mudrā* with six aspects - the position of closing six orifices in the head while humming in a type of *Bhrāmarī* practice.	78
Shannaih शन्नैः	Meaning slowly referring to slow movement	71

Ṣhaṭkarma षट्कर्म	The six internal cleansing practices of *Haṭha Yoga* tradition.	80-81, 99, 108, 110-112
Ṣhaṭkriyās षट्क्रिया	Another term used for *Ṣhaṭkarma.*	3, 56, 58, 108, 111
Śhavāsana शवासन	Corpse pose in *Haṭha Yoga* used for relaxation.	54, 105, 127, 138, 175
Śheetalī शीतली	Meaning that which is cooling, refers to the *Haṭha Yoga* breathing practice of inhaling through the mouth by curling the tongue like a straw and sucking in air, and exhaling through the nostrils.	83, 112
Seetkārī सीत्कारी	Similar practice to *Śheetalī*, except that the inhalation of the breath is below the tongue placed in the palate, and sucking is in-between the teeth.	83, 112
Śhirasāsana शिरसासन	Headstand pose of *Haṭha Yoga.*	105
Śhiva शिव	Literally meaning the one who is tranquil, refers to God in Shaivite traditions and to the spirit of dissolution in other traditions. For distinction of God from the spirit, the term often used is *ParāŚhiva* or *SadāŚhiva.*	20, 128, 132-134
Śhrī Chakra श्री चक्र	The flat diagram or illustration of five downward pointed triangles and four upward pointed triangles whose intersection create 64 triangles, encircled with circles and a square that is considered the representation of the energetic system of creation.	190
Śhrī Vidyā श्री विद्या	Literally meaning the knowledge of creation, also refers to a form of worship to the Divine Mother to attain that knowledge.	189-190
Śhrī Yantra श्री यन्त्र	A metal plate with the etching of the *Śhrī Chakra*	190
Śhvāsāyāma श्वासायाम	There is no such regular word usage. However, in this instance it is Swami Veda Bharati's special reference to distinguish regulation of breath as opposed to regulation of vitality which is *Prāṇāyāma.* In yoga we understand the distinction between breath (*Śhvāsa)* and vitality.	74
Siddhis सिद्धि	Abilities acquired -- typically referring to special abilities coming from higher meditative realization.	223
sofar	Jewish scribe of the Torah.	187
Sūkśhma सूक्ष्म	Means subtle.	137
Sthūla स्थूल	Means gross.	137
subtle body	The communicating vibrations from the causal body that enters the physical body that makes the psychosomatic profile of the individual.	25-28, 39, 137, 146

Sudarśhana सुदर्शन	Literally meaning having clear vision. It is referred to a presence experienced above the head that is considered the protector of the physical body until the purpose of the lifetime is fulfilled. It is also referred to as the Soul Star in western mysticism.	180
Sudarśhana Kriyā सुदर्शन क्रिया	Literally meaning a practice or activity that enables clear vision, is a trademarked practice of the Art of Living Foundation in recent times. While some people claim that it has origins in traditional literature, we view it as a generic concept of cyclical rhythmic exercising of breath.	56
Sūrya Bhedana Prāṇāyāma सूर्य भेदन प्राणायाम	*Haṭha Yoga* breathing practice of inhaling from the right nostril and exhaling from the left.	85, 112
Sūrya Nādi सूर्य नाडि	The communication channel that flows through the right nostril.	63, 70
Sūrya Prāṇāyāma सूर्य प्राणायाम	Inhalation and exhalation through the right nostril.	84
Sūryanamaskar सूर्यनमस्कार	Popularly translated and written in English as Sun Salutation is a twelve-step bending and stretching exercise popular among yoga practitioners, that is not from traditional *Haṭha Yoga* texts.	103
Suśhruta Samhitā सुश्रुत सम्हिता	Translates in meaning as the document of *Suśhruta* written for benefit of all and is the title of a book that is considered the Ayurvedic manual of surgery.	28 footnote
Suṣhumnā सुषुम्ना	The Central Channel through which the left and right *nādis* integrate to unfold the activity of a person.	29-30, 60, 67-68, 131, 171
Sva-dharma स्वधर्म	One's own cosmic duty. It can be understood as the unfolding through the *Suṣhumnā* when it is in perfect balance with the left and right *nādi* flows. Another way to understand it is being true to one's conscience when one has high meditative connectivity -- the concept of pure *saṅkalpa* and *Kriyā Yoga*.	23, 59, 83, 100, 125, 127, 134, 215
Svādhiṣhṭhāna स्वाधिष्ठान	Translated as the center of the self, refers to the second *chakra* behind the pubic area, that in the psychic plane refers to fulfilling of the psychosomatic need of the individual and in a somatic zone controls the reproductive organs and the kidneys.	131, 140-141
Svādhyāya स्वाध्याय	Often translated as self-learning, it refers to the process of self-inquiry which becomes the point of *Dhāraṇā* that in *Samyama* reveals intuitive understanding.	138, 150, 165
Svara Yoga स्वर योग	Yoga of Rhythm – often associated with rhythm of breath and consequent vibrations within.	52

T

Taittriya Upaniṣhad तैत्तिरीय उपनिषद	One of the many Upaniṣhads that comes from the Yajur Veda tradition.	47

Tantra Yoga तन्त्र योग	The system of yoga that focuses on vibrations to transcend the body.	3-5, 18, 37, 86, 99, 104, 126, 135, 138, 149, 179, 181-182, 185, 192, 195, 222
tapa/s तपस्	Literally translated as meaning heat, is meant in the yoga context as the purification of the human system by exhausting *kleśha-karmas*. Commonly written as austerities, it has the misleading connotation of doing penance and giving physical pain to the self.	47-48, 138, 150
torsion field	Spiraling flow that carries information of intent into the subtle plane riding on the scalar waves.	123
Tribandha त्रिबन्ध	The three lock - another name for *Mahābandha*.	118
Trikā त्रिका	The three-fold philosophical term of Kashmir Shaivism referring to *Śhiva*, *Śhaktī*, and the individual.	128
Trikonāsana त्रिकोणासन	The triangular pose of *Haṭha Yoga*.	104
Tri-pura-sundarī त्रि-पुर-सुन्दरी	Translated as the beauty of the three worlds, refers to the Divine Mother.	189
Tumo breath	Tibetan Buddhist term of a practice that is like *Kapālabhāti* practice in the yoga tradition.	80
Tyāgī त्यागी	One who gives up – associated with renunciation of worldly living, often mistakenly called *sannyāsī*	135

U

Udāna उदान	The *nādi* communication beyond the body into cosmic consciousness, that enables higher level of meditative connectivity and in the physical domain strengthens the immune system.	29-32, 111, 116-117, 140, 142, 200, 221
Uddiyāna Bandha उड्डियान बन्ध	The abdominal lock.	115, 118
Ujjayī Kumbhaka उज्जयी कुम्भक	Term used to describe the *Ujjayī Prāṇāyāma* in the *Haṭha Yoga Pradīpikā*. However, in modern application of some schools of yoga it also refers to holding the breath after *Ujjayī* inhalation.	66
Ujjayī Prāṇāyāma उज्जयी प्राणायाम	Literally meaning the higher winning *Prāṇāyāma* practice, it is supposed to enable the unfolding of one's *Sva-Dharma* and thus result in purification. The practice is done with slow and deep breathing with mild constriction and focus at the vocal cords. The stimulation is considered to permeate the area from the lower sternum area to the base of the brain.	55, 58, 65-69, 112, 176

Upaniṣhads उपनिषद	Literally meaning 'learning in close quarters' (near to the teacher), is the philosophical segment of the Vedas.	18, 47
Uṣhtrāsna उष्ट्रासन	Camel pose of the *Haṭha Yoga* tradition.	104

V

Vagus nerve	The tenth cranial nerve that travels between the brain and the abdominal region, the longest cranial nerve connecting many organs, that impacts the cardio-respiratory and digestive systems, and its stimulation has an anti-inflammatory impact.	55, 66, 79, 91
Vaiśheṣhika वैशेषिक	One of the six ancient philosophies associated with the Vedic system.	18
Vaiśhya वैश्य	Literally meaning one who seeks to control, refers to the self-centered nature.	130-131, 202
Vakrāsana वक्रासन	A sideward twisting pose	104
Valsalva sinus	Sinus space on the top of the heart at the basal edge of the aorta.	79
varṇa-āshramas वर्ण-आश्रम	Literally translated as where one's nature or duties rest, it refers to one's outlook which can be four-fold: unthinking (*kśhudra*), self-centered (*vaiśhya*), society-centered (*kśhatriya*), and existence-centered (*brāhmaṇa*).	129-130
varṇa-dharma वर्ण धर्म	One's duty being in sync with one's *varṇa-āshrama* to support the cosmic flow.	130
Vaśha वश	To control or keep in grasp.	130
Vāta वात	Ayurvedic disposition of a wandering focus.	109
Vedānta वेदान्त	Philosophy of the Vedas written by Vyasa in the *Brahma Sutras*	5, 18-20, 33, 148-149
Vedas वेद	The collection of ancient hymns compiled by Vyāsa to formalize the philosophy and practice of the Vedic religion along with integration of 33 ancient religions of India.	17-18, 222
Veerabhadrāsana वीरभद्रासन	Called warrior pose in *Haṭha Yoga* tradition	104
Vi prefix वि	The prefix stands for *Viṣheśha* or *Viparīta*. *Viṣheśha* (विशेष)means special, and *Viparīta* (विपरीत)means opposite. Examples of words with the prefix *Vi* follow: *Vigraha, Vijñyānam, Vinyasa*, etc..	
Vigraha विग्रह	Translates as special holder - idea of worshipped form that holds the connecting vibration with the subtle plane that a devotee can invoke by thought or nearness.	182-185, 187, 198
Vijñyānam विज्ञानम्	Higher knowledge of cause and effect of what is observed.	48

Vikṛiti विकृति	Deformed or malformed referring to one's orientation moving away from one's true nature, that becomes the cause of disease as understood in Ayurveda.	109
Vinyasa विन्यास	Special awareness - used to describe in recent times the form of *āsana* practice with breath awareness and movement, that was traditionally known as *Prāṇakriyā* in the *tantra* system.	104
Viśheṣha विशेष	Means special.	59, 170, 183
Viṣhnu Mudrā विष्णु मुद्रा	The finger position in the hands used in Alternate Nostril Breathing. The name of the *Mudrā* suggests that which brings awareness of the expanded existence -- idea of calmness of the mind to observe everything.	62
Viśhuddhi विशुद्धि	Literally meaning Special Purification, refers to the fifth *chakra* in the throat. In the scheme of evolving awareness, the throat is the first step of awareness ascending from the temporal domain to the subtle domain beyond. For the mind to go to that level requires enough purification.	74, 131, 141
Viśhuddhi Chakra विशुद्धि चक्र	The fifth *chakra* in the throat. See implication of *Viśhuddhi* above.	74, 131, 141
Vivekachūdāmani विवेक चूडामणि	A composition of Shankaracharya that describes the nature of existence.	134
Vṛikśhāsana वृक्षासन	Tree pose of *Haṭha Yoga.*	104
Vyāna व्यान	The communication that controls the fluids in the body and hence pervades the whole body.	29-30, 32, 111, 116, 142, 199, 221
Vyāsa व्यास	The compiler of the Vedas and the author of Vedānta philosophy.	17-18, 20, 216, 222

Y

Yajñya यज्ञ	Fire-based worshipping with offering.	183
Yama यम	Summarized as being true to one's conscience, Patajali describes five aspects of moral code, the most important of which are not wantonly hurting others (*Ahimsā*) and to be inquiring and thoughtful in one's engagement with life (*Brahmacharya*). This is the first limb of the eight-fold *Aṣhṭānga Yoga.*	2, 134, 158, 166, 197. 215-216
Yantra यन्त्र	Matter imbued with vibration.	124-125, 185, 190
Yoga Nidrā योग निद्रा	Translated as yogic deep sleep, it refers to a state of deep relaxation and internal awareness where one becomes a non-reactive observer. This is considered effective for relieving stress from unpleasant memories. This practice is considered useful for PTSD.	163

www.ingramcontent.com/pod-product-compliance
Ingram Content Group UK Ltd.
Pitfield, Milton Keynes, MK11 3LW, UK
UKHW061959290726
14090UKWH00021B/1296